MRCS Part A

MRCS Part A

500 SBAs and EMQs

Pradip K Datta MBE MS FRCS (Ed, Eng, Irel, Glas)
Honorary Consultant Surgeon
Caithness General Hospital, Wick, UK
Member of Council, Royal College of Surgeons of Edinburgh (2000–2012)

Christopher JK Bulstrode MCh FRCS (Orth)
Professor and Honorary Consultant Orthopaedic Surgeon
University of Oxford, Oxford, UK
Former Member of Council, The Royal College of Surgeons of Edinburgh
Former Elected Member of the General Medical Council of the UK

William FM Wallace BSc MD FRCP FRCA FCAI FRCSEd
Professor Emeritus of Applied Physiology
Queen's University, Belfast, UK
Former Examiner, Royal College of Surgeons of Edinburgh

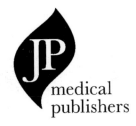

JP
medical
publishers

London • St Louis • Panama City • New Delhi

© 2013 JP Medical Ltd.
Published by JP Medical Ltd,
83 Victoria Street, London, SW1H 0HW, UK
Tel: +44 (0)20 3170 8910   Fax: +44 (0)20 3008 6180
Email: info@jpmedpub.com   Web: www.jpmedpub.com

The rights of Pradip K Datta, Christopher JK Bulstrode and William FM Wallace to be identified as authors of this work have been asserted by them in accordance with the Copyright, Designs and Patents Act 1988.

All brand names and product names used in this book are trade names, service marks, trademarks or registered trademarks of their respective owners. The publisher is not associated with any product or vendor mentioned in this book.

Medical knowledge and practice change constantly. This book is designed to provide accurate, authoritative information about the subject matter in question. However readers are advised to check the most current information available on procedures included and check information from the manufacturer of each product to be administered, to verify the recommended dose, formula, method and duration of administration, adverse effects and contraindications. It is the responsibility of the practitioner to take all appropriate safety precautions. Neither the publisher nor the authors assume any liability for any injury and/or damage to persons or property arising from or related to use of material in this book.

This book is sold on the understanding that the publisher is not engaged in providing professional medical services. If such advice or services are required, the services of a competent medical professional should be sought.

Every effort has been made where necessary to contact holders of copyright to obtain permission to reproduce copyright material. If any have been inadvertently overlooked, the publisher will be pleased to make the necessary arrangements at the first opportunity.

ISBN: 978-1-907816-33-8

British Library Cataloguing in Publication Data
A catalogue record for this book is available from the British Library

Library of Congress Cataloging in Publication Data
A catalogue record for this book is available from the Library of Congress

JP Medical Ltd is a subsidiary of Jaypee Brothers Medical Publishers (P) Ltd, New Delhi, India

Publisher:	Richard Furn
Commissioning Editor:	Hannah Applin
Senior Editorial Assistant:	Katrina Rimmer
Design:	Designers Collective Ltd

Copy edited, typeset, printed and bound in India.

Preface

e Intercollegiate MRCS examination (Member of the Royal College of Surgeons) is taken in two rts, Part A and Part B. This book is primarily meant to help those preparing for the Part A exam d covers every aspect of basic surgical knowledge that is expected of the candidate.

The book adheres to the syllabus. It is written in the format of the examination but with an sential difference. The reader is supplied with the answer and is given a detailed explanation r each one. A good explanation goes a long way in helping to understand a subject and thus ment the knowledge in one's mind. In each chapter all the questions are at the beginning, with e answers at the end. This approach helps the reader resist the temptation to look at the answer mediately; it thus acts as a personal tutorial and a self-assessment exercise.

The answers are liberally illustrated with images, clinical photographs, line drawings and jorithms. The contributors have subscribed to the dictum 'A picture is worth a thousand words'. e illustrations will help the reader to remember the clinical features, macroscopic pathology and aging as they read a particular topic.

The contributors have a wide range of experience. Some have examined in postgraduate and dergraduate examinations for several decades; others are surgical and anaesthetic trainees, on e threshold of becoming a consultant or just starting out on their chosen careers.

It is hoped that in this book the reader will find not only everything that is necessary to pass the amination, but also enough to embark on a surgical career with great enthusiasm.

Pradip K Datta
Christopher JK Bulstrode
William FM Wallace
June 2012

Contents

Contents

Contents

Contributors

Marilyn A Armstrong BSc PhD
Former Senior Lecturer in Immunology
School of Medicine and Dentistry
Queen's University, Belfast, UK

Catherine Collinson BSc(Hons)
ST4 Anaesthesia, South East Scotland
Deanery, UK

Andrew Duckworth MSc BSc(Hons)
MBChB MRCSEd
Registrar and Clinical Research Fellow
Edinburgh Orthopaedic Trauma Unit,
South-East Scotland, UK

Vasha Kaur MBChB(Hons) MRCS
ST5 General Surgical Trainee, London
Deanery, UK

Alex Laird MBChB MRCSEd
Specialty Registrar in Urological
Surgery, West of Scotland Deanery, UK

Pawanindra Lal MS DNB MNAMS
MNASc FRCS(Ed) FRCS(Glasg) FRCS(Eng)
Professor of Surgery, Maulana Azad
Medical College, (University of Delhi),
New Delhi, India

Ian Leeuwenberg FRCA
Specialty Trainee Anaesthesia, South
East Scotland, UK

Alistair May FCARCSI
ST6 Anaesthesia, West of Scotland
Deanery, UK

Iain Nixon FRCS(Ed) (ENT and Head &
Neck)
Clinical Fellow, Department of Head
and Neck Surgery, Memorial Sloan
Kettering Cancer Centre, New York, USA

Zahid Raza MBChB FRCS MD FRCSEd
Consultant Vascular Surgeon, Royal
Infirmary, Edinburgh, UK

Diptendra Sarkar MS DNB FRCS(Ed)
Associate Professor and Incharge
Breast Service, Department of Surgery,
IPGME&R, Kolkata, India

Grant Stewart BSc(Hons) MBChB
MRCS(Ed) PhD
Clinical Lecturer and Specialist
Registrar in Urological Surgery,
University of Edinburgh, Department
of Urology, Western General Hospital,
Edinburgh, UK

Ben Stutchfield BSc(Hons) MSc MRCS
ST4 General Surgery, South East
Scotland Deanery, UK

Introduction to the MRCS Part A

The Intercollegiate MRCS Part A is a 4-hour multiple choice question (MCQ) based exam, which is sat over a 1-day period. The exam takes place at each of the colleges throughout the UK at the same time, with identical questions asked.

The exam consists of two papers that cover the MRCS syllabus, including questions that cover the core applied knowledge of surgical sciences, as well as the recommended core knowledge of the nine surgical specialties. Questions will be in either a single best answer (SBA) format or in an extended matching question (EMQ) format, with equal marks available for each question. Details of the two papers are:

1. **Applied Basic Sciences**
   a. 2 hours in length
   b. 135 SBA questions with five possible answers per question
   c. Questions are clinically based but test core theoretical knowledge of surgical sciences

2. **Principles of Surgery in General**
   a. 2 hours in length
   b. 135 questions
   c. Themed EMQs consisting of 2–5 questions per theme, with a selection of potential answer options (average 8)
   d. Questions are more clinically based

On the day of the exam, remember to bring proof of identity, e.g. passport or driving licence, so you can register. Leave all personal belongings, including bags and mobiles phones (turned off), outside in the designated area. All stationery will be provided but bring in some hydration if you think you will need it.

On your table will be the exam paper, an answer sheet, a pencil and a rubber. Remember to check all these items are correct and working, and then complete your candidate details at the top of the answer sheet. You will be required to complete your answers on an electronic marking sheet, using a clear horizontal pencil line in the appropriate box on the answer sheet; for example, if you think the answer to question 15 is D, a mark should be placed in box of column D in the row labelled 15. Only one mark is allowed per question/row. The paper is not negatively marked. During the exam, you are not permitted to leave in the first 60 minutes or in the last 15 minutes.

For a candidate to progress to the MRCS Part B Objective Structured Clinical Examination (OSCE), a pass in Part A is necessary. For a pass, you need to pass both papers individually, as well as achieving the minimum overall mark set for the exam (combined mark for Papers 1 and 2).

Andrew Duckworth
June 2012

How to answer SBAs and EMQs

Firstly, always carefully check the instructions – they may be different from what you expect! The questions are based on short clinical vignettes. Read them with care, as each item of information is critical and should influence your choice. Particularly when making your final choice, perhaps between two options, do not make assumptions which are not supported by the information given. Although your general approach should be similar for the two types of question, they will now be dealt with separately because the detailed approach is somewhat different.

Single best answer

Here the situation is simple – for each vignette, you must decide which one of five answers is 'best', e.g. the **most likely diagnosis**, or the **most effective management**. It follows that the other answers are inferior. Some may be less complete, or incorrect in some aspect, but each option to be rejected is flawed, irrelevant, or just wrong. Be on the lookout for options which:

- Conflict with the information given in the vignette, including gender and age
- Require assumptions for which there is no foundation in the vignette

Once you have read the initial vignette and question, before you go to the options, think in your mind what the correct answer should be. Once you have that in your mind, look at the list of options to see if your answer is in the list. If it is, then most likely this is the correct option, but check the others carefully to make sure one is not better than your initial instinctive choice.

When you read a vignette and question and you feel that you are not comfortable with the topic and do not know a lot about it, then do not waste time in thinking about it. It will get you down mentally and you will lose valuable time. Just go ahead and answer the questions you know. Come back to the unanswered questions later.

The correct options are randomly distributed, so don't be surprised if you have a preponderance of Cs or Ds over a group of questions, and don't bother to work out whether you have the same numbers of As and Es.

Extended matching questions

With these there is a list of options which are to be used for each of a number of vignettes, but again the requirement is to pick the single best option from the list for each particular vignette. Remember, an option can be picked to match more than one vignette and some options may not be used.

With EMQs it is a good method to read the clinical scenarios first and not the list on top. Once you read a scenario, you should have an idea about the possible option, e.g. the diagnosis. Then look at the list of diagnoses. Look for the diagnosis that you made. If that is present in the list, then that is probably the correct answer. Do not start by reading all the scenarios one after another. Finish each scenario and make the diagnosis.

Tactical points

First be alert. As with any exam your mental state as you start the exam is much more important than any final revision in the last few minutes before you start. Your preparation for this alert state starts several days before.

Candidates are asked to use a pencil and the aim is to make a mark, usually horizontal, so that the answer is unequivocal when the sheet is being read by the optical marker. The test you should apply is this – would there be the slightest doubt to someone reading your completed paper about whether one and only one option is marked? Bear in mind that the machine will be faced with erased options which can still be seen faintly and it is programmed to ignore these. For this reason avoid pencils which have been sharpened to a very fine point, which may not give a readable response especially if little pressure is exerted. The box should be very clearly marked and this is best done with a worn rounded pencil, so don't hesitate to do an initial wearing down of a fine point. It's not necessary to fill 99.9% of the box area, but very slight marks may not register with the machine, resulting in no mark. Of course, there will be no mark if two or more boxes could reasonably be interpreted as filled.

You may like to mark the options on the question sheet initially and then copy them to the optically read sheet. No extra time, of course, is allowed for this, so **be very sure** you have time to do this!

Some people, if the time is not up, will re-read and modify their answers. Unless you have obviously marked a different box from the one intended, changes of mind at this stage very rarely improve results.

And, finally, of course, make sure you answer **all** the questions, or you are throwing away potential marks.

William FM Wallace
May 2011

Acknowledgements

The figures listed below have previously been published in the following books and are reproduced with permission.

Datta PK, Bulstrode CJK, Kaur, V. How to Pass the MRCS OSCE Volume 1. Oxford: Oxford University Press, 2011. Figures 34.1, 45.5, 46.1, 46.2a, 46.3a, 46.4a, 46.7, 46.10, 46.12, 47.3, 47.4, 48.2, 48.4, 48.8, 48.9, 48.10b, 48.14, 48.15, 57.2, 57.4.

Datta PK, Bulstrode CJK, Praveen BV. MCQs and EMQs in Surgery. London: Hodder Arnold, 2010. Figures 48.12, 53.1, 54.3, 57.1, 57.2, 57.3.

Misra RR, Uthappa MC, Datta PK. Radiology for Surgeons. Cambridge: Greenwich Medical Media, 2001. Figures 45.5, 45.6, 46.1, 48.2, 48.9a, 48.11, 48.12, 53.1, 57.2, 57.4.

Tunstall R and Shah N. Pocket Tutor Surface Anatomy. London: JP Medical, 2012. Figure 3.1.

Section A

Applied Basic Sciences

Chapter 1

Skull and brain

A 25-year-old man, a footballer, presents to the emergency department after having lost consciousness during a game. He is very drowsy, with a Glasgow Coma Score of 13. A CT scan shows an extradural haemorrhage.

Which blood vessel is the patient bleeding from?

A Internal carotid artery
B Middle cerebral artery
C Middle meningeal artery
D Superficial temporal artery
E Superior sagittal sinus

A 35-year-old woman with an untreated infected lesion on her face complains of severe ocular pain, fever and chemosis, and has a pulsating proptosis.

Which one of the following structures is involved?

A Cavernous sinus
B Optic nerve
C Pituitary gland
D Superior sagittal sinus
E Trigeminal nerve

A 70-year-old man, a smoker, presents with intermittent amaurosis fugax (temporary visual loss) in the form of a shutter dropping in front of his eye. He has a systolic carotid bruit on the same side.

The main artery that is affected enters the orbit through which one of the following foramina?

A Foramen rotundum
B Foramen spinosum
C Inferior orbital fissure
D Optic canal
E Superior orbital fissure

A 45-year-old woman is diagnosed with a space-occupying lesion at the cerebellopontine angle.

The lesion is arising from which one of the following structures?

A Basilar artery aneurysm
B Cerebellum

    C   Glossopharyngeal nerve
    D   Hypoglossal nerve
    E   Vestibulocochlear (8th cranial) nerve

5. A 55-year-old man presents with sudden onset of severe headache, which he liken
    to a 'hammer blow' to the back of the head. A gadolinium-enhanced MRI shows a
    haemorrhagic lesion in the anterior cranial fossa.

    Which one of the following vessels is involved

    A   Anterior communicating artery
    B   Basilar artery
    C   Internal carotid artery
    D   Middle cerebral artery
    E   Posterior communicating artery

6. A 30-year-old man presents with an extradural haemorrhage with a dilated pupil.

    Dilatation of the pupil is due to pressure on the occulomotor (3rd cranial) nerve by
    which one of the following structures?

    A   Cerebellar tonsil
    B   Crus of the cerebral peduncle
    C   Falx cerebri
    D   Mammillary body
    E   Uncus of the temporal lobe

7. A 30-year-old man, a recent immigrant from Africa, presents with an advanced
    right-sided nasopharyngeal carcinoma. A CT scan shows widespread extension
    into the right posterior base of the skull. On protruding the tongue, it deviates
    towards the side of the lesion.

    Which one of the following nerves is affected by the growth?

    A   Glossopharyngeal nerve
    B   Hypoglossal nerve
    C   Spinal part of accessory nerve
    D   Superior cervical sympathetic nerve
    E   Vagus nerve

8. A 30-year-old man presents with anosmia, after sustaining a fracture of his
    anterior cranial fossa in a road traffic accident 5 weeks ago. At that time he had
    cerebrospinal rhinorrhoea.

    Fracture of which one of the following bones is causing his anosmia?

    A   Cribriform plate of the ethmoid bone
    B   Frontal process of the zygomatic bone
    C   Nasal bones
    D   Orbital plate of the frontal bone
    E   Squamous part of the temporal bone

Answers

1. C Middle meningeal artery

The middle meningeal artery is a branch of the maxillary artery which along with the superficial temporal artery is one of the terminal branches of the external carotid artery. It enters the middle cranial fossa through the foramen spinosum and divides into an anterior and posterior branch. It is the cause of bleeding in extradural haemorrhage because it lies deep to the squamous part of the temporal bone which is a very thin part of the cranium, and therefore easily fractured. A burr hole is usually made at the level of the pterion to access the middle meningeal artery to stop the bleeding, although the ideal surgical procedure is a craniotomy.

2. A Cavernous sinus

The cavernous sinus is vulnerable to thrombosis in any serious infections of the face in the 'danger area' – upper lip, nose and medial part of cheek. This is a very serious condition and may lead to proptosis and ophthalmoplegia. The structures of the cavernous sinus are: internal carotid artery, ophthalmic division (1st division) and maxillary divisions (2nd division) of the 5th cranial nerve, 3rd, 4th and 6th cranial nerves. The other surgical condition that can occur within the cavernous sinus is an aneurysm of the internal carotid artery, resulting in a caroticocavernous fistula presenting clinically as a pulsating proptosis.

3. D Optic canal

The central artery of the retina is affected. It is a branch of the ophthalmic artery which enters the orbit through the optic canal inferolateral to the optic nerve within a common dural sheath. It supplies the extraocular muscles, the lachrymal gland and the eye. The eye is supplied by the central artery, an end artery (which supplies the optic nerve and retina) and the anterior and posterior ciliary arteries. The venous drainage from the orbit is by the superior ophthalmic vein which passes through the superior orbital fissure and the inferior ophthalmic vein that passes through the inferior orbital fissure.

4. E Vestibulocochlear (8th cranial) nerve

The lesion is arising from the vestibulocochlear nerve at its entrance to the auditory meatus. The auditory meatus is situated in the posterior cranial fossa in the petrous part of the temporal bone. In that area a cerebellopontine angle tumour arises from the nerve sheath of the 8th nerve (schwannoma, acoustic neuroma); it may press on the adjacent 7th nerve, causing facial numbness or weakness.

5. A Anterior communicating artery

This patient has a classical presentation of a ruptured berry aneurysm resulting in subarachnoid haemorrhage. The commonest site for a berry aneurysm is the anterior communicating artery. Congenital berry aneurysms (so-called because of their resemblance to the fruit) occur in the circle of Willis, particularly at the junction of the vessels where the tunica media is weakest. Patients present with features of subarachnoid haemorrhage: complaining of a severe and sudden headache, where they feel a hammer-blow on the back of the head. Patients fast become unconscious. Unless suspected by clinical awareness, promptly investigated by MRI and immediately treated as an emergency, it carries a poor prognosis.

6. E Uncus of the temporal lobe

The uncus of the temporal lobe compresses the occulomotor nerve. The extradural haematoma causes the cerebral hemisphere to move to the opposite side resulting in a midline shift. As the haematoma enlarges the cerebrum is shifted more to the opposite side causing the uncus on the temporal lobe to impinge upon the occulomotor nerve. This causes paralysis of the parasympathetic innervation of the eye resulting in pupillary dilatation. This is a serious clinical finding. The patient needs an urgent CT scan followed by intracranial decompression.

7. B Hypoglossal nerve

The hypoglossal nerve exits the posterior cranial fossa through the hypoglossal canal. This is a separate foramen seen at the edge of the foramen magnum. Direct extension of the growth into the base of the skull infiltrates the hypoglossal nerve which may also be invaded by secondary lymph nodes. The nerve supplies all the intrinsic and extrinsic muscles of the tongue except the palatoglossus because the latter is essentially a muscle of the palate and hence supplied by the pharyngeal plexus. Iatrogenic damage is known to occur and this would cause the tongue to deviate to the paralysed side with atrophy of the tongue.

8. A Cribriform plate of ethmoid bone

After recovery from a head injury, the patient suffers from anosmia. This means that the olfactory (1st cranial) nerve has been damaged as a result of fracture of the cribriform plate of the ethmoid bone. The olfactory bulb may be separated from the olfactory nerves or the nerves may be torn as a result of the fracture. Such an injury will cause cerebrospinal rhinorrhoea at the time of initial injury.

Chapter 2

Head and neck

. A 45-year-old man underwent simple excision of the submandibular salivary gland for sialadenitis. On the first postoperative day, the patient is drooling saliva from the angle of the mouth on the side of the operation.

Which of the following anatomical structures is most likely to be damaged?

A   Buccal branch of the facial nerve
B   Hypoglossal nerve (12th cranial)
C   Lingual nerve
D   Marginal mandibular branch of the facial nerve (7th cranial)
E   Spinal branch of accessory nerve (11th cranial)

2. A 35-year-old woman is undergoing a hemithyroidectomy. The surgeon is in the process of mobilising the superior pole to ligate the superior thyroid artery.

Which one of the following structures must the surgeon be very careful not to damage during this manoeuvre?

A   Ansa hypoglossi
B   Cervical branch of facial nerve
C   External laryngeal nerve
D   Pharyngeal branch of the glossopharyngeal nerve
E   Recurrent laryngeal nerve

3. A 50-year-old man presents with a recently developed pain in his face over the upper and lower jaws. This is brought on by washing, shaving, eating or cold wind blowing on the face.

Which one of the following nerves is the cause of this symptom complex?

A   Ansa cervicalis
B   Cervical plexus
C   Facial (7th cranial)
D   Spinal branch of accessory (11th cranial)
E   Trigeminal (5th cranial)

4. A 58-year-old man, a smoker, presents with severe cramp-like pains in his right upper limb, associated with fainting attacks and visual disturbances. These are particularly strong when he uses the limb vigorously, such as when painting the ceiling. Vascular investigations have shown an atheromatous obstruction to the first part of the subclavian artery, resulting in a diagnosis of subclavian steal syndrome.

From which of the following branches of the subclavian artery is blood being stolen as a result of retrograde flow?

A   Costocervical trunk
B   Dorsal scapular artery
C   Internal thoracic artery
D   Thyrocervical trunk
E   Vertebral artery

5. A 70-year-old woman is undergoing an open operation on her pharyngeal pouch. A pharyngeal pouch occurs through the Killian's dehiscence.

    Between which one of the following sites is the weakness most likely?

    A   Middle and inferior constrictor muscles of the pharynx
    B   Right and left palatopharyngeus
    C   Superior and middle constrictor muscles of the pharynx
    D   Thyropharyngeus and cricopharyngeus (two parts of the inferior constrictor) muscles
    E   Upper oesophageal musculature (circular and longitudinal fibres)

6. A 60-year-old woman is being anaesthetised for a total gastrectomy. The anaesthetist is about to insert a central venous pressure line on the right side of the neck. She is looking for the terminal part of the internal jugular vein.

    Which one of the following anatomical sites is the anaesthetist aiming for to find the target?

    A   Between angle of mandible and sternocleidomastoid
    B   Between anterior border of trapezius and posterior border of sternocleidomastoid
    C   Between the sternal and clavicular heads of sternocleidomastoid
    D   Between sternocleidomastoid and posterior belly of digastric
    E   A point 1 cm lateral and 2 cm above the sternoclavicular joint

7. A 28-year-old man undergoes an endoscopic transthoracic sympathectomy for palmar hyperhidrosis. Postoperatively, he has developed ptosis of his eye.

    This is due to iatrogenic damage to which one of the following nerves?

    A   8th cervical nerve
    B   1st thoracic nerve
    C   Lower cord of brachial plexus
    D   2nd thoracic ganglion
    E   7th cervical nerve

8. A 35-year-old man has been investigated for hypercalcaemia from primary hyperparathyroidism. A technetium-labelled sestamibi scan shows a parathyroid adenoma in the superior mediastinum.

    The adenoma has developed from which of the following sites of origin of the parathyroid?

    A   1st pharyngeal pouch
    B   4th pharyngeal pouch
    C   2nd pharyngeal pouch
    D   3rd pharyngeal pouch
    E   Ultimobranchial body

Answers

. D Marginal mandibular branch of the facial nerve (7th cranial)

The patient is drooling saliva because the depressor anguli oris has been paralysed due to damage of the marginal mandibular branch of the facial nerve. This is the most superficial nerve and can be damaged, if the skin incision is made incorrectly. To avoid damaging the nerve, a horizontal skin crease incision is made two fingers breadth below the ramus of the mandible, and the incision deepened down to the body of the gland. The superior flap consisting of the skin, platysma and fascia investing the gland is then lifted up to the ramus of the mandible. Damage to the nerve which lies between the platysma and the fascia is thus avoided (**Figure 2.1**).

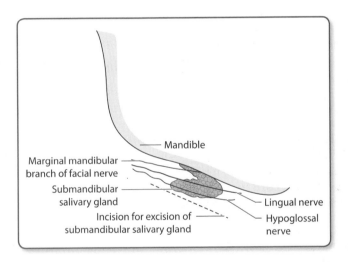

Marginal mandibular branch of facial nerve

Submandibular salivary gland

Incision for excision of submandibular salivary gland

Mandible

Lingual nerve

Hypoglossal nerve

Figure 2.1 Nerves that are vulnerable during excision of the submandibular salivary gland: the marginal mandibular branch of the facial nerve, hypoglossal nerve and lingual nerve.

2. C External laryngeal nerve

During ligation and division of the superior thyroid pedicle, a manoeuvre facilitated by using the Kocher's dissector, the external laryngeal nerve is vulnerable to injury because it lies close behind the superior thyroid artery on the inferior constrictor muscle. To avoid damage to the nerve, the pedicle is ligated as close to the gland as possible. Three ligatures are applied, two of which are left in the patient. Paralysis of the external laryngeal nerve affecting the cricothyroid may produce no disability or minimal hoarseness of voice but an inability to produce higher notes in singing.

3. E Trigeminal (5th cranial)

The three divisions (or branches) of the trigeminal nerve, ophthalmic, maxillary and mandibular supply the skin of the face in three zones. The sensations from the front, near the orbit, are carried by the ophthalmic, division; sensations from the lower lid, mid-face, nose and upper lip and gum by the maxillary division and the mandibular division carries sensations from the temporal region, both surfaces of the lower lip and gum and mucous membrane of the floor of the mouth and the lingual gum. Hence in trigeminal neuralgia the face is the most affected. The pattern of a facial capillary haemangioma (port-wine stain) and the distribution of vesicles when herpes zoster affects the trigeminal ganglion fit the pattern of sensory supply of the facial skin.

4. E Vertebral artery

Subclavian steal syndrome results from retrograde flow of blood from the vertebral artery of the vertebrobasilar system. In this condition, there is atheromatous obstruction of the first part of the subclavian artery. Therefore, when extra blood is required due to excessive use of the upper limb, particularly in any DIY (do-it-yourself) activity, blood is provided by the vertebral artery by reversal of its flow into the subclavian artery. This causes ischaemic cerebral symptoms from vertebrobasilar insufficiency.

5. D Thyropharyngeus and cricopharyngeus (two parts of the inferior constrictor) muscles

The Killian's dehiscence is a potential weakness between the cricopharyngeus (transverse fibres) and thyropharyngeus (oblique fibres) parts of the inferior constrictor muscle of the pharynx. It was first described by Gustav Killian, Director of Rhinolaryngological Clinic in Freiberg and Berlin. The inferior constrictor encloses the middle and superior constrictor muscles with its fibres, curving backwards and upwards around them. The cricopharyngeus is continuous with the circular muscle coat of the oesophagus and acts as a sphincter. It is always closed, relaxing only during deglutition. After excision of a pharyngeal pouch, cricopharyngeal myotomy is an essential part of the operation.

6. C Between the sternal and clavicular heads of sternocleidomastoid

The anaesthetist is looking for the terminal part of the internal jugular vein which lies in the triangular gap between the sternal and clavicular heads of the sternocleidomastoid muscle. It joins the subclavian vein to form the brachiocephalic vein behind the sternal end of the clavicle. This anatomical knowledge is essential to help in the insertion of a central venous pressure cannula. The procedure can be facilitated by the use of ultrasound Doppler to localise precisely the site of venous puncture. The right side is most commonly used to insert a central venous pressure line as the approach is direct to the superior vena cava and there is no danger of damage to the thoracic duct, as on the left side.

7. B 1st thoracic nerve

During this operation the 1st thoracic nerve has been inadvertently damaged resulting in division of the sympathetic fibres which ultimately supply the smooth muscle part of the levator palpebrae superioris (Muller's muscle). Paralysis of this part of the muscle causes partial ptosis. This is one of the features of Horner's syndrome, the others being constriction of the pupil and absence of sweating in the forehead. The syndrome, described in 1869 by Johann Friedrich Horner (1831–1916), Professor of Ophthalmology in Zurich, can also occur from compression of the T1 nerve root by a space-occupying lesion such as a carcinoma of the apex of the lung, carcinoma of the thyroid or oesophagus, metastatic lymph nodes or pressure from thoracic inlet/outlet syndrome.

8. D 3rd pharyngeal pouch

The inferior parathyroid gland would be the site of the adenoma. This is because, it is less constant in its position and hence more likely to be in the mediastinum. The inferior glands develop from the 3rd pharyngeal pouch. They lie within the pretracheal fascia behind the lower pole of the thyroid. The thymus also develops from the 3rd pharyngeal pouch. This close association between the two results in the inferior parathyroids descending with the thymus. Therefore, they may be found in the thorax, superior or posterior mediastinum and in front of the trachea or oesophagus. The superior parathyroids develop from the 4th branchial pouch and are much more constant in position. Therefore, the superior parathyroids are sometimes referred to as parathyroid IV and the inferior parathyroids as parathyroid III. A normal parathyroid is 50 mg in weight. The glands are very close to the anastomosis between the superior and inferior thyroid arteries on the posterior border of the thyroid gland. The superior parathyroids are usually dorsal and inferior parathyroids ventral to the recurrent laryngeal nerves.

Chapter 3

Upper limb and breast

A 29-year-old man presents complaining of pain in his left neck and shoulder region following a forced abduction injury to his arm, resulting from a fall from his motorbike at high speed. Subsequent imaging demonstrates an upper brachial plexus lesion.

Which of the following nerves is a branch of the lateral cord of the brachial plexus?

A   Axillary
B   Musculocutaneous
C   Radial
D   Thoracodorsal
E   Upper subscapular

A 35-year-old woman presents with winging of the right scapular due to paralysis of the serratus anterior muscle.

A lesion to which nerve would result in this presentation?

A   Dorsal scapular
B   Long thoracic
C   Nerve to subclavius
D   Suprascapular
E   Thoracodorsal

A 23-year-old man presents following a fall onto his left shoulder whilst playing rugby. He complains of pain throughout the shoulder and on examination has weakness when testing internal rotation of the arm compared to the contralateral side. Radiographs are negative.

Injury to which tendon would explain his symptoms?

A   Deltoid
B   Infraspinatus
C   Subscapularis
D   Supraspinatus
E   Teres minor

A 38-year-old woman presents following a twisting injury during a fall from her horse at low speed. She complains of pain in the region of the fracture and on examination has a wrist drop in the ipsilateral hand. Radiographs reveal a fracture of the humeral diaphysis.

An injury to which nerve would explain her presentation?

    A Axillary
    B Median
    C Musculocutaneous
    D Radial
    E Ulnar

5. An 18-year-old man presents following a deep penetrating stab injury to the anterior aspect of his left forearm.

   Which of the following muscles of the forearm is supplied by the ulnar nerve?

   A Flexor carpi radialis
   B Flexor carpi ulnaris
   C Flexor digitorum superficialis
   D Palmaris longus
   E Pronator teres

6. An 18-year-old man presents with a posterior dislocation of the left elbow. He complains of decreased sensation and weakness throughout the left hand. On examination, there is a weakness to abduction and adduction of the fingers.

   Which of the following nerves has been injured as a result of the dislocation?

   A Anterior interosseous
   B Posterior interosseous
   C Median
   D Radial
   E Ulnar

7. A 48-year-old woman presents with a 1-year history of numbness and tingling affecti the radial three and half digits of her left hand. On examination, she has signs of atrophy to the thenar eminence of the hand and has positive Tinel's and Phalen's tes

   Compression of which structure is causing the patient's symptoms?

   A Flexor carpi radialis tendon
   B Flexor digitorum profundus tendons
   C Flexor digitorum superficialis tendons
   D Flexor pollicis longus tendon
   E Median nerve

8. A 49-year-old woman presents for unilateral mastectomy for an isolated carcinor of the breast.

   Which of the following is the primary contributor to the arterial supply of the female breast?

   A Dorsal scapular artery
   B Internal thoracic artery
   C Suprascapular artery
   D Thoracodorsal artery
   E Transverse cervical artery

nswers

B Musculocutaneous

The brachial plexus is formed from the ventral rami of the lower four cervical nerve roots (C5–C8) and the first thoracic nerve root (T1). It provides muscular and cutaneous innervation to the pectoral girdle as well as to the rest of the upper limb. The plexus is divided into zones with roots (C5–T1), trunks (superior C5–C6, middle C7, inferior C8–T1), divisions (anterior or posterior divisions of the three trunks) and cords (lateral, posterior, medial). The cords are named according to their location in relation to the second part of the axillary artery. Branches arise from these zones as shown in **Figure 3.1**. The branches of the posterior cord include the upper subscapular nerve that supplies subscapularis, the lower subscapular nerve that supplies subscapularis and teres major, the thoracodorsal nerve that supplies latissimus dorsi, the axillary nerve that supplies teres minor and deltoid, and the radial nerve that supplies the extensors of the elbow, wrist and hand. The musculocutaneous nerve is a branch of the lateral cord, which also gives rise to the lateral pectoral nerve, along with the medial cord the median nerve.

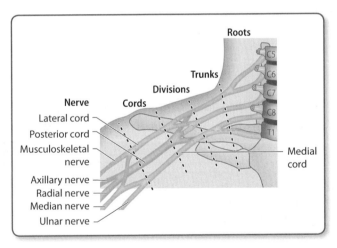

Figure 3.1 The brachial plexus. The roots are located between scalenus anterior and medius, the trunks in the posterior triangle of the neck, the divisions posterior to the clavicle and the cords in the axilla. (Reproduced from Goodfellow JA. Pocket Tutor Neurological Examination. London: JP Medical Ltd, 2012).

There are three types of injury that can occur to the brachial plexus: upper, lower or whole. Excessive lateral flexion of the neck (downward traction of arm) away from the pectoral girdle can lead to an upper plexus injury (C5/C6). The clinical presentation is known as an Erb–Duchenne paralysis with the arm in a 'waiter's tip' position due to dysfunction of the suprascapular nerve, musculocutaneous nerve and axillary nerve leading to paralysis of the rotator cuff muscles and unopposed elbow extension and forearm pronation. A forced traction injury on an abducted arm (upward traction) can lead to a lower plexus injury (C8/T1) and the clinical presentation is known as Klumpke's palsy. A characteristic sign is that of an ipsilateral clawed hand due to loss of the ulnar nerve leading to paralysis of the intrinsic muscles of the hand. T1 involvement can lead to Horner's syndrome (sympathetic chain involvement) with ptosis, miosis and anhydrosis. Such a presentation can be associated with a cervical rib or Pancoast's tumour.

The reflexes of the upper limb are:

- Biceps (C5/C6, musculocutaneous, biceps)
- Triceps (C7/C8, radial, triceps)
- Supinator (C7/C8, radial, brachioradialis)

2. B Long thoracic nerve

The serratus anterior muscle originates on the surface of the first 8–9 ribs on the lateral aspect of the chest wall and inserts on the anterior medial border of the scapula. The muscle protracts and stabilises the scapula, and also assists with arm abduction passed 120° by rotating the scapula and forcing the glenoid cavity to point superiorly. A winged scapula (scapula alata) is caused by paralysis of the serratus anterior muscle, commonly secondary to a lesion of the long thoracic nerve of Bell (C5–C7, see Figure 3.1). Injury can be traumatic (blunt trauma, subscapular bursitis, or iatrogenic, e.g. mastectomy with axillary clearance), nontraumatic (viral illness, radiculopathy, coarctation of the aorta) or idiopathic. A palsy of the accessory nerve (affecting the trapezius muscle) and dorsal scapular nerve (rhomboid) can lead to a clinical winged scapula also.

3. C Subscapularis

The rotator cuff is a mesh of four tendon insertions that insert into the greater and lesser tuberosity of the humerus, covering the shoulder capsule and reinforcing the stability of the glenohumeral joint. The four muscles of the rotator cuff are:

Table 3.1

Muscle	Origin	Insertion	Innervation	Movement
Subscapularis	Scapular subscapular fossa	Lesser tuberosity	Upper and lower subscapular nerve (C5–C6)	Internal rotation
Infraspinatus	Scapula infraspinous fossa	Greater tuberosity (middle facet)	Suprascapular nerve (C5–C6)	External rotation
Supraspinatus	Scapula supraspinous fossa	Greater tuberosity (superior facet)	Suprascapular nerve (C5–C6)	Abduction
Teres minor	Lateral border of scapula	Greater tuberosity (inferior facet)	Axillary nerve (C5)	External rotation

Table 3.1 Origin, insertion, innervation and action of the four rotator cuff muscles.

- Subscapularis
- Infraspinatus
- Supraspinatus
- Teres minor

Features of the four muscles are shown in **Table 3.1**.

4. D Radial

The radial nerve arises from the posterior cord of the brachial plexus (C5–T1), passes through the lower triangular space of the axilla, passes posteriorly between the long and medial head of triceps, enters the arm posterior to the axillary artery and branches to give the posterior cutaneous nerve of the arm. It travels on the posterior medial aspect of the humerus giving a branch to the medial head of biceps and then passes into spiral groove of the humerus, circumnavigating the humerus with the deep brachial artery and providing innervation to the lateral head of triceps. It emerges posteriorly on the lateral aspect of the distal humerus and pierces the lateral intermuscular septum, running between brachialis and brachioradialis in the anterior compartment of the arm. During this course, motor innervation to elbow extensors (anconeus, triceps), brachioradialis and extensor carpi radialis longus are provided, as well as sensory cutaneous branches to the posterior forearm and the lateral arm. It then passes anterior to the lateral epicondyle of the humerus, traversing the antecubital fossa posterior to brachioradialis, entering the forearm. The nerve divides into a deep and superficial branch, with the deep branch continuing as the posterior interosseous nerve after penetration of the supinator muscle and innervates the muscles in the posterior compartment of the forearm. The superficial branch of the radial nerve descends the forearm posterior to brachioradialis, emerges just above the wrist and then provides sensory cutaneous innervation to the lateral dorsum of the hand including the first dorsal web space.

Injury to the radial nerve predominantly occurs at two levels with a distinct clinical picture:

- At the axilla, resulting in loss of elbow extension, wrist extension and metacarpophalangeal joint (MCPJ) extension
- At the spiral groove of the humerus, resulting in loss of wrist extension and MCPJ extension, but with preservation of elbow extension

5. B Flexor carpi ulnaris

The muscles of the flexor compartment of the forearm are divided into a superficial and deep layer, as outlined in **Table 3.2**.

The muscles of the flexor compartment of the forearm are supplied by the median nerve except for:

- Flexor carpi ulnaris (ulnar nerve)
- Flexor digitorum profundus medial two digits (ulnar nerve)

Muscle	Origin	Insertion
Superficial		
Pronator teres	Medial epicondyle of humerus	Lateral body of radius
Flexor carpi radialis	Medial epicondyle of humerus	Bases of 2nd and 3rd metacarpals
Palmaris longus	Medial epicondyle of humerus	Palmar aponeurosis
Flexor carpi ulnaris	Medial epicondyle of humerus	Pisiform
Flexor digitorum superficialis	Medial epicondyle of humerus	Base middle phalanges four fingers
Deep		
Flexor digitorum profundus	Upper third of volar ulna	Base distal phalanges four fingers
Flexor pollicis longus	Middle third of volar radius	Base distal phalanx thumb
Pronator quadratus	Anteromedial surface ulna	Anterolateral surface radius

Table 3.2 The origin and insertion of the muscles of the flexor compartment of the forearm.

6. E Ulnar

The ulnar nerve arises from the medial cord of the brachial plexus (C8–T1), entering the arm medial to the axillary artery. It travels down the posterior medial aspect of the humerus (medial to brachial artery), pierces the medial intermuscular septum, and descends distally anterior to triceps, giving off no branches in the arm. It passes posterior to the medial epicondyle of the humerus, entering the anterior compartment of the forearm between the two heads of flexor carpi ulnaris. The nerve descends through the forearm alongside the ulna and ulnar artery deep to flexor carpi ulnaris, which it innervates along with the medial two digits of the flexor digitorum profundus. Approximately 5 cm above the wrist, the nerve gives off the palmar and dorsal branches of the ulnar nerve, which provide cutaneous innervation to the hand (**Figure 3.2**). At the wrist, the ulnar nerve and artery pass through Guyon's canal, superficial to the flexor retinaculum. In the hand the superficial and deep branches of the ulnar innervate the intrinsic muscles of the hand (hypothenar muscles, 3rd and 4th lumbricals, adductor pollicis, interossei). The interossei muscles are responsible for abduction (dorsal) and adduction (palmar) of the fingers. Dysfunction of the ulnar nerve in the hand can also be tested using Froment's sign (test pinch grip and patient compensates by flexing the interphalangeal joint of thumb using flexor pollicis longus, which is innervated by the median nerve).

When severe lesions of the ulnar nerve occur at the wrist a classic clawing appearance to the hand is observed. However, if the lesion is more proximal at the elbow, the claw like appearance of the hand is reduced due to the loss of innervation to flexor digitorum profundus medial two digits. This is known as the ulnar paradox.

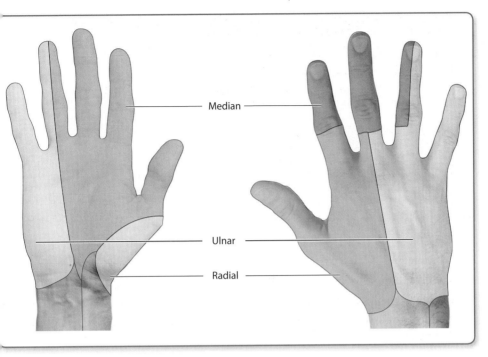

Figure 3.2 Cutaneous nerve supply to the hand. Photographs reproduced courtesy of Sam Scott-Hunter, London.

7. E Median nerve

The carpal tunnel is found on the volar or palmar aspect of the wrist and connects the anterior forearm to the volar aspect of the hand. It is formed through the flexor retinaculum and its attachments radially to the scaphoid tubercle and the trapezium, and on the ulnar side to the pisiform and hook of hamate. The contents of the carpal tunnel include the median nerve, four tendons of flexor digitorum profundus, four tendons of flexor digitorum superficialis and the tendon of flexor pollicis longus. The tendon of flexor carpi radialis is adjacent to, but not within the carpal tunnel.

The median nerve arises from the medial and lateral cords of the brachial plexus (C6–T1), entering the arm anterior to the distal third of the axillary artery. It travels down the arm lateral to the brachial artery, moving to the medial side at the mid-humeral level. The median nerve exits the antecubital fossa and passes into the forearm between the heads of pronator teres, giving off the anterior interosseous nerve. It then travels down the forearm between flexor digitorum superficialis and flexor digitorum profundus, before emerging near the wrist medial to flexor carpi radialis and entering the carpal tunnel. In the forearm the nerve innervates some of the muscles in the flexor compartment of the forearm along with one of its branches (anterior interosseous nerve). It then enters the hand via the carpal tunnel (inferior to the flexor retinaculum) and innervates some of the small muscles of the hand (thenar eminence, 1st and 2nd lumbricals). The palmar cutaneous branch of the median nerve is given off prior to the carpal tunnel and explains the preservation of sensory innervation to the central and radial aspect of the palm in patients with carpal tunnel syndrome (**Figure 3.3**).

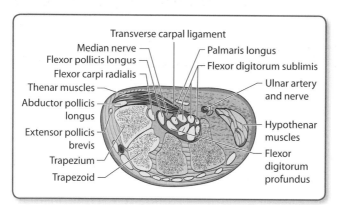

Figure 3.3 The carpal tunnel.

8. B Internal thoracic artery

The arterial supply of the female breast is through the:

- Internal mammary/thoracic artery
- Intercostal arteries
- Axillary artery (lateral thoracic and acromiothoracic)

The dorsal scapular artery arises from the subclavian artery and supplies the levator scapulae, rhomboids, and trapezius. The thoracodorsal artery is a branch of the subscapular artery and supplies the latissimus dorsi. The transverse cervical artery is an upper branch of the thyrocervical trunk and has contributions to trapezius and sternocleidomastoid. The suprascapular artery is a lower branch of the thyrocervical trunk and has contributions to supraspinatus, sternocleidomastoid and subclavius.

Chapter 4

Thoracic cavity

A female neonate is born with severe respiratory distress as a result of a congenital diaphragmatic hernia. This was diagnosed antenatally.

Through which one of the following foramina in the diaphragm has the hernia occurred?

A   Aortic hiatus
B   Bochdalek's foramen
C   Inferior vena cava hiatus
D   Morgagni's foramen
E   Oesophageal hiatus

A 60-year-old man , a smoker, presents with a 3-day history of worsening headaches and shortness of breath with swelling of his face and neck.

Which one of the following structures is compressed causing his symptoms?

A   Azygos vein
B   Bifurcation of the trachea
C   Both lung hila
D   Superior vena cava
E   Thoracic duct

A 50-year-old man complains of symptoms of heartburn and acid reflux. He is due to have an oesophagogastroduodenoscopy (OGD).

At what level will the normal gastro-oesophageal junction be found from the incisors?

A   36 cm
B   38 cm
C   40 cm
D   37 cm
E   42 cm

A 45-year-old man is due to undergo a Heller's operation of cardiomyotomy for achalasia of the cardia through the left chest.

Which one of the following structures is in danger of being damaged?

A   Hemiazygos vein
B   Phrenic nerve
C   Sympathetic trunk
D   Thoracic duct
E   Vagus nerve

5   A 35-year-old man needed a routine annual medical examination for his employment. His ECG result showed prolongation of the PR interval to more than 0.22s (normal = 0.12–0.20s).

In which one of the following sites in the heart is the abnormal conducting system situated?

A   The left atrium
B   The right atrium
C   The right ventricle
D   The left ventricle
E   The aortic sinus

6   A 35-year-old woman presents with shortness of breath and is diagnosed with mitral stenosis. On auscultation she has an opening snap with middiastolic murmur with presystolic accentuation.

At which one of the following anatomical sites will these auscultatory findings be best heard?

A   Sternal end of the 2nd left intercostal space
B   5th left intercostal space in the midclavicular line
C   Sternal end of 2nd right intercostal space
D   Left lower sternal border at the 5th intercostal space
E   Opposite the 4th left costal cartilage behind the sternum

7   A 55-year-old man requires an operation for severe gastro-oesophageal reflux disease. This is due to be carried out by the laparoscopic route.

Which one of the following levels indicates the oesophageal aperture in the diaphragm?

A   10th thoracic vertebra
B   12th thoracic vertebra
C   8th Thoracic vertebra
D   9th thoracic vertebra
E   11th thoracic vertebra

8   A 60-year-old man presents a large carcinoma of the upper left lung. A chest X-ray confirms the diagnosis and also shows marked elevation of the left hemidiaphragm.

Which one of the following nerves is affected by the carcinoma causing elevation of the left dome?

A   Greater splanchnic nerve
B   Phrenic nerve
C   Recurrent laryngeal nerve
D   Thoracic sympathetic trunk
E   Vagus nerve

Answers

. B Bochdalek's foramen

This is a congenital diaphragmatic hernia which occurs through the foramen of Bochdalek. This results from a failure of development of the pleuroperitoneal membrane. The defect is posterior and occurs much more commonly on the left side due to the presence of the liver on the right. The diaphragm develops from four sources. The septum transversum gives rise to the central tendon. This septum is invaded by the 3rd, 4th and 5th cervical myotomes which carry their own nerve supply which constitute the phrenic nerve. To these are added the mesodermal folds called the pleuroperitoneal membranes that separate the abdominal from the thoracic parts of the coelom and the oesophageal mesentery. Failure in union between the xiphoid and costal parts results in the foramen of Morgagni, a smaller hernial site.

. D Superior vena cava

This is the classical presentation of superior vena caval syndrome caused by compression of the superior vena cava by enlarged mediastinal secondary lymph nodes from a presumed carcinoma of the lung. A lymphoma from mediastinal lymph nodes can also present in a similar manner. The patient requires an urgent chest X-ray followed by a CT scan of the chest and CT guided biopsy of the enlarged lymph nodes. Treatment would be urgent radiotherapy or chemotherapy or both depending upon the histology and the outcome of a multidisciplinary team discussion.

3. C 40 cm

The normal gastro-oesophageal junction is 40 cm from the incisors. This is an important anatomical landmark on OGD. In gastro-oesophageal reflux disease, the junction will be encountered earlier indicating that the oesophagus has been shortened due to oesophagitis from reflux. Biopsies will be taken from the abnormal, inflamed mucosa to look for the presence and extent of dysplasia. The oesophagus has certain normal anatomical sites of constriction where foreign bodies may get lodged. From the incisors these sites are: commencement at the cricopharyngeal sphincter 15 cm; where it is crossed by the aortic arch 22 cm; where it is crossed by the left main bronchus 27 cm; at its entrance into the abdomen through the diaphragmatic hiatus at the level of the 10th thoracic vertebra 40 cm.

4. E Vagus nerve

The operation of Heller's cardiomyotomy (Ernst Heller 1877–1964, a German surgeon, described the operation in 1913) can be done through the chest or abdomen by open surgery or minimal access surgery. When the operation is done through the left chest, both the vagus nerves are vulnerable to inadvertent damage because of their proximity to the oesophagus. Below the pulmonary hila, the vagus nerves descend in contact with the oesophagus – the right behind and the left in front.

5. B Right atrium

This patient has a first degree atrioventricular (AV) block. This denotes that the site of abnormality is the AV node. This is situated in the right atrium on the interatrial septum above the attachment of the septal cusp of the tricuspid valve. It consists of a specialised mass of myocardial cells. It receives impulses from the sinoatrial node the pacemaker of the heart situated in the right atrium just below the superior vena cava. From the AV node runs the AV bundle of His, which divides into right and left branches that travel down the respective sides of the interventricular septum (**Figure 4.1**). The bundle is the means of conducting the contractile impulse from atria to ventricles. The right branch becomes subendocardial on the right side of the septum. The left branch breaks up into a sheaf of subendocardial fibres. Abnormalities of heart rhythms are due to malfunctioning of the conducting system.

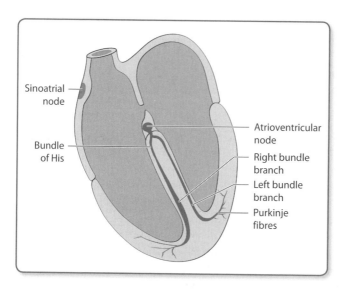

Figure 4.1
Diagrammatic representation of the conduction system of the heart.

6. B 5th left intercostal space in the midclavicular line

This patient has mitral stenosis. Hence the mitral valve needs to be auscultated to maximum benefit. The mitral valve sounds are best heard over the apex of the heart at the 5th left intercostal space in the midclavicular line (**Figure 4.2**). The sites of auscultation for the heart valves do not correspond to the surface anatomy of the valves because the intensity of the sounds is influenced by the direction of blood

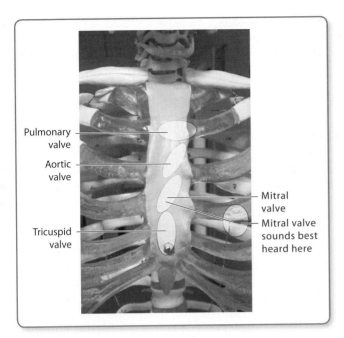

Pulmonary
valve

Aortic
valve

Tricuspid
valve

Mitral
valve

Mitral valve
sounds best
heard here

Figure 4.2 Surface markings of the heart valves. Mitral valve sounds are best heard over the apex of the heart at the 5th left intercostal space in the midclavicular line circled in yellow and arrowed.

flow. The sites for hearing the other sounds are: pulmonary sternal end of 2nd left intercostal space; aortic – sternal end of 2nd right intercostal space and tricuspid – left lower sternal border at the 5th intercostal space.

7. A 10th thoracic vertebra

The oesophageal hiatus is at the level of the 10th thoracic vertebra. At the level of the 12th thoracic vertebra is the aortic opening through which also passes the thoracic duct. At the level of the 8th thoracic vertebra ascends the inferior vena cava. The oesophageal hiatus is an important anatomical landmark because hiatus hernia occurs at this site. There are three types – sliding (commonest) where the oesophagogastric junction moves up into the chest causing gastro-oesophageal reflux, para-oesophageal (rolling) where the greater curve of the stomach rolls into the chest alongside the oesophagus with the cardio-oesophageal junction remaining in the abdomen and a mixed variety which is a combination of the two.

8. B Phrenic nerve

Elevation of the left hemidiaphragm denotes paralysis of the left dome. The motor supply of the diaphragm is from the phrenic nerve which has been paralysed by infiltration with the lung cancer (**Figure 4.3**). The nerve arises in the neck from the 3rd, 4th and 5th cervical rami, the main contribution coming from the 4th. Approximately, two-thirds of the nerve fibres are motor to the diaphragm; the remainder of the nerve is sensory to the diaphragm, mediastinal

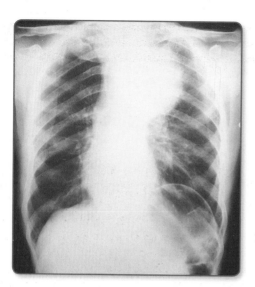

Figure 4.3 Chest X-ray showing large carcinoma of left lung with raised left hemi-diaphragm from infiltration of left phrenic nerve.

and diaphragmatic pleura, serous and fibrous pericardium and diaphragmatic peritoneum. Pain from irritation of the diaphragmatic peritoneum, as in perforation of a hollow viscus, collection of blood or pus in the subphrenic space is referred to the shoulder tip (C4).

Chapter 5

Abdomen

A 55-year-old chronic alcoholic man presents to the outpatient clinic complaining of upper abdominal discomfort and swelling. He recovered from an attack of recurrent acute pancreatitis 6 weeks ago. On examination, he has a smooth fixed lump in his epigastrium, confirmed on ultrasonography to be a fluid-filled cyst of 6 cm in diameter.

In which one of the following anatomical spaces is this fluid collection most likely to be situated in?

A   Left anterior subphrenic space
B   Left posterior subphrenic space
C   Left subhepatic space
D   Right anterior subphrenic space
E   Right subhepatic space

A 60-year-old man presents following two bouts of upper gastrointestinal haemorrhage, from which he recovered with conservative management. oesophagogastroduodenoscopy (OGD) shows a puckered ulcer in the first part of the duodenum penetrating posteriorly with a large blood clot in the middle of the floor of the ulcer.

Which one of the following arteries is the most probable cause of the bleeding?

A   Aberrant right hepatic artery
B   Gastroduodenal artery
C   Right gastric artery
D   Right gastroepiploic artery
E   Superior pancreaticoduodenal artery

3. A 50-year-old man presents with severe acute upper gastrointestinal haemorrhage. After resuscitation, an OGD shows a large penetrating gastric ulcer on the posterior wall in the middle of the body of the stomach with pulsatile arterial blood.

Which one of the following vessels is the cause of the bleeding?

A   Coeliac artery
B   Left gastric artery
C   Left gastroepiploic artery
D   Splenic artery
E   Superior mesenteric artery

4. A 70-year-old woman presents with painless obstructive jaundice and a distended gallbladder. Ultrasound has shown a solid 3 cm mass arising from the head of the pancreas.

Which part of the extrahepatic biliary tree is being compressed by the mass?

A   Common hepatic duct
B   Infraduodenal common bile duct
C   Left extrahepatic duct
D   Right extrahepatic duct
E   Supraduodenal common bile duct

5. A 45-year-old man presents with a lump protruding from his abdomen into his groin and the upper part of the scrotum.

Through which one of the following spaces would the lump have extruded out of the peritoneal cavity?

A   Deep inguinal ring
B   Femoral ring
C   Inguinal triangle
D   Interparietal space
E   Superficial inguinal ring

6. A 55-year-old woman has been diagnosed with an advanced carcinoma of the stomach. She complains of a discharging swelling over her belly button.

Which one of the following intra abdominal ligaments is the portal of cause of this ulcer?

A   Coronary ligament of the liver
B   Left triangular ligament
C   Lesser omentum
D   Ligamentum teres
E   Urachus

7. A 25-year-old man, a cyclist, presents after being hit on the left side of his lower chest when involved in a collision with a car. He complains of pain in his left lower chest, left upper abdomen and left shoulder tip. He has full range of movements of his left upper limb. A FAST (focused abdominal sonography in trauma) scan shows free fluid under the left hemidiaphragm.

Which one of the following anatomical factors is the most likely cause of his left shoulder tip pain?

A   Diaphragmatic rupture causing pain through the intercostobrachial nerve
B   Left acromion fracture causing pain through the long thoracic nerve
C   Left kidney rupture causing pain through the vagus nerve
D   Left lower rib fractures causing pain from the lower six intercostal nerves
E   Splenic rupture causing pain through the phrenic nerve

3. A 70-year-old man is undergoing an elective open repair of an infrarenal abdominal aortic aneurysm.

Which one of the following structures is most adherent to the aneurysm neck?

A Left renal vein
B Neck of pancreas
C Third part of duodenum
D Portal vein
E Pylorus of stomach

Answers

1. C Left subhepatic space

This collection is a pancreatic pseudocyst which is most commonly located in the left subhepatic space. Pancreatic pseudocysts (nonepithelial lined, hence pseudo) are granulation tissue-lined collections that occur as a consequence of moderate to severe acute pancreatitis. Acute pancreatitis results in disruption of the pancreatic parenchyma and ductal system, consequent extravasation of pancreatic enzymes and autodigestion of surrounding tissue. This results in a collection rich in pancreatic enzymes, blood and necrotic tissue. These collections are usually peripancreatic and typically found in the subhepatic space.

The left subhepatic space (lesser sac or omental bursa) is an irregular potential space found posterior to the stomach and lesser omentum, and anterior to the pancreas, left kidney, left adrenal gland and diaphragm. It is bounded superoanteriorly by the liver including the caudate lobe and inferiorly by the transverse mesocolon. On the right it is bounded by the liver and duodenal bulb, while on the left the spleen and gastrocolic ligament form its border. It is a closed space except on its right side where it communicates with the greater sac though an opening, the epiploic foramen of Winslow. To drain a pseudocyst, the subhepatic space can be accessed by:

1. Percutaneously, under radiological guidance
2. Endoscopically, either transpapillary via the pancreatic duct or transmurally, via the posterior gastric wall and
3. Surgically either open or laparoscopically, the last procedure being called cystogastrostomy.

2. B Gastroduodenal artery

A duodenal ulcer penetrates posteriorly into the gastroduodenal artery. An anterior duodenal ulcer, on the other hand, perforates into the general peritoneal cavity. The gastroduodenal artery is a short but large branch of the common hepatic artery. It lies between the first part of the duodenum and the pancreas and supplies the pylorus and upper half of the duodenum. It terminates at the lower border of the T1 when it branches into the right gastroepiploic artery and the superior pancreaticoduodenal artery, which supplies the upper half of the duodenum and pancreas.

The foregut and its derivatives are supplied by the coeliac trunk, which gives rise to the following branches – left gastric artery, common hepatic artery and the splenic artery. The right gastric artery arises from the common hepatic artery. The right gastric artery courses along the lower half of the lesser curve while the left gastric artery courses along the upper half of the lesser curve. Both these arteries anastomose along the lesser curve within layers of the lesser omentum. The fundus of the stomach and upper part of the greater curvature is supplied by the short gastric arteries from the splenic artery that lie in the gastrosplenic ligament. The left and right gastroepiploic arteries supply the greater curve and lie within the layers of the greater omentum. The left gastroepiploic artery arises from the splenic artery while the right gastroepiploic artery is a branch of the gastroduodenal artery.

3. D Splenic artery

This patient is bleeding from the splenic artery which forms one of the constituents of the stomach bed. Posteriorly, the bed of the stomach is related to a number of clinically important structures, which form the posterior wall of the omental bursa. These structures include left crus and dome of the diaphragm, left kidney and adrenal gland, pancreas, spleen, splenic artery, the transverse mesocolon and colon. From the position of the artery and endoscopic findings, the cause of the bleeding in this patient is penetration of the ulcer into his splenic artery. It is important that the splenic artery as the source of bleeding is appreciated early by the position of the ulcer and the rate and amount of bleeding. This ulcer is at high risk of re-bleeding and may necessitate emergency surgery to control the bleeding.

4. B Infraduodenal common bile duct

The infraduodenal common bile duct lies in close relationship to the pancreatic head and hence is compressed early in a carcinoma of the pancreatic head. The right and left hepatic ducts correspondingly drain the right and left lobes of liver. Shortly after leaving the porta hepatis, the right and left hepatic ducts converge to form the common hepatic duct (CHD), which carries on inferiorly for approximately 2 cm. The CHD then unites with the cystic duct to form the common bile duct (CBD). The CBD is approximately 8 cm long and can be divided into four parts – supraduodenal, retroduodenal, infraduodenal and intraduodenal parts.

The supraduodenal part lies in the free margin of the lesser omentum with the portal vein posteriorly and the hepatic artery on its left. The retroduodenal part lies posterior to the first part of the duodenum and anterior to the portal vein. The gastroduodenal artery lies to its left. The infraduodenal part, the narrowest part of the CBD, terminates in the posteromedial aspect of the second part of the duodenum at the hepatopancreatic ampulla of Vater, surrounded by the sphincter of Oddi. The confluence of the infraduodenal CBD and the main pancreatic duct form the hepatopancreatic ampulla of Vater. The infraduodenal CBD lies within the concavity of the duodenum in a groove on the posterior aspect of the pancreatic head. A small mass within the pancreatic head will compress the infraduodenal CBD causing obstructive jaundice. However, it is very important to be aware of the variations in the anatomy of the extrahepatic biliary tree. In 7% the cystic duct is long and can enter the CBD low down either in front or behind in which case the growth would envelop both the CBD and cystic duct.

5. A Deep inguinal ring

The groin lump in this patient has extruded out of the deep inguinal ring. The description of the lump is such that it represents an indirect inguinal hernia. Inguinal hernias are protrusions of abdominal cavity contents into the inguinal canal and may be classified as either direct or indirect. An indirect inguinal hernia may be seen in adults or children. They emerge through the deep inguinal ring, lateral to the inferior epigastric artery. Indirect inguinal hernias are covered by the spermatic fascia and traverse the inguinal canal, to varying degrees. Large indirect inguinal hernias may traverse the entire length of the inguinal canal and emerge from the superficial inguinal ring into the scrotum – inguinoscrotal hernias. Direct inguinal hernias emerge through a weakness of the posterior wall, medial to the inferior epigastric artery, in the inguinal triangle. It is usually an acquired defect and hence is seen in adults. Direct inguinal hernias may exit via the superficial inguinal ring but do not extend into the scrotum, even when large. The inguinal triangle (Hesselbach's triangle) is bounded by the lateral border of the rectus muscle medially, the inferior epigastric artery laterally and the inguinal ligament inferiorly.

6. D Ligamentum teres

The carcinoma has spread through the ligamentum teres, the condition being referred to as Sister Mary Joseph's nodule. Sister Mary Joseph Dempsey (1856–1939, surgical assistant to William Mayo at St Mary's Hospital) was the first to note the presence of a firm, non-tender reddish umbilical nodule in patients with advanced intra-abdominal malignancy (commonly gastric, colonic, pancreatic and ovarian cancers). These nodules, eponymously named Sister Mary Joseph's nodule, represents metastatic cutaneous tumour deposits (**Figure 5.1**). The most common route for tumour spread to the umbilicus is from contiguous extension of the tumour through peritoneum folds, falciform ligament and ligamentum teres. Ligamentum teres is a fibrous remnant of the foetal umbilical vein and lies within the free edge of the falciform ligament. It runs on the anterior abdominal wall and inserts around the umbilicus. Similarly, Cullen's sign, periumbilical ecchymosis, is seen in patients with haemoperitoneum where diffusion of blood along the ligamentum teres to the umbilicus results in periumbilical bruising. Cullen's sign is typically seen in acute haemorrhagic pancreatitis and tubal rupture in patients with ectopic pregnancy.

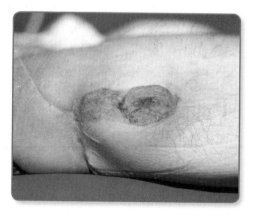

Figure 5.1 Sister Mary Joseph's nodule.

E Splenic rupture causing pain through the phrenic nerve

This patient's shoulder tip pain is caused by referred pain through the phrenic nerve as a result of diaphragmatic irritation from free blood under the diaphragm. In any patient with left sided upper abdominal and lower chest trauma, there should be a high index of suspicion for splenic injury. This index of suspicion should be heightened further in a patient with these symptoms and acute left shoulder tip pain. This sign, a left sided Kehr's sign, is classically described in patients with a ruptured spleen. This occurs due to the presence of blood in the subdiaphragmatic space causing irritation of the diaphragm. The phrenic nerve provides the motor supply and most of the sensory supply of the diaphragm except peripherally where the sensory supply is from the subcostal and intercostal nerves. The phrenic nerve is formed from the 3rd, 4th and 5th cervical nerves. The dorsal nerve roots of C3, C4 and C5 supplies cutaneous sensation to the dermatomes around the shoulder. Although, the mechanism is unclear, the brain appears to perceive the signals coming from the internal organ as originating from the somatic supply, resulting in diaphragmatic irritation causing shoulder tip pain. This phenomenon, of pain being felt remote from the location of the offending structure, is called referred pain.

C Third part of duodenum

While dissecting the neck of the aneurysm to put on a clamp, the third part of the duodenum is the most vulnerable. It is particularly in danger in an inflammatory aneurysm, where the duodenum is extremely adherent to the neck.

The abdominal aorta is a retroperitoneal structure. It enters the abdomen at the level of T12 through the aortic hiatus of the diaphragm and terminates at the level of L4 when it bifurcates into paired common iliac arteries. It courses just to the left of the midline and descends anterior to the bodies of the L1 to L4 vertebrae and the anterior longitudinal ligament.

Anteriorly, the abdominal aorta is closely related to a number of upper abdominal structures. Intra-operatively, these structures usually have to be retracted or dissected to allow access to the aorta. During aortic aneurysm surgery, after division of the ligament of Treitz, the 3rd part of the duodenum is dissected off the neck of the aneurysm and the duodenum retracted to the right to allow adequate exposure. The left renal vein and pancreas may also need to be retracted superiorly to expose the aneurysm neck. The left ureter may be dangerously adherent to the aneurysmal sac making it liable to iatrogenic damage.

Chapter 6

Pelvis

A 30-year-old woman is to have postoperative analgesia by means of a nerve block following an operation for a fistula-in-ano.

Which one of the following nerves is the anaesthetist going to block by local anaesthetic?

A   Common peroneal nerve
B   Lumbosacral trunk
C   Nerve to levator ani and external anal sphincter
D   Obturator nerve
E   Pudendal nerve

A 42-year-old man, a labourer, while at work, suddenly develops severe pain in his lower back radiating to the buttocks, back of thigh, lower leg and sole of foot. He cannot feel when he sits as he has diminished sensation on his buttocks.

Which one of the following nerves is most likely affected?

A   L5
B   S1
C   S2
D   S3
E   S4

A 65-year-old woman presents with severe pain on the inside of her thigh, which began 1 week ago. The pain radiates along the inside of the thigh to the knee. It is relieved by bending the hip and rotating it outwards. In that position a soft lump is palpable.

Which one of the following nerves is causing the pain?

A   Femoral
B   Genitofemoral
C   Ilioinguinal
D   Lateral femoral cutaneous
E   Obturator

A 30-year-old man presents with left ureteric colic. A spiral CT scan shows a stone impacted at the pelvic brim.

At which of the following anatomical sites would the stone be impacted?

A   Common iliac artery bifurcation
B   Fifth lumbar transverse process

C   Ischial spine
D   Pelviureteric junction
E   Vas deferens crossing above the ureter

5. A 35-year-old woman is undergoing a hysterectomy with preservation of ovaries.

During the operation which one of the following anatomical structures is vulnerable to iatrogenic damage?

A   Fallopian tubes
B   Ovaries
C   Rectum
D   Ureters
E   Urinary bladder

6. A 25-year-old man presents following a straddle injury to his perineum having fallen astride on the beam in the gymnasium. Clinically there is a perineal haematoma with blood on his external urinary meatus.

Which anatomical structure is most likely to be injured?

A   Bladder neck
B   Bulbar urethra
C   Membranous urethra
D   Prostatic urethra
E   Urinary bladder

7. A 16-year-old boy presents with a condition, where he passes urine from a meatus on the underside of his glans penis, a situation he finds embarrassing.

Which one of the following congenital anatomical abnormality does he suffer from?

A   Coronal hypospadias
B   Epispadias
C   Glandular hypospadias
D   Penile hypospadias
E   Perineal hypospadias

8. A 35-year-old man is recovering from a severe motorcycle injury where he sustained major pelvic fractures and bladder and urethral injuries. He did not suffer any head injuries. Six months after his accident his urethral catheter is removed. He is completely incontinent.

Which one of the following anatomical structures has been irreparably damaged, causing his incontinence?

A   External urethral sphincter
B   Internal urethral sphincter
C   Membranous urethra
D   Puboprostatic ligaments
E   Urinary bladder rupture

Answers

1. E Pudendal nerve

The pudendal nerve (S2, S3 and S4) in the perineum is the one that can be blocked by local anaesthetic. The nerve is accessed through the lateral wall of the vagina to produce anaesthesia to the perineal and anal skin. The nerve is formed by the anterior divisions of the ventral rami of the 2nd, 3rd and 4th sacral nerves. After its origin, it leaves the pelvis through the greater sciatic foramen to enter the gluteal region near the ischial spine. The nerve accompanies the internal pudendal vessels into the pudendal (Alcock's) canal on the lateral wall of the ischiorectal fossa. In the posterior part of the canal it gives off its branches – inferior rectal nerve, the perineal nerve and the dorsal nerve of clitoris or penis.

The common peroneal nerve is formed by L4, L5 and S1 and S2. The lumbosacral trunk is constituted by L4 and L5, and joins the sacral plexus. S4 contributes to the nerve supplying the levator ani and external anal sphincter. The obturator nerve arises from the lumbar plexus from the anterior divisions of L2, L3 and L4. None of these nerves is the target of the caudal block.

2. D S3

The S3 nerve root is responsible for the sensation of the sitting area of buttock. It is a constituent of the sacral plexus. The most important nerve arising from the sacral plexus is the sciatic nerve. It arises from L4, L5, S1, S2 and S3 roots of the sacral plexus. At its origin it is 2 cm wide and is the thickest nerve in the body. It enters the gluteal region from the pelvis through the greater sciatic foramen. At a variable level in the back of the thigh proximal to the popliteal fossa it divides into the common peroneal (fibular, L4, L5, S1, S2 and tibial, L4, L5, S1, S2, S3) nerves. The surface anatomy is an imaginary line drawn from the midpoint of the ischial tuberosity and greater trochanter to the apex of the popliteal fossa formed by the junction of the semimembranosus and semitendinosus medially and biceps femoris laterally. As an aid to remember the dermatome levels, we stand mainly on S1 (sole of foot), sit on S3 (buttocks) and wipe S4 (immediate perianal area).

The commonest cause of damage to the sciatic nerve is iatrogenic misplaced gluteal injection. It may be affected in pelvic disease, severe hip trauma (7% of dislocations and 16% of fracture dislocations), or after total hip replacement (1%). Complete sciatic nerve palsy is rare and results in a flail foot and severe difficulty in walking. Because of its anatomical location in close proximity to the fibular head, the common peroneal nerve is the commonest nerve to be damaged in the lower limb. This results in a foot drop, high stepping gait and sensory loss over the lower lateral part of the leg and dorsum of the foot.

3. E Obturator

The obturator nerve is causing this patient's pain. She has the clinical features of an obturator hernia. The pain is referred to the knee by the geniculate branch of the obturator nerve (anterior divisions of L2, L3 and L4). The pain is much more pronounced in a strangulated hernia. Arising from the lumbar plexus, the obturator nerve lies on the psoas muscle and enters the obturator foramen. In the obturator canal it divides into anterior and posterior branches.

In an obturator hernia, a swelling is not often palpable unless the hip is abducted, flexed and externally rotated. The hernia can sometimes be felt as a tender swelling on rectal or vaginal examination.

4. A Common iliac artery bifurcation

The stone is impacted at the bifurcation of the common iliac artery where it leaves the psoas muscle. This is one of the points of natural narrowing where a stone may get arrested. The other points of natural narrowing are: pelviureteric junction, where it is crossed by the vas deferens or broad ligament and at the ureterovesical junction.

Knowledge of the relationships of the ureter is very important, so as to prevent iatrogenic damage. On the left it underlies the apex of the sigmoid mesocolon. It then runs over the external iliac artery and vein and then down the side wall of the pelvis in front of the internal iliac artery and behind the ovary. On the right it will be in close proximity to a pelvic appendix. Further distally at the level of the ischial spine it travels forwards and medially to enter the bladder base. Here the vas deferens in the male crosses above the ureter and in the female it crosses the lateral vaginal fornix.

5. D Ureters

The ureters are vulnerable to iatrogenic damage by virtue of their close relationship to the structures in the female pelvis. Once the ureters descend to the pelvis, at the level of the ischial spine they travel forwards and medially above the pelvic floor to enter the bladder base at its upper lateral angle. Here the ureter lies at the base of the broad ligament where the uterine artery crosses it in the upper part. Under the broad ligament the ureters penetrate the lateral cervical ligaments in close proximity to the lateral vaginal fornix being no more than 2 cm from the cervix before entering the bladder anterior to the fornix. This is where the ureters are at greatest danger of damage, whilst ligating vessels and dividing ligaments.

The position of the ureters is of huge applied importance as they can be inadvertently damaged in operations of right hemicolectomy, sigmoid colectomy, anterior resection, abdominoperineal excision of rectum, hysterectomy and oophorectomy. In these operations the ureters should always be identified in their entire length by noting peristalsis, particularly when pinched with a forceps, and by noting the white shiny tubular structure with overlying longitudinal arterial anastomosis.

6. B Bulbar urethra

This patient has injured his bulbar urethra (sometimes referred to as the anterior urethra) in the perineum. This injury involves the junction of the membranous with the bulbar portion of the urethra. The anatomy of this region is such that extravasation of urine occurs, unless recognition of the injury and treatment is carried out promptly. Urine leaks between the perineal membrane and the membranous layer of the perineal fascia (Colles' fascia). As both these layers are firmly attached to the ischiopubic rami posteriorly, urine extravasates anteriorly into the loose connective tissue around the scrotum, penis and anterior abdominal wall. Should the posterior urethra be injured, urine leaks into the pelvic extraperitoneal tissues. Tear of the perineal membrane results in extravasation in the perineum.

Anatomically, the membranous urethra is the shortest (1.5 cm) and least dilatable part of the male urethra (which is 18–20 cm long). The anterior urethra (16 cm) has a proximal perineal and a distal penile component. The posterior urethra is subdivided into preprostatic, prostatic and membranous parts. The female urethra is 4 cm long and 6 mm wide.

Injury to the bladder neck, membranous and prostatic urethra can occur in fractures of the pelvis. Bladder rupture, extra- or intraperitoneal, is highly unlikely with such an injury. The clinical findings are not those of a bladder rupture.

7. C Glandular hypospadias

This boy has glandular hypospadias, the most common type of hypospadias. The urethra proximal to the ejaculatory ducts is developed from the lower ends of the mesonephric ducts and the ureters. The remainder of the urethra is derived from the pelvic and phallic parts of the urogenital sinus and the genital tubercle. The ventral section of the penile part of the urethra is formed by the fusion of the urogenital folds. Failure of complete fusion of the urogenital folds results in hypospadias. The degree of lack of fusion results in the various types of hypospadias, the incidence of which is 1 in 300 boys. The type of hypospadias depends upon the placement of the meatus: in coronal the meatus is at the junction of the underside of the glans and the body of the penis; in penile and penoscrotal the opening is on the underside of the penile shaft; in perineal, the most severe type, the urethra opens between the two halves of a bifid scrotum. There may be an additional abnormality of the prepuce which may be longer dorsally and absent ventrally with chordee (ventral curvature of the penis). In epispadias, a very rare abnormality, the urethral opening on the dorsum is associated with an upward penile curvature.

8. A External urethral sphincter

This person's urinary incontinence is due to damage to the external urethral sphincter. The internal urethral sphincter surrounding the proximal prostatic urethra is not responsible for urinary continence. This helps to prevent retrograde ejaculation by closing off the bladder neck during ejaculation.

The urethral sphincter mechanism extends from the perineum through the urogenital hiatus into the pelvic cavity. The mechanism consists of the striated and smooth muscle of the urethra and the pubourethral part of levator ani; this surrounds the membranous urethra in the male. The fibres also reach up to the lowest part of the bladder neck. The muscles are of the slow twitch variety. The innervation is from the perineal branch of the pudendal nerve and the pelvic splanchnic nerves. All these nerves originate in the S2, S3 and S4 spinal segments.

The urethral sphincter mechanism compresses the urethra when the bladder contains urine. It is located around the region of the highest urethral closing pressure, thus playing an important role in maintaining urinary continence. It relaxes during micturition and contracts to expel final drops of urine or semen from the bulbar urethra.

Chapter 7

Lower limb

A 62-year-old man presents with shock, secondary to acute pancreatitis. A decision is made to place a femoral line as part of his initial resuscitation in the emergency department.

Which one of the following lies outwith the femoral sheath?

A   Cloquet's node
B   Femoral artery
C   Femoral canal
D   Femoral nerve
E   Femoral vein

A 75-year-old woman attends 6 months following left total hip arthroplasty through a lateral approach. She is found to have a left sided Trendelenburg gait with weakness of the ipsilateral abductors.

Which one of the following nerves is most likely to be injured, and explains the examination findings?

A   Femoral nerve
B   Inferior gluteal nerve
C   Obturator nerve
D   Sciatic nerve
E   Superior gluteal nerve

A 45-year-old man presents with a chronic swelling in the popliteal fossa consistent with a Baker's cyst.

Of the following muscles that comprise the borders of the popliteal fossa, which one has an insertion on the head of the fibula?

A   Biceps femoris
B   Gastrocnemius
C   Plantaris
D   Semimembranosus
E   Semitendinosus

A 25-year-old man presents with significant pain and swelling to the anterior aspect of the leg following a direct blow during a football match. Clinical examination and compartment pressure monitoring confirm the diagnosis of acute compartment syndrome of the leg.

Which of the following structures is found within the lateral compartment of the leg?

A   Anterior tibial artery
B   Deep peroneal nerve
C   Peroneus tertius
D   Superficial peroneal nerve
E   Tibialis anterior

5.   A 68-year-old woman presents with a bimalleolar fracture of the right ankle. Operative fixation is undertaken using a direct lateral approach to the lateral malleolus, with a direct incision used for the medial malleolus.

Which one of the following structures is found anterior to the medial malleolus?

A   Flexor digitorum longus tendon
B   Posterior tibial artery
C   Saphenous nerve
D   Tibial nerve
E   Tibialis posterior tendon

6.   A 43-year-old woman presents with lumbar back pain and sciatica, with associated numbness over the lateral border of the right foot and ankle, along with an absent ipsilateral ankle jerk.

Which spinal nerve distribution does this represent?

A   L4
B   L5
C   S1
D   S2
E   S3

Answers

. D Femoral nerve

The femoral sheath is 3–4 cm long (from the inguinal ligament) and is formed from a prolongation of the transversalis fascia (anteriorly) and iliacus fascia (posteriorly). It encompasses the femoral artery, femoral vein and femoral canal.

The femoral triangle is formed by the:

- Inguinal ligament (superiorly)
- Medial border of adductor longus (medially)
- Medial border of sartorius (laterally)
- Fascia lata (anteriorly/roof)
- Pectineus, iliopsoas, adductor longus (posteriorly/floor)

The femoral triangle is of major clinical significance, e.g. for arterial access in angioplasty, venous access in the shutdown patient. The following structures are contained within the femoral triangle (lateral to medial):

- Femoral nerve
- Femoral artery
- Femoral vein
- Femoral canal

Mnemonic: **NAVY** = Nerve, Artery, Vein, Y-fronts

The femoral artery is located at the mid-inguinal point (midpoint between the anterior superior iliac spine and the pubic symphysis). The femoral canal superiorly contains fat, lymphatic vessels and nodes (deep inguinal lymph nodes, Cloquet's node). The entrance to the femora canal is known as the femoral ring, through which a femoral hernia can occur. The borders of the femoral ring are the inguinal ligament (anteriorly), pectineal ligament (posteriorly), lacunar ligament (medially) and femoral vein fascia (laterally).

2. E Superior gluteal nerve

When using the lateral approach to the hip the patient is in the lateral decubitus position. A lateral incision is made through skin, subcutaneous fat and the tensor fascia lata. The fibres of gluteus medius are then split (excess splitting to be avoided), along with the fibres of vastus lateralis, and an anterior flap is developed providing access to the hip capsule and then joint. The superior gluteal nerve (L4–S1) arises from anterior sacral foramina of the sacral plexus, exiting the pelvis through the greater sciatic foramen above piriformis (only structures above), travelling adjacent to the superior gluteal artery and vein. It then transverses between gluteus medius and gluteus minimus, passing approximately 4 cm above the greater trochanter. Muscular innervation is to gluteus medius, gluteus minimus and tensor fascia lata. Damage to the superior gluteal nerve can occur following excess splitting of gluteus medius and results in paralysis of the abductor muscles of the ipsilateral hip. A Trendelenburg gait is seen when the pelvis sags on the contralateral side of the lesion due to the lack of the abductor pull on the ipsilateral side.

The inferior gluteal nerve (L5–S2) arises from the sacral plexus, exiting the pelvis through the greater sciatic foramen below piriformis. From there it provides muscular innervation to the gluteus maximus. The sciatic nerve (L4–S3) exits the pelvis through the greater sciatic foramen below piriformis. It then transverses posterior to gluteus maximus and descends the thigh anterior to adductor magnus and posterior to the hamstrings. It supplies muscular innervation to biceps femoris, semitendinosus, semimembranosus, and adductor magnus. Sensory innervation is to the posterior aspect of the thigh and gluteal regions. The nerve divides, often just superior to the popliteal fossa, to give rise to the common peroneal and tibial nerves. The sciatic nerve is at risk during the posterior approach to the hip, with damage leading to paralysis and paraesthesia below the knee joint (sensory innervation spared medial aspect ankle and foot supplied by saphenous nerve). The femoral nerve (L2–S4) arises from the ventral rami of the lumbar plexus, passing through psoas major and emerging on the inferior lateral aspect where it then passes into the thigh posterior to the inguinal ligament. Approximately 5 cm inferior to the ligament, it provides terminal muscular (quadriceps femoris, Sartorius, pectineus), sensory (intermediate cutaneous nerve, medial cutaneous nerve) and articular (hip and knee joint) branches.

3. A Biceps femoris

The popliteal fossa is a diamond shaped depression that forms the posterior aspect of the knee and is made through the following borders (**Table 7.1**):

Table 7.1

Muscle	Origin	Insertion	Innervation
Semimembranosus	Ischial tuberosity	Medial aspect of tibia	Sciatic (tibial)
Semitendinosus	Ischial tuberosity	Upper part of tibia	Sciatic (tibial)
Biceps femoris			
Long head	Ischial tuberosity	Head of fibula	Sciatic (tibial)
Short Head	Linea aspera femur	Head of fibula	Sciatic (common peroneal)
Gastrocnemius	Distal femur		
Medial head	Medial condyle	Achilles tendon	Sciatic (tibial)
Lateral head	Lateral condyle		
Plantaris	Supracondylar ridge femur (lateral)	Achilles tendon	Sciatic (tibial)

Table 7.1 The origin, insertion and innervation of the muscles that border the popliteal fossa.

- Semimembranosus and semitendinosus (superomedially)
- Biceps femoris (superolaterally)
- Medial head of gastrocnemius (inferomedially)
- Lateral head of gastrocnemius and plantaris (inferolaterally)
- Skin and superficial/deep fascia (roof)
- Posterior aspect of femur/knee joint and popliteus muscle (floor)

The first three muscles make up the posterior compartment of the thigh (hamstrings – semimembranosus, semitendinosus, biceps femoris). Semitendinosus, gracilis and sartorius (posterior to anterior) insert via a conjoined tendon into an area on the anteromedial aspect of the proximal tibia known as the pes anserinus. This insertion can become inflamed and can be a source of chronic knee pain. It is also the source of tendon harvesting for anterior cruciate ligament reconstruction.

The contents of the popliteal fossa (the deepest to the most superficial) include:

- Popliteal artery
- Popliteal vein
- Sciatic nerve (superiorly)
- Tibial and common peroneal nerves (inferiorly)
- Lymph nodes
- Fat
- Popliteus bursa

D Superficial peroneal nerve

The leg is divided into four distinct fascial compartments (**Table 7.2**) through the interosseous membrane, the transverse intermuscular septum and the posterior intermuscular septum.

Table 7.2			
Compartment	Contents	Neurovascular supply	Movement
Anterior	Tibialis anterior	Deep peroneal nerve	Dorsiflexors of ankle and toes
	Extensor hallucis longus	Anterior tibial artery	
	Extensor digitorum longus		
	Peroneus tertius		
	Deep peroneal nerve		
	Anterior tibial vasculature		

Table 7.2 The contents, neurovascular supply and action of the four leg compartments. *Contd...*

Table 7.2 Contd...

Compartment	Contents	Neurovascular supply	Movement
Lateral	Peroneus longus	Superficial peroneal nerve	Ankle/foot eversion and plantarflexion
	Peroneus brevis	Peroneal artery	
	Superficial peroneal nerve		
Deep posterior	Tibialis posterior	Tibial nerve	Ankle/foot plantarflexion
	Flexor hallucis longus	Posterior tibial artery	
	Flexor digitorum longus		
	Popliteus		
	Tibial nerve		
	Posterior tibial vasculature		
Superficial posterior	Gastrocnemius	Tibial nerve	Ankle/foot plantarflexion
	Soleus	Posterior tibial artery	
	Plantaris		
	Medial sural cutaneous nerve		

Injury to the tibial nerve leads to loss of ankle/foot plantar flexion with an associated loss of sensation on the plantar aspect of the foot. Injury to the common peroneal nerve can lead to foot drop with loss of ankle/foot dorsiflexion (deep peroneal nerve), loss of ankle/foot eversion (superficial peroneal). Loss of sensation is over the dorsum of the foot (deep peroneal = 1st dorsal web space, superficial peroneal nerve = dorsum of foot; **Figure 7.1**).

5. C Saphenous nerve

Important structures that pass anterior to the medial malleolus are the saphenous nerve and saphenous vein. This is a useful site of peripheral access in a patient with circulatory collapse, i.e. saphenous cut down. The structures that are posterior to the medial malleolus are:

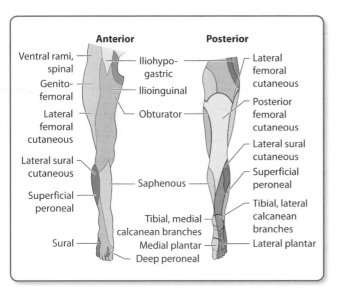

Figure 7.1 Cutaneous nerve supply of the leg and foot.

- Tibialis posterior tendon
- Flexor digitorum longus tendon
- Posterior tibial artery
- Tibial nerve
- Flexor digitorum hallucis tendon

Anterior

↓

Posterior

NB: Mnemonic is **T**om, **D**ick **A**nd a **N**ervous **H**arry

The ankle joint is a synovial hinge type mortise joint with an articulation between the body of the talus and the distal aspects of the tibia and fibula. The ligaments of the ankle joint include:

- The medial deltoid ligament
  - Origin: medial malleolus of tibia
  - Insertion: medial aspect of the talus, sustentaculum tali of the calcaneus, calcaneonavicular ligament, navicular tuberosity
- Lateral
  - Anterior talofibular ligament
  - Posterior talofibular ligament
  - Calcaneofibular ligament

C S1

The sciatic nerve (L4–S3) arises from the sacral plexus. Sciatica describes a constellation of symptoms and signs associated with neural compression, due to intervertebral disc compression, of one of the five spinal nerve roots that give rise to the sciatic nerve. The most frequently affected sites are L4/L5 and L5/S1.

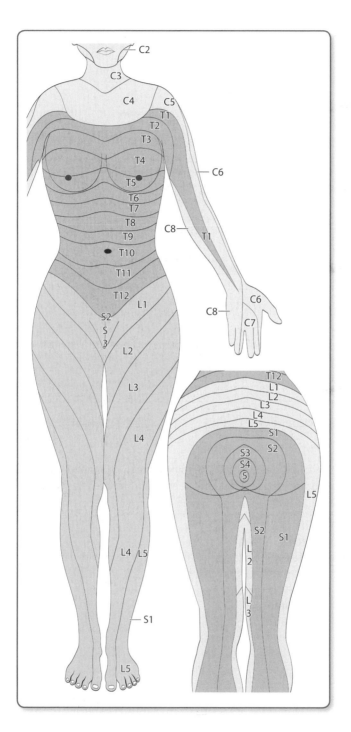

Figure 7.2
Dermatomes.

The dermatome distribution is shown in **Figure 7.2**. The reflexes in the lower limb are:

- Knee (L3/L4, femoral nerve, quadriceps femoris)
- Ankle (S1, sciatic nerve/tibial division, gastrocnemius)

The myotomes of the lower limb are shown in **Table 7.3**.

Table 7.3

Joint movement	Muscle	Root (nerve)
Hip abduction	Gluteal muscles	L4–S1 (sciatic)
Hip adduction	Adductors	L2/L3 (obturator)
Hip flexion	Iliopsoas (anterior compartment muscles)	L1–L3 (femoral)
Knee extension	Quadriceps femoris	L3/L4 (femoral)
Hip extension	Gluteal and posterior compartment muscles	L5/S1 (sciatic)
Knee flexion	Hamstrings	L5–S1 (sciatic)
Ankle dorsiflexion	Anterior tibial	L4/L5 (common peroneal)
Hallux extension	Extensor hallucis longus	L5/S1 (common peroneal)
Ankle plantar flexion	Gastrocnemius and soleus	S1/S2 (tibial)
Hallux flexion	Flexor hallucis longus	S2/S3 (tibial)

Table 7.3 The myotomes of the lower limb. (Adapted from Duckworth AD, Porter D, Ralston SH. Churchill's Pocketbook of Orthopaedics Trauma and Rheumatology. Edinburgh: Churchill Livingston, 2009.)

Chapter 8

Homeostasis, coagulation and bleeding

1. A 60-year-old man has been admitted to hospital unconscious after a car crash with multiple injuries and excessive bleeding in relation to his injuries. He is found to have atrial fibrillation and another occupant of the car (without serious injuries) reports that the unconscious man was taking treatment to prevent complications of his irregular heartbeat.

    Which of the following is most likely to have caused the excessive bleeding?

    A   Deficient heparin level in the blood
    B   Deficient prothrombin level in the blood
    C   Excessive calcium level in the blood
    D   Excessive haematocrit
    E   Excessive vitamin D level in the blood

2. A 60-year-old woman is having open cholecystectomy which has been prolonged by technical difficulties. It is noted that her core temperature has fallen by over a degree since the start of surgery.

    Which of the following is most likely to have caused the fall in core temperature?

    A   Reaction to propofol administered by the anaesthetist
    B   An operating theatre temperature in the range 25–30°C
    C   Intravenous fluids administered at around 35°C
    D   Loss of homeostasis due to the anaesthetic
    E   The patient's increased metabolic rate

3. A 60-year-old man has been admitted for repair of an inguinal hernia. He has been on insulin therapy for many years and now suffers from orthostatic hypotension due to diabetic autonomic neuropathy. His arterial blood pressure when lying down is 130/80 mmHg, but when he stands for five minutes it falls to 105/70 mmHg and he feels somewhat light-headed.

    Which of the following is most likely to have caused the fall in his blood pressure on standing?

    A   Excessive blood pressure homeostasis
    B   Excessive variability of his resting heart rate due to sinus arrhythmia
    C   Excessive venoconstriction
    D   Impaired sympathetically-induced peripheral vasoconstriction
    E   Impairment of his renin-angiotensin system

4. A 24-year-old man undergoes an uncomplicated appendicectomy for acute appendicitis. Shortly after the end of surgery, in the recovery room, he develops violent shivering and becomes cyanotic.

Which of the following is most likely to have caused this condition?

A   Depression of the reflex control of blood oxygen saturation
B   Exaggeration of the reflex control of body temperature
C   Low temperature in the recovery room
D   Septicaemia related to the appendicitis
E   Undiagnosed cyanotic heart disease

5. A 30-year-old man, a sportsman, presents for cruciate ligament repair in his right leg. He is otherwise a fit young man, but mentions that after minor cuts he thinks he bleeds rather longer than normal. This has not bothered him and it has not been investigated.

Which of the following is the most appropriate investigation?

A   Measure his factor VIII level
B   Measure his haemoglobin level
C   Measure his INR (international normalised ratio)
D   Measure his plasminogen level
E   Measure his platelet count

6. A 55-year-old woman presents with clear evidence of a postoperative myocardial infarction, developing after an uneventful laparoscopic cholecystectomy. She had been otherwise healthy prior to surgery and there is no evidence of other postoperative complications.

Which of the following is the most effective management?

A   Administer a plasminogen activator urgently
B   Administer a thrombin antagonist urgently
C   Await a neurological opinion next day on the risk of cerebral haemorrhage
D   Await serial troponin measurements
E   Monitor the blood pressure at hourly intervals

7. A 64-year-old man treated previously with warfarin for postoperative deep venous thrombosis (target INR 2–2.5), presents with a recurrence 6 months after stopping treatment. Low dose heparin is started and his INR is checked before recommencing warfarin. When told his initial INR is 1.1, he is very concerned because 2–2.5 was the previous target.

Which of the following statements is the best way to relieve his anxiety?

A   Initial INR test was to exclude likely liver disease
B   Initial low dose heparin gives only slight protection
C   Treatment of recurrent embolism differs from that of the previous embolism
D   Treatment was important to prevent fatal embolism
E   Value of 1.1 is completely normal before warfarin treatment

A 55-year-old woman with multiple injuries has developed disseminated intravascular coagulation leading to hypofibrinogenaemia and a risk of excessive haemorrhage.

Which of the following is most likely to have caused this condition?

A   Activation of the extrinsic clotting pathway by a drug (extrinsic agent) administered to her

B   Activation of the extrinsic clotting pathway by products of tissue damage

C   Activation of the intrinsic clotting pathway by excess factor VIII levels

D   Activation of the intrinsic clotting pathway by excess calcium ions

E   Excess production of prothrombin (factor II)

Answers

1. B Deficient prothrombin level in the blood

A deficient prothrombin level is a common cause of a haemorrhagic state. The prothrombin deficiency may be due to the effect of warfarin treatment, or to serious liver disease. This man is likely to be on treatment with warfarin which suppresses hepatic production of prothrombin. This treatment reduces the risk of thrombi forming in his fibrillating atria and throwing off emboli either from the right atrium to the lungs, or from the left atrium to the systemic circulation, including the cerebral circulation to cause a stroke. Two things must be dealt with in this case. Firstly, the risk of excessive bleeding must be dealt with before surgical intervention. Secondly, the risk of emboli from the atria must also be addressed perhaps by some other treatment which can minimise it without causing unacceptable bleeding.

Options D and E are not associated with haemorrhage; the changes in A and C are the reverse of those which cause haemorrhage.

2. D Loss of homeostasis due to the anaesthetic

Depression of brain function during anaesthesia leads to loss of various homeostatic reflexes (which maintain constancy of blood pressure, core temperature, etc). Vasodilation produced by anaesthetic drugs leads to excessive heat loss by bringing increased flow of warm blood to the peripheries (warm operating theatres, B, help to reduce the heat loss). With loss of temperature-regulating reflexes, the vasodilation is unopposed and increased heat production by shivering is not possible. The resting metabolic rate falls somewhat, partly due to decreased brain metabolism (reverse of E). Warming intravenous fluids (C) to around core temperature helps to reduce cooling. Gentle heating of limbs helps to combat inevitable heat loss from exposed parts, including evaporative heat loss. Reactions to anaesthetic drugs are more likely to cause hyperthermia than hypothermia (A), though this is a rare problem. Even a degree fall below normal core temperature has an adverse effect on recovery, since mechanisms like haemostasis and healing are impaired.

3. D Impaired sympathetically-induced peripheral vasoconstriction

Blood pressure stability (homeostasis), when standing, relies heavily on increased sympathetic vasoconstriction, as blood pressure usually falls when changing from a horizontal to a vertical posture. Diabetic autonomic neuropathy implies progressive loss of function in autonomic nerves, including sympathetic nerves, so, on standing, the fall in cardiac output cannot be adequately compensated for by increased peripheral resistance. Thus blood pressure stability [homeostasis (A)] is compromised. Sympathetic nerves also produce venoconstriction (C) so this also is impaired, which contributes to the postural fall in arterial blood pressure.

Sinus arrhythmia (B) is a normal phenomenon due to variation in vagal tone with breathing and it too is impaired in diabetic neuropathy. The renin-angiotensin system (E) is hormonal, and not affected in diabetic neuropathy. It would compensate in this man for his poor reflex compensation in the standing posture, and treating him with inhibitors of this system (angiotensin-converting enzyme inhibitors which antagonize the angiotensin converting enzyme which produces angiotensin II) could be catastrophic.

A Depression of the reflex control of blood oxygen saturation

The violent, cyanotic, shivering in the recovery room, as this man recovers from the effects of his anaesthetic suggests that, during the anaesthetic, the loss of body temperature homeostasis due to suppression of brain function allowed his core temperature to fall. With recovery of reflex control of core temperature, vigorous shivering is initiated. However, recovery of homeostatic control of arterial blood oxygenation has lagged behind that of core temperature, due to residual suppression of ventilation, so oxygen intake is unable to keep up with the very large oxygen consumption associated with shivering. Thus, the shivering is normal in relation to restoring body temperature (B). There is no evidence for the other options.

E Measure platelet count

This man gives a vague suggestion of excessive bleeding after minor injury. This suggests the possibility of inadequate initial closure (spasm) of local small blood vessels. Platelets have a major role in this initial closure, favouring both vascular spasm by release of 5-hydroxytryptamine (5-HT or serotonin) and by adhering to damaged blood vessel endothelium. Factor VIII deficiency [haemophilia (A)] produces a different pattern. It impairs clotting, so, with normal vascular closing, bleeding may stop initially but then develop persistently when the initial spasm wears off. Measuring the INR (C) and plasminogen levels (D) does not fit his history, and there is no suggestion that he has become anaemic (B).

A Administer a plasminogen activator urgently

The aim is to reopen a coronary end artery by dissolving the recent blood clot which has obstructed it. This is affected by increasing the thrombolytic ('clot-busting') ability of the blood by converting inactive plasminogen into plasmin which is active in breaking down the offending clot provided the plasminogen activator is administered very promptly. Awaiting a neurological opinion (C) or serial troponin measurements (D) and hourly measurement of blood pressure (E) would involve unacceptable delay. A thrombin antagonist (B) would tend to prevent further clotting but is inappropriate as the definitive treatment is thrombolysis.

7. E Value of 1.1 is completely normal before warfarin treatment

The intention is to reassure him that his anxieties about having an initial INR of 1.1 are false. The basis of doing the test can be briefly explained – a routine check on the INR before adjusting it with warfarin. The other options are likely to increase rather than decrease anxiety.

8. B Activation of the extrinsic clotting pathway by products of tissue damage

With multiple injuries this woman is a typical candidate for the generation of products which activate the extrinsic (extravascular) clotting pathway. These products then enter the blood stream and activate the final stages of the clotting pathway, by passing the initial intrinsic (intravascular) pathway. Fibrin is laid down widely in the circulation, depleting circulating fibrinogen so that, paradoxically, excessive clotting leads to a risk of excessive bleeding.

Chapter 9

Temperature regulation

A 25-year-old woman presents with gangrenous changes in both legs. She reports that she has been living rough and has suffered greatly from the recent extremely cold spell (around –10°C at night).

Which of the following is most likely to have caused this condition?

A   Abnormal temperature-regulating centre in the basal ganglia
B   Cerebrally-induced hypothermia
C   Core temperature maintained by peripheral vasoconstriction
D   Disorder of the autonomic nerves
E   Leg skin temperature has been only 20–25°C

Two 40-year-old men have just been admitted to the emergency department, one with immersion hypothermia and the other with haematemesis. Both have relatively cool peripheries and contracted superficial veins, from which it is difficult to obtain a blood sample.

Which of the following is most likely to differ between the two men?

A   The level of activity in peripheral sympathetic nerves
B   The part of the brain initiating vasoconstriction
C   Heat exchange between forearm arteries and venae commitantes
D   Peripheral catecholamine receptors
E   Total forearm and hand blood flow

An 18-year-old woman presents with severely excessive sweating in her hands, which interferes with her daily activities.

Which of the following is most likely to have caused this condition?

A   Emotional instability
B   Over-activity of cholinergic parasympathetic nerves
C   Over-activity of cholinergic sympathetic nerves
D   Over-activity of temperature sensitive receptors in her hands
E   Under-activity of noradrenergic sympathetic nerves

A 30-year old woman is attending the gastroenterology clinic with a complaint of severe diarrhoea and weight loss. While waiting in the clinic, she is sweating profusely. Her temperature is normal and pulse rate 110 beats per minute. The temperature in the clinic room is 22°C.

Which of the following is the most likely diagnosis?

A   Anxiety neurosis
B   Hyperhidrosis
C   Inflammatory bowel disease
D   Primary thyrotoxicosis
E   Sepsis

5. A 25-year-old woman suffers intermittently from cold white hands, particularly in cold weather. During a test period of body warming in a cool environment her hand skin temperature rises, after some time, from 20°C to 35°C on both sides, her pulse rate rises from 65 to 90 beats per minute, and her blood pressure from 115/80 mmHg to 135/80 mmHg.

What is the most likely diagnosis?

A   Bilateral arterial disease in the arms
B   Early heart failure
C   Excessive and dangerous body warming
D   Intermittent vasospasm related to sympathetic nervous activity
E   Thyrotoxicosis

6. A 16-year-old man is one of a group of young people who have been rescued from a hill walk after they were caught in mist, rain and wind, the environmental temperature being about 5°C. He has cold peripheries and looks exhausted, but can answer questions rationally.

Which of the following is most likely to have caused his condition?

A   Early stage of infection
B   Frostbite
C   Hypoglycaemia
D   Hypothermia
E   Ventricular fibrillation

7. A 40-year-old woman has been on holiday in a warm locality, where the humidity is low. While sitting in the shade in the garden of her hotel, she began to feel seriously light-headed and nauseated and is advised by an attendant to lie down.

What is the most likely diagnosis?

A   Cardiac arrhythmia
B   Excessive alcohol intake
C   Heat syncope
D   Internal haemorrhage
E   Myocardial infarction

8. A 20-year-old man presents following a bare foot run in a city park on a bright frosty morning. He developed severe pain in the soles of his feet one hour after returning home. His feet show areas resembling partial thickness burns and these are extremely tender.

What is the most likely diagnosis?

A   Abrasion trauma due to rough ground
B   Alcoholic intoxication
C   Frostbite
D   Syringomyelia
E   Peripheral neuropathy

Answers

1. C Core temperature maintained by peripheral vasoconstriction

This woman is able to respond to questions and to give a history, so her cerebral temperature has been maintained close to normal values (B). The changes in her legs are consistent with cold injury. This is to be expected in the extremely cold circumstances in which she has been living as the temperature-regulating centres in the hypothalamus (A) have maintained core temperature by intense activity in sympathetic vasoconstrictor nerves in her peripheries. The damage is likely to be due to freezing of the superficial tissues – ice crystals produce irreversible damage. Peripheral nerves cannot conduct their impulses at such low temperatures, so intense pain is not experienced until the peripheries have warmed and the pain fibres resume function, stimulated by the products of tissue damage. 20–25°C is normal peripheral skin temperature in a cold environment.

2. B The part of the brain initiating vasoconstriction

In the man with hypothermia it is the temperature regulating centre that initiates the peripheral vasoconstriction. In the man with haematemesis it is the blood pressure regulating centre that initiates the peripheral vasoconstriction. The peripheral mechanisms are similar for the two men.

Both these men have life-threatening conditions and in both cases their initial survival depends on reducing peripheral blood flow. The physiological mechanism for this is intense motor sympathetic activity to their peripheral blood vessels (augmented by circulating adrenaline and noradrenaline). The sympathetic nerves release noradrenaline, which acts on the predominant α-receptors at the surface of vascular smooth muscle cells. The result is constriction of arterioles, venules and veins.

For the man with early hypothermia this almost arrests the blood flow through hands and feet so that core heat is retained. The small amount of blood flow sustaining tissues in the arms and legs returns in the deep venae commitantes and there is counter-current heat exchange, so that blood in the distal arteries is well below core temperature and returning venous blood picks up heat from the proximal arteries.

For the man with haematemesis peripheral vasoconstriction maximises the blood volume in the central circulation, reducing the fall in arterial pressure and maintaining the vital cerebral and coronary blood flow. The features mentioned in the other options are similar in the two men.

3. C Over-activity of cholinergic sympathetic nerves

This young woman has hyperhidrosis which interferes with her daily life and should be helped greatly by bilateral cervical sympathectomy. There are no parasympathetic nerves in the limbs (B). Nerves which activate sweat glands are sympathetic nerves which release acetylcholine to cholinergic receptors as an important mechanism for body cooling in a hot environment. Noradrenergic sympathetic nerves (E) are important for promoting peripheral vasoconstriction in a cold environment and also for maintaining arterial blood pressure, particularly in the upright posture. Sympathectomy also severs these constrictor nerves, so that the hand is usually noticeably warmer after sympathectomy. The effects of sympathectomy are immediate dryness and warmth of the corresponding periphery. With time, the effects may decline. There is no evidence for emotional instability (A) or over-activity of temperature receptors (D).

4. D Primary thyrotoxicosis

A history of diarrhoea, weight loss, excessive sweating and tachycardia in a female should always alert one to the first possibility of primary thyrotoxicosis or Graves' disease. This is an autoimmune disease whereby serum immunoglobulin G (IgG) antibodies are produced. These bind to and activate thyroid stimulating hormone receptors, leading to release of excess thyroid hormones – tri-iodothyronine (T3) and thyroxine (T4). In thyrotoxicosis, there is increase in the basal metabolic rate which makes the patient very sensitive to heat. As a result, there is increased sympathetic activity to sweat glands thus making the patient sweat profusely. This is the most effective mechanism to remove heat from the body. Thyroid function tests should confirm the diagnosis – a rise in T3 and T4 and fall in thyroid stimulating hormone.

Anxiety neurosis (A) is highly unlikely, hyperhidrosis (B) usually affects limbs, inflammatory bowel disease (C) should not produce tachycardia and the septic patient (E) would usually be very ill with pyrexia.

5. D Intermittent vasospasm related to sympathetic nervous activity

This is a relatively common problem in young women, and it may be relieved by cervical sympathectomy. A sympathetic release test can help to predict the result of sympathectomy and exclude vascular narrowing as a cause of poor blood flow. It is carried out in a cool environment which causes a reflex rise in sympathetic tone to the extremities. The patient's body is then warmed, with the arms kept exposed. In the cool environment hand skin temperature is well below core temperature. Body heating releases the sympathetic tone (a normal response) and hand skin temperature rises towards core values. Such a test confirms that the blood vessels in the arms are normal and that a sympathectomy has a good chance of relieving symptoms. The tachycardia and increased pulse pressure are normal responses to body warming. Thus, there is nothing to support the other options.

6. D Hypothermia

With prolonged rain and wind, particularly if clothing protection is not fully adequate, there is a considerable risk of hypothermia. The chilling wind and evaporation of damp clothing increase heat loss. With serious exhaustion the ability to generate internal heat by activity and increased muscle tone is lost. Frostbite (B) requires freezing of tissues and does not occur at an environmental temperature of 5°C. Ventricular fibrillation (E) is a risk with hypothermia but is not present when the individual is conscious. The picture described does not suggest hypoglycaemia (C) as the primary problem, though exhaustion of energy stores in skeletal muscle is likely. Again the features of early infection (A) do not need to be invoked as the cause of his condition. Careful monitoring to detect cardiac arrhythmias is needed and to avoid early peripheral vasodilation which may carry cold skin blood to the core, depressing core temperature.

7. C Heat syncope

This is a classic case of heat syncope. When experiencing a holiday with relaxing heat it is easy to avoid adequate fluid intake, and blood volume becomes depleted. This effect is augmented by considerable sweat loss which may not be noticed when the sweat evaporates rapidly due to low humidity. This is a vital mechanism for avoiding a serious rise in core temperature. Meanwhile profound reflex vasodilation in the peripheries to maintain heat loss demands a considerable rise in cardiac output. Thus, the two components of arterial blood pressure (cardiac output and total peripheral resistance) are reduced and blood pressure tends to fall. This tends to reduce cerebral blood flow in the upright posture.

The combination of mild cerebral ischaemia and a developing vasovagal reflex produce presyncopal symptoms with eventual loss of consciousness and a fall, unless remedial action is taken rapidly. This remedial action consists of adopting the horizontal posture (ideally the head-down position with the feet raised to augment venous return), drinking a considerable quantity of fluid and getting into a cool environment. With this remedial action symptoms should rapidly improve, making the other options unlikely.

8. C Frostbite

On a bright frost morning ground temperature can be well below freezing point. With bare foot running, the soles will be cooled, firstly, to a temperature where the local nerves are no longer able to initiate impulses to the afferent nerves, including pain fibres. Thus, as with frostbite generally, an initial sensation of cold is replaced with the false security of numbness. As the exposed part cools further, freezing of the superficial tissues occurs, with formation of ice crystals which produce irreversible damage to the cells. Huge amounts of highly painful products are released from the damaged cells, but these fail to initiate impulses in afferent nerves so no pain is experienced. As the peripheral temperature in the feet rises, the pain fibres start to transmit again and intense pain is experienced. The other options do not fit the symptoms reported by the young man.

Chapter 10

Metabolic pathways and abnormalities

1. A 40-year-old woman is advised to lose 30 kg of body weight prior to surgery.

   Which of the following is the most effective dietary management of this woman?

   A   Energy intake equal to metabolic requirements plus 10%
   B   Her present food intake plus weight-losing drugs
   C   Less energy intake than metabolic requirements
   D   Most of her energy should be derived from fat
   E   She should eat only carbohydrate and protein

2. A 10-year-old boy with insulin-dependent diabetes mellitus has developed vomiting and is becoming drowsy and confused. His pulse is weak, with a rate of 100 beats per minute; blood pressure is 80/60 mmHg.

   Which of the following best explains his condition?

   A   Blood osmolality is rising due to increased sodium and chloride levels
   B   Cellular energy is derived from an excessive fat to carbohydrate ratio
   C   His pH is above 7.5 and is rising steadily
   D   Intracellular volume is falling, while extracellular volume is rising
   E   Vomiting is adding directly to his acid-base disturbance

3. A 55-year-old man undergoes a transfusion with 15 units of blood, following catastrophic bleeding from a gastric ulcer. He develops pulmonary damage and is transferred to the intensive care unit for ventilation with an increased oxygen concentration. His PO_2 is 8 kPa, PCO_2 4 kPa and pH 7.31.

   Which of the following is most likely to have caused these results?

   A   Anaemic hypoxia
   B   Brain damage causing under ventilation
   C   Ketoacidosis
   D   Hypoxic hypoxia with lactic acidosis
   E   Widespread haemolysis

4. A 20-year-old man presents following a car crash and is in a relatively stable state after initial resuscitation.

   Which of the following is most likely to maintain life after this severe physical stress?

    A   A negative sodium balance
    B   A positive nitrogen balance
    C   Depression of adrenocorticotrophic hormone secretion
    D   Glucocorticoid induced gluconeogenesis
    E   Hormonal reduction of breakdown of muscle proteins

5.   A 40-year-old man presents with established hepatic disease and a preoperative coagulation screen shows an INR of 2.0.

Which of the following metabolic disturbances is most likely to have caused this result?

    A   Decreased conjugation of bilirubin
    B   Decreased formation of prothrombin
    C   Decreased cholesterol in the bile
    D   Increased formation of bile acids
    E   Increased formation of fibrinogen

6.   A 75-year-old woman with non-insulin dependent diabetes mellitus is on long-term diuretic therapy. She has had a difficult postoperative period after a partial colectomy, and is still on intravenous fluids. Recently, she has become increasingly confused and her blood osmolality is below normal.

Which of the following is most likely to have caused her confusion?

    A   A blood glucose level of 10 mmol/L
    B   A blood urea level of 10 mmol/L
    C   A raised plasma sodium level
    D   Both blood urea and glucose elevated to 10 mmol/L
    E   Cerebral cellular overhydration

7.   A 30-year-old woman presents with a fractured femur after a road traffic accident. For some years previously she had been receiving parenteral nutrition following surgical removal of a large portion of small bowel.

Which of the following is the most appropriate management of her parenteral nutrition?

    A   Decreased amino acid content
    B   Decreased lipid content
    C   Increased energy content
    D   Increased sodium content
    E   No change in her usual nutrition

8.   A 50-year-old man with chronic liver failure presents with bleeding oesophageal varices, which is treated successfully. Next day he is stable, apart from moderate drowsiness. His outstretched arms show irregular flapping.

Which of the following is most likely to have caused his drowsiness?

A   Absorption from the gut of altered blood
B   An increased blood urea level
C   Cerebral damage related to hypotension
D   Continued oesophageal bleeding
E   Hypoglycaemia

Answers

1. C Less energy intake than metabolic requirements

It is essential for weight loss that energy use should exceed energy intake. The exte
of the reduction can be related to the urgency of the situation. During dieting, all o
the basic nutrients – fat, carbohydrate, protein, vitamins, trace elements and fibre a
required for health. Energy for metabolic requirements, plus an additional 10% (A)
would lead to weight increase; weight-losing drugs (B) also breach the requirement
for decreased energy intake, and there are many and serious side-effects of using
such drugs. A high fat diet (D) does not allow the normal Krebs cycle to take place
in mitochondria and carries the danger of ketoacidosis. The other unbalanced
intake (E) would lead to deficiency of fat-soluble vitamins and an unpalatable and
unhealthy diet. Normally energy is derived from a blend of fat and carbohydrate.

2. B Cellular energy is derived from an excessive fat to carbohydrate ratio

This boy is suffering from diabetic ketoacidosis. The problem is a lack of insulin
action to promote uptake of glucose into most energy-consuming cells, including
skeletal muscle (but not brain cells which do not require insulin for glucose uptake).
Cells must then derive most of their energy from fat and this leads to ketoacidosis
which involves production of a huge excess of hydrogen ions. Infusion of insulin is
required to restore uptake of glucose and redevelop normal metabolism and energy
production in the mitochondria.

Acidosis implies that the pH has fallen below 7.35 (C); in severe cases it can fall belov
7.0 so this is incorrect. Blood osmolality (A) is rising due to increased blood glucose.
Glucose normally contributes about 5 mmol but this rises typically to 20–30 becaus
glucose is not entering the cells. The greatly increased blood glucose level causes
an osmotic diuresis, which depletes all compartments of body water (D), including
the circulation, so arterial blood pressure falls dangerously, with compensatory
tachycardia. Vomiting, by loss of gastric acid, compensates in a minor way for the
acidosis (E) but any benefit in this direction is small and is overwhelmed by further
serious loss of body fluid, with inability to take oral replacement, so intravenous
fluids as well as insulin are required immediately.

3. D Hypoxic hypoxia with lactic acidosis

This man developed pulmonary damage secondary to severe blood loss and massive
blood transfusion (defined as a volume of transfusion equal to or greater than the
patient's blood volume). Oxygen transport is severely impaired and this is one cause of
hypoxic hypoxia (the other being a reduced inspired oxygen level). With severe hypoxia
mitochondrial oxygenation and generation of ATP may be inadequate, so anaerobic
glycolysis can increase ATP to a just adequate level for survival. Anaerobic glycolysis
produces lactic acidosis, a metabolic (or nonrespiratory) acidosis. A 5–10-fold increase

in blood lactic acid is typical. There is no suggestion of residual anaemia (A) or of brain damage with under ventilation (B). Ketoacidosis (C) and widespread haemolysis (E) also are not supported by information given.

D Glucocorticoid induced gluconeogenesis

A major component of the stress response is a surge of endogenous cortisol which dwarfs the normal daily surge. This is produced by release from the hypothalamus of corticotrophin releasing hormone which in turn releases adrenocorticotrophic hormone from the anterior pituitary (C). This releases cortisol from the adrenal cortex. If this mechanism fails at any point (long-term suppression exogenous glucocorticoid medication is now a common cause) survival after severe physical stress is only possible by appropriate administration of exogenous glucocorticoid such as hydrocortisone.

The cortisol surge favours survival in various ways, but a major component is mobilisation of glucose for energy by diverting amino acids from protein repair to glucose synthesis in the liver. Thus body protein, particularly in skeletal muscle, is broken down to ensure survival but leaving a legacy of muscle wasting (E). The excess nitrogen is excreted in the urine, giving a negative rather than a positive nitrogen balance (B). High levels of cortisol also contribute by their secondary mineralocorticoid action on the kidneys to retain sodium and chloride (A) and secondarily water, thus helping to maintain the circulation.

B Decreased formation of prothrombin

A major cause of a prolonged coagulation time and hence excessive bleeding in patients with liver disease is inadequate synthesis of prothrombin and other vitamin K dependent coagulation factors. Bilirubin metabolism (A) does not affect coagulation, nor does cholesterol (C). In liver disease formation of bile acids may be reduced, not increased (D) and this may hinder vitamin K absorption and prothrombin synthesis. This is also a problem in obstructive jaundice where bile acids as well as bilirubin may fail to reach the gut. Fibrinogen deficiency, not excess (E) is also a cause of bleeding.

E Cerebral cellular overhydration

The disturbances in blood glucose (A), urea (B), plasma sodium (C) and blood glucose and urea combined (D) all cause increased blood osmolality. A decreased blood osmolality implies an excess of body water in relation to dissolved components. This applies in all body fluids, since cell membranes and capillary walls in general are freely permeable to water. The most serious effects are experienced in the brain, because swelling of brain cells raises intracranial pressure, progressive and potentially fatal loss of brain function. This woman has had prolonged treatment with intravenous fluids and diuretics leading to over-dilution of body fluids. Low sodium and chloride levels make a major contribution to the low blood osmolality. Similar problems occur in infants who receive hypotonic fluids. Even some sports people have ingested excessive water (following the misleading fashion 'you can't drink too much during prolonged exercise') leading to confusion and even death.

7. C Increased energy content

During the stress reaction the resting metabolic rate increases due to the various energy-consuming activities associated with survival. This requires a corresponding increase in the overall energy content of her diet, with increased, rather than decreased amino acids (A). Decreasing the lipid content (B) would risk inadequate total energy content.

8. A Absorption from the gut of altered blood

With bleeding oesophageal varices a variable amount of the blood proceeds along the gut and is absorbed. This constitutes a high protein load from broken down haemoglobin and plasma proteins. People with liver failure have impaired ability to deal with the products of a high protein meal, due to impaired conjugation and metabolism of toxins derived, with the help of bacteria, from protein. These products depress brain function and produce a typical 'liver flap' of the outstretched arms. Urea formation from ammonia tends to be one of the detoxication functions that are depressed, so increased blood urea level (B) is inappropriate. No evidence is given to support the other options.

Chapter 11

Fluid balance

1. A 5-year-old boy presents to the paediatric surgery department with a 24-hour history of abdominal pain. His history and examination findings are consistent with a diagnosis of acute appendicitis. He is dehydrated with an estimated fluid deficit of 15%.

   Which of the following is the most appropriate resuscitation fluid?

   A   Packed red blood cells
   B   5% dextrose and 0.45% sodium chloride
   C   10% dextrose and 0.18% sodium chloride
   D   0.9% sodium chloride
   E   3% sodium chloride

2. A 67-year-old woman weighing 50 kg undergoes mastectomy for breast cancer. Intraoperative blood loss is 525 mL.

   What percentage is this blood loss of her estimated blood volume?

   A   5%
   B   10%
   C   15%
   D   20%
   E   25%

3. A 43-year-old man who has been involved in a road traffic accident is hypotensive and tachycardic in the resuscitation area of the emergency department. A CT scan shows a ruptured spleen with an estimated 1500 mL blood in the abdominal cavity.

   In the response to acute hypovolaemia, which of the following acts to restore an adequate circulating volume?

   A   Decreased antidiuretic hormone release
   B   Increased activation of the carotid bodies
   C   Increased activation of the parasympathetic nervous system
   D   Increased renin release
   E   Redistribution of blood from the renal medulla to the renal cortex.

4. A 34-year-old man presents to the surgical admissions department with a history suggestive of acute gallstone pancreatitis. Intravenous rehydration with Hartmann's solution is commenced.

   Which of the following is the most likely ionic composition of Hartmann's solution?

A   Calcium 20 mmol/L
B   Chloride 111 mmol/L
C   Lactate 10 mmol/L
D   Potassium 15 mmol/L
E   Sodium 154 mmol/L

5.   A 64-year-old man presents with symptoms of a perforated gastric ulcer. He was dehydrated on admission and received 3 L of 0.9% sodium chloride for fluid resuscitation.

Which of the following is the most likely biochemical derangement in this patient?

A   Hyperchloraemic metabolic acidosis
B   Hyperchloraemic metabolic alkalosis
C   Hypernatraemic metabolic acidosis
D   Hypochloraemic metabolic acidosis
E   Hypochloraemic metabolic alkalosis

6.   A 24-year-old healthy man weighing 70 kg is awaiting elective circumcision. The theatre list has been delayed so he has been given 1000 mL of 5% dextrose on the ward whilst he was waiting.

Which of the following volumes is the interstitial fluid compartment most likely to increase?

A   80 mL
B   250 mL
C   330 mL
D   670 mL
E   1000 mL

7.   A 49-year-old man is oliguric 12 hours following a Whipple's resection for pancreatic cancer. Clinical assessment and review of the observation charts suggest that this patient is not hypovolaemic.

Which of the following is the most likely cause of oliguria in this patient?

A   Decreased antidiuretic hormone secretion
B   Decreased metabolic rate
C   Decreased urinary nitrogen excretion
D   Potassium retention
E   Sodium retention

Answers

1. D 0.9% sodium chloride

The most appropriate choice of fluid is 0.9% sodium chloride. This remains within the extracellular compartment. In the past, fluid prescribers have been advised to limit the sodium load in children, but the National Patient Safety Agency issued an alert in 2007 highlighting the dangers of hyponatraemia in children resulting from the administration of large volumes of hypotonic fluids, e.g. 0.18% and 0.45% sodium chloride. There is an argument for using these as maintenance fluids in some groups of patients. Packed red cells may be necessary but with only a 15% fluid deficit, the risks outweigh the benefits in this case. Whilst there has been some interest in using hypertonic saline for fluid resuscitation, there is not enough evidence for it to have become an established practice especially in the paediatric population.

The British Consensus Guidelines on Intravenous Fluid Therapy for Adult Surgical Patients (GIFTASUP) published in 2009, contain 28 recommendations for assessment of fluid requirements, perioperative fluid and nutrition management. They recommend that although 4%/0.18% dextrose/saline and 5% dextrose are important sources of free water for maintenance, these should be used with caution in children because of the risk of dangerous hyponatraemia with excessive amounts, and that with some provisos they are not appropriate for replacement therapy.

2. C 15%

In this patient, estimated blood volume should be calculated using 70 mL/kg, i.e. 3500 mL so 525 mL is 15% of the patient's estimated blood volume. In obese patients, this would lead to an overestimate of blood volume so a value of 45–55 mL/kg of actual body weight should be used. Young children have a higher blood volume by weight approximately 80–90 mL/kg.

It is important to consider blood loss in the context of estimated blood volume so its full significance can be understood. A similar blood loss (525 mL) in an 8-year-old, 25 kg child would probably put the child into class III hypovolaemic shock. This should be taken in the clinical context as intraoperative blood loss is difficult to estimate so heart rate, blood pressure, capillary refill time, peripheral perfusion, urine output, etc. should be considered in conjunction with any estimated blood loss. Postoperatively a drain can be useful in gauging ongoing blood loss but remember that drains can become blocked or be dislodged so they may not fill even in the context of significant bleeding.

3. D Increased renin release

The decreased venous return and cardiac preload seen in acute hypovolaemia cause a reduction in cardiac output and blood pressure falls. The first response is a shift in the balance between the sympathetic and parasympathetic nervous systems such that the sympathetic becomes more dominant in order to attempt to maintain perfusion of vital structures and restore cardiac output. The increase in sympathetic discharge caused by a reduction in blood pressure is mediated by a decrease in the afferent activity of the carotid sinus baroreceptors to the pressor area in the dorsal hypothalamus. (Carotid bodies are involved with the chemical control of breathing not blood pressure.) The decrease in parasympathetic discharge occurs as a result of decreased output to the depressor centre from low-pressure baroreceptors situated within the atria and great veins.

The hypothalamo-pituitary-adrenal response is slower. Renin release is triggered by decreased renal blood flow and ultimately leads to the formation of angiotensin II within the lung. This is not only a potent arteriolar vasoconstrictor but also stimulates release of antidiuretic hormone from the posterior pituitary and aldosterone from the adrenal cortex. Antidiuretic hormone and aldosterone both enhance water and sodium reabsorption at the distal renal tubule. Redistribution of blood from the cortex to the medulla [not the other way round] enhances sodium and water reabsorption.

4. B Chloride 111 mmol/L

Hartmann's solution is a balanced electrolyte solution, which is isotonic with plasma and is a useful crystalloid for extracellular fluid compartment replacement. As shown in **Table 11.1**, it has a lower chloride and sodium content than 0.9% sodium chloride so helps to avoid problems with hyperchloraemic acidosis when large volumes are infused. It was developed in the 1930s by Alexis Hartmann, an American biochemist and paediatrician, who recognised the need for a type of fluid with proportionately more sodium than chloride for the treatment of children with metabolic acidosis.

It is important to be aware of its other constituents for its safe use:

- lactate (29 mmol/L)
- calcium (2 mmol/L)
- potassium (5 mmol/L)

Table 11.1

	Ionic composition (mmol/L)					
	Sodium	Potassium	Calcium	Chloride	Lactate	pH
0.9% sodium chloride	154	0	0	154	0	5.0
Hartmann's solution	131	5	2	111	29	6.5

Table 11.1 Comparison of the ionic composition of 0.9% sodium chloride and Hartmann's solution.

Lactate is metabolised by the liver to produce bicarbonate. Some groups advocate avoiding Hartmann's solution in patients with diabetes because of the risk of metabolism of one of the lactate isomers to glucose but in clinical practice, this effect is minimal. In addition, patients in hepatic failure may be at risk of lactate accumulation and acidosis if hepatic lactate metabolism is impaired. The calcium is postulated to cause accelerated clotting of packed red cells if the same fluid giving set is used for administration without flushing the line first with saline. Potassium may accumulate in patients with significant renal failure.

5. A Hyperchloraemic metabolic acidosis

The most likely biochemical derangement seen after large volumes of 0.9% saline are administered is hyperchloraemic metabolic acidosis. The British Consensus Guidelines on Intravenous Fluid Therapy for Adult Surgical Patients (GIFTASUP) point out the risk of inducing this, when crystalloid resuscitation or replacement is indicated. They recommend that 0.9% saline should be replaced with a balanced salt solution, such as Hartmann's solution or Ringer's lactate/acetate (except when there is hypochloraemia, e.g. from vomiting or gastric drainage). Stewart's theory of acid-base balance can be used to explain the mechanism behind this. Stewart's theory says that the strong ion difference, the total concentration of weak acids in the plasma and $PaCO_2$ are the three independent variables, which determine acid base balance. A reduction in strong ion difference, an increase in $PaCO_2$ or an increase in the total concentration of weak acids in the plasma will acidify the plasma. Strong ion difference can be calculated by subtracting the sum of the chloride and lactate concentrations from the sum of the sodium and potassium concentrations. An increase in the concentration of chloride ions as seen after infusion of 0.9% sodium chloride will decrease the strong ion difference and cause a metabolic acidosis to develop.

6. B 250 mL

Dextrose 5% is a way of administering free water because the glucose is rapidly taken up into cells. Dextrose 5% can be used for rehydration of the intracellular compartment, but will have negligible effect on the intravascular volume. As shown in **Figure 11.1**, in men, 60% of body weight (3/5) is water so in a 70 kg male, total body water is approximately 42 L; two-thirds of this is intracellular and one-third extracellular. Dextrose 5% will equilibrate throughout all of the fluid compartments so two-thirds or approximately 670 mL will enter the intracellular space and one-third or approximately 330 mL will enter the extracellular space. The extracellular space comprises the interstitial fluid, which accounts for 75% by volume and the intravascular space, which accounts for 25% by volume. Therefore, approximately 250 mL will enter the interstitial fluid leaving only 80 mL in the intravascular compartment. Dependent on the type of colloid, colloids may remain within the plasma for up to 24 hours before equilibrating with the remainder of the body fluid compartments. Isotonic crystalloids (e.g. Hartmann's and 0.9% sodium chloride) will redistribute within the extracellular compartment but not the intracellular compartment within 10–20 minutes.

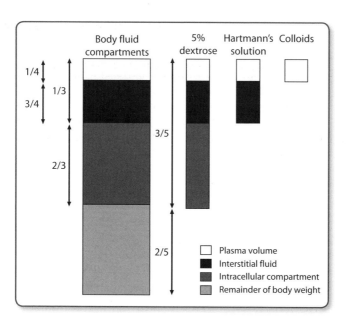

Figure 11.1 Body fluid compartments and distribution of some infusion fluids (not to scale).

7. E Sodium retention

Following surgery or significant trauma, a patient's ability to excrete a salt and water load and maintain normal serum osmolarity is compromised as part of a complex widespread neuroendocrine response which aims to conserve body fluid and release endogenous fuel via an increase in metabolism. The magnitude of this state of antidiuresis and oliguria produced by catecholamines, antidiuretic hormone, and the renin–angiotensin–aldosterone system (RAAS) is related to the degree of surgical stress or the extent of surgery or trauma. Water and salt are therefore retained even in the presence of overload. In addition, intracellular sodium and fluid retention may occur due to failure of the cellular Na/K ATPase pump. Cortisol levels also increase rapidly after a surgical insult. This has complex effects on carbohydrate, fat and protein metabolism to play a major role in the breakdown of protein and liberation of energy without which patients may not survive.

The ability to excrete free water is limited and the ability to dilute urine is impaired so the administration of hypotonic fluid risks dilutional hyponatraemia. If normal saline is infused, the additional problem of chloride overload is seen and this can cause renal vasoconstriction and reduced glomerular filtration rate. The ability to excrete a sodium load is further compromised by depletion of potassium stores due to RAAS activation and the cellular loss of potassium, which accompanies protein catabolism.

Metabolic rate is significantly increased with increased protein breakdown, gluconeogenesis and lipolysis such that urinary nitrogen excretion increases. Since the ability to concentrate urine is impaired, urea competes with sodium and chloride for excretion and the minimum urine volume required to excrete the urea, sodium and chloride load increases by 200–300%. If this does not occur, interstitial oedema may result.

Following a Whipple's resection, hepatorenal syndrome is another cause for oliguria and deteriorating renal function.

Knowledge of this stress response to surgery reminds us that postoperative oliguria should be assessed in the context of volume status, i.e. that the patient may not be hypovolaemic and that the low urine output may be in spite of adequate filling. If this is not clear based on clinical examination, there may be a requirement for invasive arterial and central venous pressure monitoring.

Chapter 12

Sepsis and shock

A 24-year-old woman presents to the emergency department with right iliac fossa pain. Her heart rate is 100 beats per minute, blood pressure is 88/62 mmHg and respiratory rate is 19 breaths per minute. Her temperature is 37.7°C. The results of her blood tests are unremarkable, aside from a white cell count of 3.9×10^9 cells/L.

Which of the following is part of the criteria for systemic inflammatory response syndrome?

A   Presence of infection
B   Respiratory rate 19 breaths per minute
C   Systolic blood pressure 88 mmHg
D   Temperature 37.7°C
E   White cell count 3.9×10^9 cells/L

A 32-year-old man is in the resuscitation bay of the emergency department. He is complaining of abdominal pain after being a restrained passenger in a road traffic accident. His heart rate is 128 beats per minute, blood pressure is 91/72 mmHg and respiratory rate is 38 breaths per minute. There are no obvious signs of head injury, but he appears confused. He has passed 10 mL of urine in the last hour via the urinary catheter

How much blood loss is likely as a percentage of blood volume?

A   Up to 15%
B   15–30%
C   30–40%
D   At least 40%
E   Not enough information to determine this

A 49-year-old woman with known rheumatoid arthritis on immunosuppression therapy presents with a 2-day history of a painful, red and swollen knee joint. Urgent gram staining of fluid aspirated from the knee reveals gram-positive cocci. The patient is developing septic shock.

Which of the following factors is most closely associated with lower mortality in septic shock?

A   Advanced age
B   Gram-positive sepsis
C   Presence of three or more organ failures
D   Prior immunocompromise
E   Unidentified source of sepsis

4. A 24-year-old man has fallen two storeys from the roof of a house. He has a
    Glasgow coma scale 15 and is complaining of pain in his back. On arrival in the
    emergency department, he is hypotensive with warm peripheries despite 2 L of
    Hartmann's solution. Following primary and secondary survey, the only injury
    identified on a CT scan is a burst fracture of T10 with significant impingement of
    the spinal canal.

    In neurogenic shock, which is the most important contributor to hypotension?

    A   Decreased parasympathetic tone
    B   Decreased circulating volume
    C   Increased sympathetic tone
    D   Increased systemic vascular resistance
    E   Increased venous capacitance

5. An 84-year-old man is in the surgical high dependency unit the morning following
    laparotomy for a perforated duodenal ulcer. He had an episode of chest pain and
    dyspnoea overnight and is now hypotensive and tachycardic with cool peripheries
    and a raised jugular venous pressure. He is thought to be in cardiogenic shock and
    is awaiting transfer to the intensive care unit.

    Which is the most common postoperative cause of cardiogenic shock?

    A   Hypovolaemia
    B   Myocardial infarction
    C   Pericardial tamponade
    D   Pulmonary embolus
    E   Ventricular fibrillation

6. A 23-year-old woman is under general anaesthesia for tonsillectomy. The
    anaesthetist requests that surgery does not commence, since the patient is
    tachycardic and hypotensive, and the anaesthetist is concerned that the patient is
    anaphylactic shock.

    Which is the most common cause of anaphylaxis under anaesthesia?

    A   Antibiotics, e.g. co-amoxiclav
    B   Colloids, e.g. gelofusine
    C   Induction agent, e.g. thiopentone
    D   Latex, e.g. surgical gloves
    E   Muscle relaxants, e.g. suxamethonium

7. A 67-year-old man presents to the emergency department with abdominal
    pain, jaundice and pyrexia suggestive of acute cholangitis. He is tachycardic and
    hypotensive. The consultant asks for the Surviving Sepsis Resuscitation bundle to
    be commenced.

    Which of the following is the most appropriate initial management?

    A   Administer broad spectrum antibiotic within 24 hours of admission
    B   Blood cultures are not essential if broad spectrum antibiotics are used

C Consider vasopressors if hypotension does not respond to minimum 20 mL/kg initial fluid resuscitation

D Maintain central venous pressure >12 mmHg

E Measure lactate on an arterial blood sample

Answers

1. E White cell count 3.9 x 10^9 cells/L

This systemic inflammatory response syndrome (SIRS) is a constellation of clinical findings in which one or more of a seemingly endless list of causes has activated a cytokine cascade. These insults include trauma, burns, surgery, blood product transfusion and pancreatitis.

Criteria for SIRS were established in 1992 as part of the American College of Chest Physicians/Society of Critical Care Medicine Consensus Conference.

SIRS can be diagnosed in the presence of at least two of the following:

- Body temperature: < 36°C or > 38°C
- Heart rate: > 90 beats per minute
- Respiratory rate: > 20 breaths per minute (or $PaCO_2$ < 4.3 kPa)
- White blood cell count: < 4 x 10^9 cells/L or > 12 x 10^9 cells/L

There is no identifiable pathogen, no requirement for cardiovascular organ suppor and end organ damage has not yet developed. The inflammatory response involve a number of interleukins 1, 5, 6, 8, 11, 15 and TNF-α and platelet activating factor. Management is supportive.

2. C 30–40%

Shock is a term used to describe a state where organ and tissue perfusion is inadequate. Hypovolaemic shock can be haemorrhagic or non-haemorrhagic in aetiology. Causes of non-haemorrhagic hypovolaemic shock include pancreatitis and intestinal obstruction. Haemorrhagic shock can follow rupture of an abdomina aortic aneurysm or trauma. The source of bleeding may not always be obvious – remember to think about femoral fracture, chest injury , abdominal injury and blood loss onto the floor or at the scene. A significant percentage of blood volume can be lost before a young fit patient is no longer able to compensate and displays abnormal physiology. **Table 12.1** helps to estimate the percentage of circulating volume lost based on the physiological parameters observed.

3. B Gram-positive sepsis

Overall mortality from septic shock is approximately 50%. Gram-negative sepsis is associated with a higher mortality than gram positive sepsis. Having an unidentifie source of sepsis is also associated with an increased mortality because source control is not possible. Unsurprisingly, the more organ systems which are failing, advancing age, co-morbidity and immunosuppression all increase mortality.

In septic shock, hypotension persists despite adequate fluid resuscitation and ther is evidence of inadequate end organ perfusion, e.g. lactic acidosis, oliguria, etc. Initially the circulation may be hyperdynamic and cardiac output increased but in

Table 12.1

	Class I	Class II	Class III	Class IV
Percentage blood volume	<15	15–30	30–40	>40
Heart rate (beats per minute)	<100	>100	>120	>140
Blood pressure	Normal	Normal	↓	↓
Pulse pressure	Normal or ↑	↓	↓	↓
Respiratory rate (breaths per minute)	14–20	20–30	30–40	>35
Urine output	>30 mL/h	20–30 mL/h	5–15 mL/h	Negligible
Cognitive state	Slight anxiety	Mild anxiety	Anxiety, confusion	Confusion, lethargy
Fluid response	Good response	Good response	Transient responder	No response

Table 12.1 Recognising different classes of hypovolaemic shock.

latter stages hypotension with vasoconstriction may be seen especially in cases where the myocardium becomes ischaemic or there is hypovolaemia.

Septic shock is characterised by increased endothelial and capillary permeability, decreased systemic vascular resistance with relative hypovolaemia, impaired oxygen extraction and utilisation despite normal oxygen delivery and decreased myocardial contractility.

Management is largely supportive and efforts should be made to identify and treat the underlying cause. Few specific therapies exist, activated protein C had shown promise in recent years, but recently has been withdrawn as there is insufficient evidence to support its safe use.

4. E Increased venous capacitance

Neurogenic shock results from the loss of sympathetic outflow and consequent vasodilatation. Sympathetic tone and systemic vascular resistance are decreased, and venous capacitance is increased leading to hypotension. If the spinal cord injury is above the cardiac sympathetic supply (T1–T4) severe bradycardia and hypotension are likely to occur. However, both bradycardia (resulting from unopposed vagal activity or hypoxia) and tachycardia (from relative intravascular depletion) may be seen. Spinal cord injury, severe head injury and high spinal anaesthesia are all potential causes of neurogenic shock. The terms spinal and neurogenic are not interchangeable; spinal shock describes a neurological deficit with no haemodynamic embarrassment characterised by flaccidity and loss of reflexes.

Neurogenic shock should be suspected in patients who behave as transient responders to fluid challenges with no source of bleeding and an appropriate mechanism of injury. Spinal cord injury should be managed in the same way as any trauma with close attention paid to airway compromise and maintenance of adequate circulation and oxygenation to maintain organ perfusion and to minimise any secondary injury. Intubation and mechanical ventilation may be required if the injury is above C3–C5 or if there is an associated head injury for airway protection or manipulation of PaO_2 and $PaCO_2$ if there are concerns regarding raised intracranial pressure.

5. B Myocardial infarction

Cardiogenic shock occurs when the heart fails to generate adequate cardiac output to maintain tissue perfusion due to failure of the ventricles to function effectively. Causes can either be intrinsic, e.g. acute myocardial infarction, or extrinsic, e.g. massive pulmonary embolism, tension pneumothorax, and pericardial tamponade. In this case myocardial infarction is most likely. It is quite early in the postoperative course for massive pulmonary embolus. If the patient was in ventricular fibrillation, he would be in cardiorespiratory arrest not cardiogenic shock. It is important to remember tension pneumothorax and pericardial tamponade as potential causes, but these are much rarer in this group of patients.

Treatment is generally supportive whilst the cause of ventricular failure is treated, e.g. percutaneous coronary intervention or drainage of a tamponade. Cardiogenic shock is a low cardiac output state with high cardiac filling pressures and high systemic vascular resistance. Supportive management of cardiogenic shock includes optimising preload, cardiac contractility, and afterload.

An intra-aortic balloon pump is a mechanical device that increases myocardial oxygen perfusion while at the same time increasing cardiac output. It is of particular use in patients awaiting or following cardiac revascularisation. A pneumatic antishock garment will increase systemic vascular resistance further and is contraindicated in cardiogenic shock.

6. E Muscle relaxants, e.g. suxamethonium

The most common cause of anaphylaxis under anaesthesia is neuromuscular blocking agents. Other common causes include latex, antibiotics and colloids. Anaphylaxis is a Type 1 IgE-mediated immune response, which leads to release of histamine and other compounds from mast cells and basophils. Its onset is acute and causes life-threatening compromise of airway, breathing and circulation. An anaphylactoid reaction is as a result of non-specific histamine release without prior sensitisation.

The approach to a patient with suspected anaphylaxis should be in an ABC manner as described by the Resuscitation Council guidelines. Whilst histamine mediates many of the clinical signs and symptoms, initial treatment should be with adrenaline; either 0.5–1 mg intramuscularly or 50–100 µg increments intravenously, with an antihistamine and steroid being administered as part of ongoing management. A fluid challenge should also be given but colloid should be stopped as this may be the cause of anaphylaxis. Consideration should be given to securing the airway with an endotracheal tube early because of worsening laryngeal oedema, but this should not delay administration of adrenaline.

Working Group of the Resuscitation Council (UK). Emergency treatment of anaphylactic reactions. Guidelines for healthcare providers. London: Resuscitation Council (UK), 2012. http://www.resus.org.uk/pages/reaction.pdf. Last accessed 9 August 2012.

7. C Consider vasopressors if hypotension does not respond to minimum 20 mL/kg initial fluid resuscitation

The Surviving Sepsis Campaign is a global initiative, which aims to reduce mortality from sepsis. The first 6-hour resuscitation bundle includes obtaining blood cultures prior to antibiotic administration, the measurement of serum lactate (from either venous or arterial sample) and the administration of broad-spectrum antibiotics administered within 2 hours of admission/diagnosis. For every hour antibiotic therapy is delayed after the onset of septic shock, the patient's chance of survival is reduced by almost 8%.

A large, randomised (but unblinded) study demonstrates that early resuscitation with clear targets including central venous pressure, central venous oxygen saturation, lactate and mean arterial pressure achieved a reduction in in-hospital mortality from 44% to 29%.

The early goal directed therapy component of the resuscitation bundle requires if mean arterial pressure < 65 mmHg or lactate > 4 mmol/L, treatment should be targeted such that:

- central venous pressure > 8 mmHg
- central venous oxygen saturation > 70%
- Mean arterial pressure > 65 mmHg and a urine output of > 0.5 mL/kg/h (achieved by an initial minimum fluid bolus of 20 mL/kg of crystalloid or 5 mL/kg of colloid followed by vasopressors, e.g. noradrenaline, if required)

Improvement in haemodynamic parameters following a fluid bolus can be sustained, transient or nonexistent. A transient response to a fluid bolus suggests that there is some ongoing bleeding which may require definitive management but at present fluid resuscitation can keep pace with that loss. No improvement in haemodynamic status suggests catastrophic bleeding requiring urgent intervention or consideration given to other causes of hypotension, e.g. tension pneumothorax, neurogenic shock.

Rivers E et al. Early goal-directed therapy in the treatment of severe sepsis and septic shock. NEJM 2001; 345: 1368–77.

Chapter 13

Central nervous system

A 34-year-old man is admitted to the intensive care unit. He has been assaulted and sustained a significant head injury. He is normally fit and well.

Which of the following parameters is most likely to increase cerebral blood flow?

A Core temperature 37.4°C
B Central venous pressure 18 mmHg
C Mean arterial pressure 90 mmHg
D $PaCO_2$ 4.0 kPa
E PaO_2 6.7 kPa

An 18-year-old woman with a ventriculoperitoneal shunt which was inserted in childhood for hydrocephalus presents with acute onset confusion. A sample of cerebrospinal fluid is taken from the device for sending to the laboratories for analysis.

Which of the following results is abnormal?

A White cell count: 2×10^6/L
B Glucose: 4.4 mmol/L (plasma value is 4.7 mmol/L)
C Opening pressure: 22 mmHg
D Protein: 0.3 g/L
E Red blood cell count: 2×10^6/L

A 49-year-old man presents to the emergency department. The patient's history is unclear but he was found to be unresponsive by his wife when she awoke this morning so she called an ambulance. He has a recent history of worsening headache. His heart rate is 43 beats per minute, blood pressure is 170/90 mmHg and respiratory rate 14 breaths per minute. On examination, there are no localising signs but papilloedema is present.

Which systemic effect is most commonly seen in patients with severely raised intracranial pressure?

A Decreased blood pressure
B Decreased heart rate
C Decreased pulse pressure
D Increased respiratory rate
E Nausea but no vomiting

4. A 63-year-old woman is admitted with a Gustilo grade III open fracture of her right ankle. She is taken to theatre that evening for debridement of the wound and definitive fixation under spinal anaesthesia. She returns to theatre 48 hours later for wound inspection and delayed closure. On the evening ward round, she is found to be agitated and confused.

   Which of the following is the most likely cause of her postoperative cognitive dysfunction?

   A   Higher level of education
   B   Perioperative hypotension
   C   Preoperative benzodiazepine use
   D   Regional rather than general anaesthetic technique
   E   Repeat surgery

5. A 77-year-old man is in the surgical ward one day following laparoscope-assisted anterior resection for bowel cancer. His family report that he seems confused. On review of the patient's drug chart, it is observed that he has received a number of drugs in the previous 24 hours.

   Which of the following drugs is the most likely cause of his postoperative cognitive dysfunction?

   A   Atropine
   B   Donepezil
   C   Levobupivacaine
   D   Paracetamol
   E   Remifentanil

6. A 64-year-old woman presents to the emergency department with a 2-week history of headache, fluctuating conscious level and slurred speech. She has a history of alcohol excess and hypertension for which she is not compliant with treatment. A CT scan reveals a subacute subdural haematoma.

   How is cerebral blood flow autoregulation most likely to be affected by chronic hypertension?

   A   Autoregulation curve is shifted to the left
   B   Autoregulation curve is shifted to the right
   C   Impaired at high mean arterial pressures
   D   Impaired at low mean arterial pressures
   E   Unchanged

7. A 24-year-old man is admitted to the intensive care unit following a bicycle accident where he sustained an isolated head injury. There has been some concern regarding raised intracranial pressure so a monitor has been inserted. Current observations show: blood pressure 115/78 mmHg (MAP 90 mmHg), heart rate 78 beats per minute, SpO_2 98% with FiO_2 0.35, central venous pressure +10 mmHg and intracranial pressure 20 cmH$_2$O (15 mmHg).

What is his cerebral perfusion pressure?

A   60 mmHg
B   65 mmHg
C   70 mmHg
D   90 mmHg
E   100 mmHg

Answers

1. E PaO$_2$ 6.7 kPa

The brain receives 14% of cardiac output, which equates to 50 mL/100 g brain tissue per minute. The grey matter receives twice as much blood flow than the white matter. When intracranial pressure is raised, it can be helpful to reduce cerebral blood volume to provide a temporary reduction in intracranial pressure.

Cerebral blood flow (CBF) is determined by a number of factors:

- **PaCO$_2$**: a reduction in CO$_2$ from 5.3–4 kPa reduces cerebral blood flow by 30%. There is a linear relationship between PaCO$_2$ and CBF between 4 and 12 kPa (**Figure 13.1**).
- **PaO$_2$**: when PaO$_2$ decreases below 8 kPa there is a rapid increase in CBF to 110 mL/100 g/min. In the patient in this scenario, efforts should be made to increase PaCO$_2$ (**Figure 13.1**).
- **Mean arterial pressure (MAP)**: a MAP of 90 mmHg falls well within the limits of cerebral autoregulation so CBF is independent of MAP in a normal brain. However in head injury this may be disrupted.
- **Temperature**: CBF drops by 5% per degree celsius drop in temperature hence the interest in therapeutic hypothermia in head injury.
- **Central venous pressure**: helps to determine cerebral perfusion pressure but this will not directly affect CBF.

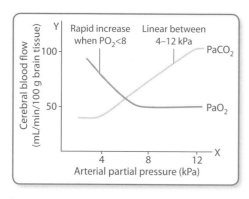

Figure 13.1 Effect of arterial oxygen and carbon dioxide tension on cerebral blood flow. When hypoxaemi (PaO$_2$ < 8 kPa) occurs, cerebral blood flow markedly increases in an attempt to maintain cerebral oxygenation. There is a linear relationship between PaCO$_2$ and cerebral blood flow between 4 and 12 kPa. When PaCO$_2$ is <4 kPa, maximal vasoconstriction has occurred so cerebral blood is independent of PaCO$_2$. When PaCO$_2$ is >12 kPa maximal vasodilatation has occurred, so no further increase in cerebral blood flow is seen.

2. C Opening pressure: 22 mmHg

Hydrocephalus refers to an increased cerebrospinal fluid (CSF) volume due to increased production (rare) or impaired drainage. To relieve hydrocephalus, ventriculoperitoneal shunts can be inserted into the lateral ventricle to drain CSF into the peritoneum via a catheter tunneled under the skin. The shunt can become blocked or infected leading to symptoms and signs of raised intracranial pressure or central nervous system infection. There is usually a valve through which a sample can be obtained using a needle and the opening pressure of the system can be measured to aid diagnosis. Normal CSF parameters are shown in **Table 13.1**.

Table 13.1	
White cell count	$0–5 \times 10^6$ cells/L (lymphocytes only, no neutrophils)
Red cell count	$0–10 \times 10^6$ cells/L
Glucose	3.3–4.4 mmol/L or $\geq$60% of plasma
Protein	0.2–0.4 g/L
Opening pressure	7–18 cmH$_2$O

Table 13.1 Normal cerebrospinal fluid values.

Cerebrospinal fluid occupies the space between the arachnoid mater and the pia mater and also is contained within the ventricles, cisterns and sulci of the brain and the central canal of the spinal cord.

It serves several main purposes:

- **Buoyancy**: mass of the human brain is approximately 1.4 kg; however, the effective weight of the brain suspended in the CSF 50 grams.
- **Protection**: CSF cushions the brain tissue from injury when jolted or hit.
- **Chemical stability**: CSF maintains a constant ionic environment for the cells of the central nervous system and may act as a transport system for neurotransmitters and hormones. CSF flow facilitates provision of nutrients for neuronal and glial cells and clearance of the metabolic waste from the central nervous system.
- **Prevention of brain ischemia**: CSF can partially buffer changes in intracranial pressure by redistribution from the intracranial to extracranial subarachnoid space.

. B Decreased heart rate

The Monro–Kellie hypothesis views the skull as a rigid box, which contains brain tissue, blood and cerebrospinal fluid. There is little scope for compensation but if one component increases in volume, there must be a corresponding decrease in another otherwise intracranial pressure increases. Once this increases above a certain threshold, perfusion will be compromised and critical ischaemia will eventually develop.

Symptoms and signs depend on whether the rise in intracranial pressure has occurred acutely or is a more chronic process. Systemic signs include hypertension and reflex bradycardia as part of Cushing's reflex. Pulse pressure is increased. Cushing's triad is constituted by papilloedema, bradycardia and abnormal respiration (usually a decrease in respiratory rate). Symptoms of raised intracranial pressure are usually worse in the morning due to increased hydrostatic pressure effects and because $PaCO_2$ may be elevated, these include headache and vomiting without nausea. Intracranial pressure can reach a critical point at which cerebral contents are forced out of the cranium, e.g. central herniation in which the cerebellar tonsils herniate through the foramen magnum and compress the medulla.

4. E Repeat surgery

In a cohort of 1200 postoperative patients of greater than 60 years of age, the incidence of postoperative cognitive dysfunction (POCD) was around 25% at 1 week and 10% at 3 months postoperatively. It is more common in patients with pre-existing cognitive dysfunction and a higher level of education seems to be protective. Surprisingly, preoperative benzodiazepine use is protective and perioperative hypotension and hypoxaemia have not been demonstrated to be risk factors. Types of surgery, which are higher risk, include cardiac, carotid and neurosurgery especially prolonged or repeat surgery. A study in which older patients undergoing lower limb joint replacement were randomised to receive either regional or general anaesthesia gave the following results: in the first week following surgery, the incidence of cognitive dysfunction was less in the regional anaesthesia group (12.7 vs. 21.2%); however, this difference did not persist at 3 months. Reducing the incidence of early POCD may make initial rehabilitation easier and hospital stay shorter.

In 40% of cases, there is no identifiable cause for POCD. Early causes within hours of surgery include residual anaesthetic agents, pain and opioid analgesia, hypoxaemia, hypotension, hypoglycaemia and intraoperative stroke. Causes which account for the development of POCD in the days following surgery include sepsis and organ failure, withdrawal from alcohol, nicotine or regular drugs and sleep deprivation or disruption.

5. A Atropine

Atropine is the most likely of these drugs to cause postoperative confusion. It crosses the blood brain barrier and has central anticholinergic actions, which have an adverse effect on cognitive function. Glycopyrrolate is a quaternary amine so will not cross the blood brain barrier, making it is less likely to cause confusion than the other anticholinergic agents atropine and cyclizine. Remifentanil has a very short half-life even after prolonged infusion so it is unlikely to contribute to postoperative confusion on the day following surgery, but other opioids are well recognised causes. Levobupivacaine can cause neurological dysfunction in toxic doses but not postoperative confusion. Regional and local anaesthetic techniques are associated with a lower incidence of postoperative cognitive dysfunction than general anaesthesia. Donepezil is a treatment for dementia. It is a centrally acting reversible acetylcholinesterase inhibitor, which is unlikely to cause postoperative confusion, but cognitive impairment may be exacerbated if doses are missed and patients taking donepezil are at increased risk of postoperative cognitive dysfunction because of their preoperative cognitive dysfunction. Paracetamol is not known to have any effects on cognitive function and in fact avoiding pyrexia can reduce the incidence of postoperative cognitive dysfunction.

B Autoregulation curve is shifted to the right

Autoregulation describes the process by which cerebral blood flow is maintained at a constant level in a normal brain despite fluctuations in blood pressure between a mean arterial pressure of 50 and 150 mmHg. This may be impaired by drugs, e.g. anaesthetic agents or disease states, e.g. head injury in the acute phase of subarachnoid haemorrhage.

There are a number of theories about how autoregulation occurs. The myogenic theory is based on the presence of stretch receptors in the vascular smooth muscle cells so that increased stretch associated with increased blood flow causes vasoconstriction and reduced flow. The metabolic theory is based on the accumulation of metabolites, e.g hydrogen ions, nitric oxide and adenosine at low cerebral blood flow rates leading to vasodilatation and increased cerebral blood flow. In chronic hypertension, the whole curve is shifted to the right. In treated hypertension, with time the autoregulation curve returns towards normal values. This is important because in patients with chronic hypertension, a higher mean arterial pressure may need to be achieved to maintain adequate cerebral perfusion. Under general anaesthesia, the whole curve is shifted to the left as illustrated in **Figure 13.2**.

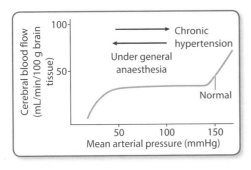

Figure 13.2 Effect of mean arterial blood pressure (MAP) on cerebral blood flow. Cerebral blood flow is independent of mean arterial pressure between 50 and 150 mmHg. Above 150 mmHg, cerebral blood flow increases passively with MAP. Below a MAP of 50 mmHg, the autoregulation mechanisms are unable to maintain normal cerebral blood flow so it decreases markedly.

B 65 mmHg

The equation used to calculate cerebral perfusion pressure is:

Cerebral perfusion pressure =
    mean arterial pressure – (intracranial pressure + central venous pressure).

- Normal cerebral perfusion pressure is 70–75 mmHg.
- Critical ischaemia occurs at a cerebral perfusion pressure of 30–40 mmHg
- Localised ischaemia may occur at a higher cerebral perfusion pressure than this
- The units should all be in mmHg.

It is important to maintain cerebral perfusion pressure after brain injury to prevent secondary brain insult occurring. This can be achieved by raising the mean arterial pressure or reducing the intracranial pressure. Once normovolaemia is achieved, agents such as noradrenaline can be used to augment mean arterial pressure. Mortality is increased by approximately 20% for each 10 mmHg reduction in cerebral perfusion pressure. It is not clear whether raised intracranial pressure in the context of normal cerebral perfusion pressure has an adverse effect on outcome.

Chapter 14

Cardiovascular system

1. A 70-year-old man on surgical high-dependency unit has been admitted with a 2-day history of vomiting and upper abdominal pain. He is hypotensive and hypovolaemic, he has cool peripheries and increased capillary refill. His hypotension is being treated by increasing cardiac preload with a fluid challenge of 500 mL crystalloid solution.

   Which of the following most accurately describes this patient's cardiac preload?

   A   Central venous pressure
   B   End diastolic ventricular volume
   C   Pulmonary artery occlusion pressure
   D   Ventricular myocyte length
   E   Ventricular myocyte tension

2. A 65-year-old man on the surgical high-dependency unit has been complaining of chest pain for the past hour. Cardiac ischaemia is suspected since the patient has a history of angina and his ECG shows ST depression in the lateral leads.

   What is the main determinant of his coronary blood flow?

   A   Autonomic nervous system
   B   Blood viscosity
   C   Coronary artery diameter
   D   Diastolic blood pressure
   E   Myocardial oxygen demand

3. A 58-year-old man on the postoperative surgical ward has hypotension. He underwent a laparoscopic cholecystectomy earlier today. The patient has a history of ischaemic heart disease. To treat the hypotension his cardiac output will be optimised.

   To increase cardiac output with least impact on myocardial oxygen demand which of the following physiological variables should be optimised?

   A   Afterload
   B   Contractility
   C   Heart rate
   D   Preload
   E   Serum calcium

4. A 38-year-old woman underwent a laparoscopic biopsy of a vascular lesion. The biopsy results are being reviewed. On the histopathology report, there is no

mention of the site of the biopsy, however, the biopsy is found to contain a large proportion of elastic tissue.

Based on this report, where is the elastic tissue most likely to originate from?

A   Aorta
B   Arteries
C   Arterioles
D   Veins
E   Vena cava

5. A 56-year-old man is being assessed for repair of a large aortic aneurysm. As part o his assessment he is going to undergo cardiopulmonary exercise testing.

Which organ receives the greatest proportion of cardiac output before the start of the test?

A   Brain
B   Heart
C   Liver
D   Kidneys
E   Skeletal muscle

6. A 65-year-old woman on the surgical high-dependency unit is peri-arrest. Her heart rate is 30 beats per minute, SpO_2 of 80% and the monitor is unable to measure a systolic blood pressure. High flow oxygen and IV fluids are being administered. The house officer asks if IV adrenaline should be given.

Which one of the following adrenoreceptors causes vasoconstriction by adrenaline?

A α_1
B α_2
C β_1
D β_2
E β_3

7. A 21-year-old man is brought in by ambulance to the emergency department with an abdominal stab wound. He is in class 3 hypovolaemic shock and is being resuscitated by the emergency team. The carotid baroreceptors are some of the main sensors of intravascular volume status.

What is the afferent nerve supply of the carotid baroreceptors?

A   Glossopharyngeal nerve
B   Phrenic nerve
C   Recurrent laryngeal nerve
D   Sympathetic chain
E   Vagus nerve

Answers

. D Ventricular myocyte length

It has been known for almost 150 years that myocardial contractility is related to filling pressure. The initial length of a cardiac myocyte determines its contractility. It is, however, usually impossible to measure this directly in vivo and therefore surrogate measurements, such as left ventricular end diastolic pressure (LVEDP), are used. It is assumed, providing ventricular compliance is normal, that LVEDP reflects ventricular volume and hence myocyte length. Classically a Frank–Starling curve is drawn with central venous pressure on the x-axis and stroke volume/cardiac output on the y-axis. Increasing preload (i.e. central venous pressure) leads to increased cardiac output until the myocyte becomes overstretched and cardiac output falls as occurs in cardiac failure. The position of the Frank–Starling curve is influenced by inotropic status (**Figure 14.1**).

In order for the heart to eject against the total peripheral resistance, tension needs to be generated in the myocytes. Myocyte tension therefore relates more closely to the concept of afterload.

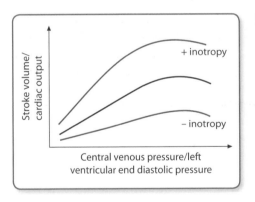

Figure 14.1 The Frank–Starling curve.

. C Coronary artery diameter

The Hagen–Poiseuille equation (in a straight tube the value of resistance is inversely proportional to the fourth power of the radius) describes laminar flow through tubes. Flow is proportional to the pressure gradient along the tube (i.e. the gradient between aortic pressure and ventricular pressure). During systole left ventricular pressure is greater than aortic pressure and there is no blood flow to the left ventricle. As it is primarily the duration of diastole that shortens when the heart rate increases, the importance of avoiding tachycardia in patients with ischaemic heart disease becomes apparent. It is also important to avoid bradycardia however, as diastolic blood pressure falls as diastole lengthens and this also compromises coronary blood flow.

The cross sectional area of the tube is of greatest importance as flow is proportional to the fourth power of the radius. Small changes in vessel diameter therefore have a large influence on flow; doubling the radius increases flow 16 times. The radius of coronary arteries is matched to myocardial oxygen demand; as oxygen demand increases vessel radius increases. The mediators for this are adenosine and nitric oxide and the process is an example of autoregulation. Flow is inversely proportional to the length of the tube and viscosity of the fluid. The autonomic nervous system has little influence on coronary artery diameter.

3. D Preload

The main determinant of myocardial oxygen demand is the amount of myocardial work performed. Myocardial work is increased by increasing heart rate, contractility and afterload. Preload also increases contractility but, because of the Laplace relationship it produces a much smaller increase in O_2 demand than the other factors. Laplace's law applies for spheres, when applied to a human ventricle, gives the following equation: ventricular wall tension = pressure x $\sqrt[3]{volume}$. Doubling the intraventricular pressure by increasing contractility or afterload will double myocardial wall tension and therefore double myocardial work. Doubling the heart rate will also roughly double the myocardial work. If preload is increased by doubling end diastolic ventricular volume however, the tension generated is only increased by approximately 26%.

4. A Aorta

One of the key functions of the aorta is to maintain blood flow and pressure during diastole. It achieves this by acting as an elastic reservoir. During systole it expands to accommodate the blood ejected from the ventricle. One-third of the stroke volume flows through the arteries to perfuse tissues but most remains in the aorta, stretching the vessel wall and storing potential energy. During diastole this energy is used as the aorta contracts due to elastic recoil and blood flow is thus maintained. This is termed the windkessel effect. For this to work effectively a nonregurgitant aortic valve and the presence of a peripheral resistance are required. As the aorta ages it loses elastic tissue and therefore becomes less compliant. A consequence of this is that there will be greater pressure variations during the cardiac cycle. This is one of the contributing factors to hypertension.

5. C Liver

Regional blood flow is regulated by the arterioles which contain a large proportion of smooth muscle in their walls. During exercise local metabolites produced in muscle and stimulation of β_2-adrenoreceptors cause vasodilatation in skeletal muscle vascular beds. Simultaneously sympathetic nervous system activation leads to vasoconstriction of splanchnic and renal arterioles. Myocardial oxygen supply increases primarily by increasing coronary blood flow as oxygen extraction is already 80% in the resting heart. Skin blood flow initially increases to promote heat loss from exercising muscle but at high cardiac outputs cutaneous vasoconstriction occurs in order to maintain muscle blood flow. This will lead to an increase in body temperature. **Table 14.1** below demonstrates the changes in distribution of blood flow in a patient going from rest to heavy exercise.

Table 14.1

	Resting blood flow (mL/min)	Light exercise blood flow (mL/min)	Vigorous exercise blood flow (mL/min)
Cerebral	650 (13%)	650 (7%)	650 (2.5%)
Coronary	250 (5%)	450 (5%)	1250 (5%)
Renal	1000 (20%)	900 (10%)	250 (1%)
Splanchnic/liver	1250 (25%)	1100 (12%)	250 (1%)
Skeletal muscle	1000 (20%)	4200 (47%)	22000 (88%)
Skin	300 (6%)	1350 (15%)	500 (2%)
Other	550 (11%)	350 (4%)	100 (0.5%)
Total cardiac output	5000	9000	25000

Table 14.1 Distribution of blood flow in a 70 kg person during rest and exercise. The percentage in parentheses is the proportion of the cardiac output received by the organ at the given level of exercise.

A α_1-receptors

Adrenoreceptors exert their effects via intracellular secondary messenger systems. They have widespread effects on the human body and can be grouped into α- and β-receptors. Adrenaline at low doses primarily affects β-receptors but in higher doses, including the dose used in cardiac arrest it has α effects also. Its onset is around 30 seconds and duration of effect a few minutes. **Table 14.2** details some of the effects of the adrenoreceptor subtypes.

Table 14.2

Receptor	Effect
α_1	Vasoconstriction
α_2	Inhibition of noradrenaline release from nerve endings
	Platelet aggregation
β_1	Increased chronotropy and inotropy
	Increased renin secretion
β_2	Bronchodilatation
	Vasodilatation
β_3	Lipolysis in fat cells

Table 14.2 Effects of adrenoreceptor subtypes.

β_2-receptors increase chronotropy and inotropy but to a lesser extent than β_1-receptors. They assume greater importance in heart failure when β_1-receptors are downregulated.

7. A The glossopharyngeal nerve

The neurohumoral response to acute hypovolaemia is complex and can be divided into an early phase where maintenance of tissue perfusion is the priority and a later phase aimed at restoring a normal circulating volume.

Carotid and aortic baroreceptors are stretch receptors that are stimulated by increased distention of the vessel. Following acute blood loss venous return decreases and due to the Frank–Starling mechanism blood pressure falls. Decreased intra-arterial pressure causes less vessel wall stretch and hence reduced activation of the baroreceptors. Afferent neurones from the carotid baroreceptors (also known as the carotid sinuses) travel in the glossopharyngeal nerves and from the aortic baroreceptors via the vagus. These afferent neurones synapse with cardiovascular control centres in the brainstem. Decreased firing of these afferent neurones will lead to inhibition of central parasympathetic outflow and increased central sympathetic outflow. Increased sympathetic outflow causes vasoconstriction and an increase in heart rate and myocardial contractility thereby maintaining perfusion to vital organs.

Other components of the early phase include an increase in serum levels of antidiuretic hormone (ADH), causing retention of water and vasoconstriction (ADH is also known as vasopressin). The renin–angiotensin–aldosterone system (RAAS) is also activated causing vasoconstriction and sodium and water retention. Atrial natriuretic peptide secretion is inhibited and together with ADH and the RAAS this leads to restoration of circulating volume. Increased erythropoiesis returns haemoglobin levels to normal over a few weeks.

The phrenic nerves supply motor function to the diaphragm and sensation to the mediastinal pleura and most of the diaphragm. The recurrent laryngeal nerve supplies the intrinsic muscles of the larynx (except cricothyroid) and sensation below the vocal cords.

Chapter 15

Respiratory system

. A 33-year-old woman is admitted to the surgical high-dependency unit with acute pancreatitis. She is breathing 15 L/min of oxygen through a standard face mask. Her oxygen saturation reading is 91%.

What most affects the actual oxygen percentage inspired by the patient?

A   Inspiratory flow rate
B   Oxygen consumption
C   Respiratory rate
D   Tidal volume
E   Ventilation–perfusion matching

. A 72-year-old man presents for elective repair of unilateral inguinal hernia associated with pain. He has a history of chronic obstructive pulmonary disease with long standing type 2 respiratory failure and poor exercise tolerance. A venous blood gas taken by the house officer shows a $PaCO_2$ of 8.5 kPa.

In this patient's venous blood, how is most of the carbon dioxide (CO_2) transported?

A   As bicarbonate
B   As carbamino compounds
C   As carbonic acid
D   Bound to haemoglobin
E   Dissolved in solution

. A 70-year-old man has been admitted to the intensive care unit for invasive ventilation. He aspirated gastric contents during upper GI endoscopy for investigation of dyspepsia. The working diagnosis is acute respiratory distress syndrome secondary to aspiration pneumonitis. The family are asking about something they read on the internet called pulmonary surfactant treatment.

What is the main constituent of pulmonary surfactant?

A   Apolipoprotein
B   Carbohydrate
C   Cholesterol
D   Lipid
E   Protein

. A 52-year-old woman on high-dependency unit has undergone open repair of aortic aneurysm 2 hours ago. She has sickle cell trait but is otherwise healthy.

She received 14 units of blood intraoperatively and is now adequately resuscitated.

What is the most likely factor impairing liberation of oxygen from haemoglobin for delivery to her tissues?

A   Alkalosis
B   Hypothermia
C   Presence of haemoglobin S
D   Reduced 2, 3-diphosphoglycerate activity
E   Residual fetal haemoglobin

5. A 42-year-old woman on a surgical ward 36 hours post laparoscopic cholecystectomy presents with breathlessness. She was previously fit and well. On examination, she has a painful and swollen left calf. There are no other abnormal clinical findings. Her partial pressure of oxygen (PaO_2) is 6.1 kPa (46 mmHg).

What does the PaO_2 signify?

A   Hypoxaemia
B   Insufficient haemoglobin to carry oxygen
C   The patient is on oxygen
D   Tissue hypoxia
E   Type 1 respiratory failure

6. A 62-year-old man on the surgical high-dependency unit is recovering following a paraumbilical hernia repair. There is a history of chronic obstructive pulmonary disease. He is breathing humidified oxygen 60% with a rate of 34 breaths per minute and has a PaO_2 of 7.4 kPa and $PaCO_2$ of 7.4 kPa.

What is the most likely cause of his hypoxia?

A   Excess oxygen administration
B   High $PaCO_2$
C   Humidification
D   Impaired lung diffusion
E   Pulmonary shunting

Answers

1. A Inspiratory flow rate

The inspired concentration of oxygen depends on the relative contributions of oxygen from the mask (100% oxygen) and entrained room air (21% oxygen). Inspiratory flow rate at rest can be estimated by thinking about the tidal volume (500 mL) and the respiratory rate. With a respiratory rate of 15 breaths per minute and equal inspiratory and expiratory times (in reality inspiration time is normally about half of expiration time), the time for each inspiration would be 2 seconds. This gives a flow rate of 0.25 litres per second or 15 litres per minute. Although 15 litres per minute oxygen flow could theoretically deliver 100% oxygen to a patient breathing at rest, room air is inevitably entrained. If either respiratory rate or tidal volume increases, the inspiratory flow rate will exceed the maximum oxygen flow rate and room air must be entrained. In fact, maximum breathing capacity can be up to 170 litres per minute. This is why a tight fitting face mask with a reservoir bag (e.g. 'trauma mask') using high flow oxygen (15 Lmin^{-1}) will deliver more oxygen to the patient.

2. A As bicarbonate

Venous blood carries the CO_2 from cellular respiration back to the lungs (via the right heart) for excretion. Around 60% is in the form of bicarbonate (HCO_3^-) through the reaction with water ($H_2O + CO_2 = H_2CO_3 = H^+ + HCO_3^-$), the first part of which being catalysed by carbonic anhydrase. Amino groups in proteins in the blood (mainly haemoglobin) combine with CO_2 to form carbamates which account for around 5% in arterial blood and 30% in venous blood. Deoxygenated haemoglobin in the venous blood carries more CO_2 which is part of the Haldane effect. CO_2 is more soluble than oxygen but only accounts for around 10% in venous blood (5% in arterial). This patient has raised $PaCO_2$ and is at increased risk of postoperative respiratory complications. If the patient decides to go ahead with the surgery, he may benefit from having the procedure carried out under local or regional anaesthesia.

3. D Lipid

Surfactant is produced by Type 2 alveolar cells and consists mainly of the lipid dipalmitoylphosphatidylcholine (DPCC) and other phospholipids. The pathophysiology of respiratory distress syndrome involves alveolar cell dysfunction and therefore inadequate surfactant production. Surface tension of the fluid lining the alveolar air spaces acts as a collapsing force. The law of Laplace tells us that the pressure (force) required to keep the alveolus open is proportional to the surface tension, and indirectly proportional to the radius of the alveolus (pressure = 2 x surface tension/radius). This means that as the alveolus reduces in size as expiration occurs, the pressure required to prevent collapse increases. Correspondingly, it requires more pressure (and therefore energy) to inflate a small alveolus with high surface tension. Surface tension of water is around 70 dyn/cm whereas surfactant is between 0–20 dyn/cm. The effect of surfactant is more pronounced at lower lung volumes (<1dyn/cm at <40% total lung capacity). Surfactant therefore increases lung compliance, particularly at low lung volumes, and minimises atelectasis. Surface tension also draws fluid into the lungs, and so surfactant helps to keep the lungs dry. There is no clear evidence supporting the use of synthetic surfactant in ARDS and it is not a recognised treatment in the UK.

4. D Reduced 2, 3-diphosphoglycerate activity

A left shift in the oxygen-haemoglobin dissociation curve equates to increased affinity for oxygen. Thinking about the curve, the P_{50} (the oxygen partial pressure whereby haemoglobin is 50% saturated) moves further to the left, i.e. haemoglobin is less likely to release oxygen for any given PaO_2. This is caused by alkalosis, reduced 2, 3-diphosphoglycerate activity, hypothermia, fetal haemoglobin, and carbon monoxide. She is adequately resuscitated which implies adequate blood oxygenation, circulating volume, normothermia, and absence of acidosis (a marker of hypoperfusion). She may have an insignificant amount of fetal haemoglobin. She may have some haemoglobin S but this causes a right shift in the curve. Transfused blood has reduced 2, 3-diphosphoglycerate activity and it takes time to replenish this by glycolysis following transfusion.

5. A Hypoxaemia

A decreased partial pressure of oxygen (PaO_2) in the blood is generally described as hypoxaemia. PaO_2 is not a measure of oxygen *total content of blood,* which is largely dependent on haemoglobin. Normal PaO_2 breathing room air would be 10–14 kPa (75–105 mmHg). For a normal adult breathing oxygen it should be considerably higher than this. PaO_2 6.1 kPa is very concerning and oxygen should be applied if it has not already. There is a possibility that this could be an inadvertent venous blood gas, but other values such as pH and $PaCO_2$ would indicate whether this was possible and compatible. Tissue hypoxia could be inferred by reduced arterial pH and raised lactate, not PaO_2. We need to know the $PaCO_2$ to distinguish Type 1 (normo- or hypocapnic) from Type 2 (hypercapnic) respiratory failure. This patient may have a pulmonary embolism and should be resuscitated and then investigated accordingly.

6. E Pulmonary shunting

Breathing room air (21% or around 21 kPa), gas must be fully humidified by the time it reaches the lung. This accounts for a 1 kPa drop in the inspired partial pressure of oxygen. The inspired gas is then mixed with the alveolar gas, which contains CO_2, further reducing the oxygen concentration. Normal lungs have a negligible diffusion barrier, accounting for a small drop in oxygen, although this is increased in lung disease. Blood shunting through unventilated parts of the lung leads to a further drop in oxygen, which in the healthy lung is <2 kPa but can account for large differences in inspired and arterial oxygen. This oxygen cascade explains why a normal PaO_2 is 12–14 kPa when breathing room air at 21 kPa. This patient is probably breathing between 40–60 kPa of oxygen and pulmonary shunting is the only one of these factors that can explain the situation. This may be due to atelectasis or consolidation. Although the patient has chronic obstructive pulmonary disease and type 2 respiratory failure, the respiratory rate is high and supplementary oxygen is vital. The patient needs ventilatory support urgently.

Chapter 16

Gastrointestinal system

A 66-year-old man presents with severe widespread tooth decay. This began some 6 months ago when he developed generalised disease of his salivary glands.

Which of the following best explains the rampant decay?

A   Decreased aqueous secretion from the sublingual salivary glands
B   Increased acid secretion from the parotid salivary glands
C   Loss of calcium-rich watery salivary secretions
D   Loss of potassium-rich watery salivary secretions
E   Reflex sympathetic vasoconstriction

A 20-year-old man, a motorcyclist, is being nursed in the semi-prone recovery position to prevent regurgitated acid gastric contents from entering his lower airways while he is in coma (Glasgow coma scale 9).

Which of the following neurological reflexes prevents regurgitation during vomiting?

A   Reflex bronchoconstriction with centre in the medulla oblongata
B   Reflex bronchoconstriction with centre in the pons
C   Reflex elevation of the larynx with centre in the medulla oblongata
D   Reflex elevation of the larynx with centre in the pons
E   Reflex pyloric constriction with centre in the hypothalamus

A 35-year-old man presents with a duodenal peptic ulcer.

Which of the following best explains how his pain can be relieved?

A   Changing the pH of the fluid bathing the ulcer from 5 to 2
B   Changing the pH of the gastric contents from 2 to 5
C   Changing the pH of the gastric contents from 5 to 2
D   Severing the nerve supply to the duodenum
E   Stimulating gastric H_2 receptors.

A 62-year-old woman with difficulty swallowing and a tendency to choke has a percutaneous endoscopic gastrostomy inserted for enteral feeding.

Which of the following best describes the fluid to be used in this feeding?

A   Carbohydrate nutrition should be in the form of glucose only
B   Daily energy content should be around 400 kcal (1.68 MJ)
C   Fat content should be as low as possible
D   Milk would be an appropriate constituent
E   Protein nutrition should be in the form of a mixture of essential amino acids

5. A 58-year-old man presents with obstructive jaundice, the cause of which has been diagnosed as cancer in the head of the pancreas.

Which of the following best explains the reason for his jaundice?

A   Bile salts are failing to reach the duodenum
B   Duodenal pH has changed due to a failure of pancreatic bicarbonate to reach the duodenum
C   The bile duct and the pancreatic duct have a common opening into the duodenum
D   The pancreatic duct is obstructed
E   There is failure of excretion of conjugated bilirubin

6. A 48-year-old woman presents with a high jejunal fistula.

Which of the following best describes why her condition is not a low (terminal) ileal fistula?

A   Fistula content has a much greater acidity
B   Fistula content has a higher amount of bile acids
C   Fistula content has a higher concentration of nutrients
D   Fistula has a lower vitamin B_{12} content
E   Fistula has a lower volume

7. Two 34-year-old men have a stoma – one a colostomy in the left iliac fossa after rectal surgery, and the other an ileostomy in the right iliac fossa after a panproctocolectomy for ulcerative colitis. Contents of the colostomy bag in the left iliac fossa are relatively small in volume and consist of well-formed stools. Contents of the ileostomy bag in the right iliac fossa are relatively copious non-smelly fluid.

What is the best explanation for the difference?

A   More than 75% of fluid absorption from the entire gut takes place in the colon
B   Random variation
C   The caecum absorbs more fluid than the small intestine
D   There is net secretion of fluid in the left (descending) colon
E   The colon absorbs a small but significant proportion of ingested plus secreted fluid in the gut

8. A 50-year-old man presents with a 6-month history of projectile vomiting. For over 30 years he has suffered from indigestion for which he has self-medicated with drugs across the chemists counter. On examination, he is extremely dehydrated, with visible gastric peristalsis and succussion splash. His blood results are as follows:

pH	7.50
PCO_2	40 mmHg (5.3 kPa)
Bicarbonate	30.1 mmol/L
Haemoglobin	17 g/dL

Urea	18 mmol/L
Creatinine	190 µmol/L

Which of the following is most likely to have caused this condition?

A   A metabolic alkalosis due to gastric outlet obstruction
B   Chronic renal failure leading to vomiting
C   Chronic respiratory failure with secondary polycythaemia
D   Compensated respiratory alkalosis
E   Renal failure as a side effect of medication for his indigestion

Answers

1. C Loss of calcium-rich watery salivary secretions

A healthy mouth and healthy teeth depend on a steady flow from the serous (watery) secreting parotid glands, with some contribution from the seromucous submandibular glands. Saliva has antiseptic properties, helping to control pathogenic bacteria. However, the copious watery output from the parotid glands, being rich in calcium and phosphate ions, is particularly important in countering erosion of the teeth by acid-forming bacteria and healing minor surface abrasions in the enamel. Rampant caries can also occur in children who constantly bathe their teeth in sweet/acidic drinks when given these in feeding bottles to pacify them.

The sublingual glands (A) are mucous. The parotid secretions help to buffer acid (B). Like gastric and intestinal secretions generally, saliva is relatively rich in potassium (D), but this is not significant in preventing tooth decay. Neither is reflex sympathetic vasoconstriction (E) a contributory factor.

2. C Reflex elevation of the larynx with centre in the medulla oblongata

During swallowing and also during vomiting, the entrance to the larynx and hence the airways is reflexly closed by elevation of the larynx (the elevation is easily seen in most males during swallowing) so that its entrance (which faces obliquely upwards and backwards) is jammed firmly against the base of the tongue. Thus swallowed (or regurgitated) material must pass from pharynx to oesophagus (or vice versa). The epiglottis is not an essential part of this mechanism (if the epiglottis is removed, the reflex still works). Reflexes for swallowing and vomiting have their centres in the medulla oblongata, not the pons (D).

Bronchoconstriction (A, B) narrows the airways during coughing, thus increasing air velocity for expulsion of mucus. Pyloric constriction (E) is part of the vomiting reflex, whereby gastric contents pass into the oesophagus rather than into the duodenum.

3. B Changing the pH of the gastric contents from 2 to 5

Peptic ulcers become more painful the greater the acidity of the fluid bathing them. The acid comes from the acid/pepsin secretion of the stomach. Normal gastric pH is around 2, enormously more acidic than most biological fluids, and considerably more acidic than the most acid normal urine (around 4–5). Each unit of pH indicates a 10-fold change in hydrogen ion concentration. A change in pH from 2 to 5 (B) indicates a 1000-fold decrease in hydrogen ion concentration (pH is the negative log of the hydrogen ion concentration and pH 7 is neutrality, with blood pH around 7.4).

A reduction in gastric acidity (i.e. a rise in pH) is directly and effectively produced by blocking the hydrogen ion pump which pumps hydrogen ions from the parietal cells to the gastric lumen. H_2 receptors mediate stimulation of the parietal cells to produce acid, so blockade of these receptors reduces ulcer pain (E wrong). Cutting the vagal nerve supply of the parietal cells (vagotomy) also reduces acid secretion, therefore cutting the nerve supply of the duodenum (D) is not an option. Changing the pH of both the fluid bathing the ulcer (A) and the gastric contents (C) from 5 to 2 would increase hydrogen ion content and hence acidity 1000-fold and would hugely increase ulcer pain.

D Milk would be an appropriate constituent

Enteral nutrition is essentially a good oral diet in liquid form; milk is a good starting point. Advantages of enteral rather than parenteral nutrition are that the fluid is administered into the gut; normal digestion takes place, elemental diets are not required and the gut remains in use and healthy rather than suffering atrophy. The daily energy content should be related to the recipient's daily requirements – in the sedentary state 4–5 times the value given in B would be appropriate. Elemental diets containing glucose (A) and amino acids (E) (plus fat, minerals, vitamins) are not required here. Fat content (C) should not be restricted to low levels.

E There is failure of excretion of conjugated bilirubin

Obstructive jaundice implies an obstruction to the excretion of conjugated bilirubin into the gut for elimination in the faeces. In this man's case the cancer in the head of the pancreas is causing the obstruction by compression of the nearby duodenum including the bile duct which conveys bile into the duodenum.

In this condition bile salts may also fail to reach the duodenum (A), but they are colourless so do not contribute to jaundice (where the pigment bilirubin causes the typical spectrum of skin colour abnormalities). Failure of pancreatic bicarbonate reaching the duodenum (B), a common opening of the bile and pancreatic ducs into the duodenum (C) and obstruction of the pancreatic duct (D) do not of themselves interfere with excretion of bilirubin.

B Fistula content has a higher amount of bile acids

Bile acids are required for emulsification in the jejunum and are reabsorbed and recycled to the liver via portal venous blood draining the terminal ileum. This reduces the metabolic cost to the body of synthesising all the bile acids required for emulsification and hence digestion of fats. Vitamin B_{12} is also absorbed actively, rather than secreted (D) in the terminal ileum.

The upper jejunum, rather than the upper ileum, is the main site of final digestion into amino acids and monosaccharides (C) and also the main site of absorption of these nutrients and also fat. Gut contents have to be around neutrality (pH 7) for the final digestion and absorption, rather than acidic (A). Bicarbonate is added in the duodenum via the pancreatic duct and from local duodenal glands (E).

7. E The colon absorbs a small but significant proportion of ingested plus secreted fluid in the gut

In 24 hours 500 mL of intestinal contents pass through the ileocaecal valve and this is reduced to 150 mL after water absorption in the colon (the volumes are influenced by dietary fibre content). The typical smell of faeces is due to chemicals produced by bacteria in the colon (subsequent to the exit of ileal fluid).

By the time the gut contents reach the start of the colon in the right iliac fossa, most of the ingested plus secreted fluid has been absorbed (A). Most of this is absorbed in the small intestine, mainly in the jejunum (not the caecum (C)). There is net absorption (not secretion) as the fluid passes along the colon (D) so by the time the contents reach the left iliac fossa they have changed from the fluid to the formed faecal state. This effect hugely exceeds random variations (B) in colostomy and ileostomy bag contents.

Patients with an ileostomy are liable to have electrolyte disturbances in the long run because of the electrolyte content of the relatively large amount of fluid lost.

8. A A metabolic alkalosis due to gastric outlet obstruction

This man's pH is raised, indicating an alkalosis; the bicarbonate is also raised, indicating that the alkalosis is metabolic in origin. For a respiratory alkalosis the PCO_2 would be low (D). (For a respiratory acidosis, compensated, or uncompensated, the PCO_2 would be raised, whereas it is norma). This man gives a clear picture of gastric outlet obstruction from long-standing peptic ulcer. Obstruction is caused by scar tissue related to repeated healing and exacerbations of the ulcer. Large amounts of relatively concentrated hydrochloric acid produced in the stomach are lost in the vomitus. Loss of hydrogen ions leads to alkalosis. Loss of chloride ions leads also to hypochloraemia. Like all intestinal fluids, gastric contents have a relatively high potassium content, hence hypokalaemia may also be present. His raised bicarbonate could be due in part to bicarbonate-containing medications for his dyspepsia.

With loss of fluid by vomiting, and inability to take oral fluids, the man is suffering from severe dehydration. This is confirmed by the raised haemoglobin concentration [haemoconcentration, rather than secondary polycythaemia (C)]. Dehydration would also account for the raised urea and creatinine levels (so no need to postulate chronic renal failure (B) or as a side-effect of the antacid medication (E).

This man requires urgent resuscitation with intravenous fluids prior to surgery to relieve the gastric outlet obstruction.

Chapter 17

Genitourinary system

A 19-year-old, 70 kg man presents with epigastric pain. He is haemodynamically stable and his abdomen is soft with minimal epigastric tenderness. He is managing normal fluid intake orally. A junior in the emergency department catheterises him and asks for hourly urine output monitoring.

What is the hourly urine output most likely to be?

A   15 mL/h
B   20 mL/h
C   60 mL/h
D   100 mL/h
E   150 mL/h

A 32-year-old man falls 20 m while washing windows. He fractures his 10th to 12th ribs on the left. On presentation to the emergency department he complains of left upper quadrant abdominal pain. His pulse is 120 beats per minute, and blood pressure is 90/50 mmHg. His abdomen is peritonitic. He is taken for emergency laparotomy and the diagnosis of splenic rupture is confirmed. He undergoes splenectomy and has a total blood loss of 1500 mL. Postoperatively he has reduced urine output.

Which mechanism is most likely to result in his reduced urine output?

A   Angiotensin II reduction
B   Antidiuretic hormone reduction
C   Nitric oxide increase
D   Natriuretic peptide increase
E   Sympathetic stimulation

A 73-year-old woman with ischaemic heart disease and hypertension is commenced on an angiotensin converting enzyme inhibitor. She attends the

Test	Result	Reference range
Urea	27.0 mmol/L	2.5–6.6 mmol/L
Creatinine	320 µmol/L	60–120 µmol/L
Sodium	135 mmol/L	135–145 mmol/L
Potassium	6.3 mmol/L	3.6–5.0 mmol/L

emergency department feeling unwell. Blood tests and renal function tests are done; the result of her renal function test is displayed in the table below. Her ECG is normal. The patient is prescribed insulin and dextrose to treat the hyperkalaemia.

What is the most likely mechanism of action?

A   Increased gastrointestinal loss of potassium
B   Increased intracellular uptake of potassium
C   Increased renal excretion of potassium
D   Myocardial stabilisation
E   Reduced gastrointestinal absorption of potassium

4. A 66-year-old woman presents with minimal urine output for 2 days and suprapubic discomfort. She has a bladder ultrasound scan which shows 650 mL c urine in her bladder. Pelvic and neurological examinations are normal. Pelvic an renal tract ultrasounds are both normal.

What is the most likely cause of this woman's urinary retention?

A   Bladder cancer
B   Fibroids
C   Multiple sclerosis
D   Rectal cancer
E   Urethral stenosis

5. A 78-year-old man is referred as an emergency with a 3-day history of minimal urine output, nocturnal incontinence and a palpable bladder. After reviewing the patient a urethral catheter is inserted, which drains 1650 mL of urine initially and then 200–400 mL every hour following insertion. An ultrasound of the renal tract immediately following catheterisation shows bilateral hydroureter and hydronephrosis. His renal function is shown below.

Test	Result	Reference range
Urea	23 mmol/L	2.5–6.6 mmol/L
Creatinine	696 µmol/L	60–120 µmol/L
Sodium	134 mmol/L	135–145 mmol/L
Potassium	6.7 mmol/L	3.6–5.0 mmol/L

What is the most likely diagnosis?

A   Bilateral ureteric stones
B   High pressure chronic urinary retention
C   IgA nephropathy
D   Low pressure chronic urinary retention
E   Upper tract urothelial carcinoma

. A 30-year-old man presents to the emergency department with a 3-day history of left loin pain, nausea and vomiting. He has no fever. He denies urinary or bowel symptoms. His abdomen is soft and urinalysis shows microscopic haematuria only. He has no past medical history and takes no regular medication.

His blood results are detailed in the table below. A CT of kidneys, ureters and bladder (CTKUB) is performed and this shows normal kidneys bilaterally with a 5 mm left ureteric calculus with minimal proximal dilatation.

Test	Result	Reference range
Urea	14.3 mmol/L	2.5–6.6 mmol/L
Creatinine	173 μmol/L	60–120 μmol/L
Sodium	140 mmol/L	135–145 mmol/L
Potassium	4.0 mmol/L	3.6–5.0 mmol/L

Which of the following is the most likely cause of his renal failure?

A Contrast nephropathy
B Dehydration
C Glomerulonephritis
D Obstructive nephropathy
E Reflux nephropathy

Answers

1. C 60 mL/h

The kidneys receive 25% of cardiac output, approximately 1300 mL/min. Combined blood flow in the renal veins is approximately 1299 mL/min. The difference is the urine output 1 mL/min. Minimum expected urine output is 0.5 mL/kg/min.

2. E Sympathetic stimulation

Blood loss stimulates the sympathetic nervous system, causing release of adrenaline and noradrenaline, which act on α-receptors in the afferent arterioles to cause vasoconstriction. This results is decreased renal blood flow and glomerular filtration. Angiotensin II also causes vasoconstriction of the arterioles and increases sodium and water reabsorption. Angiotensin II stimulates ADH secretion, which also causes vasoconstriction and collecting duct permeability. Both cause reduced renal blood flow and urine output. Nitric oxide and natriuretic peptide cause vasodilation and increased renal blood flow.

3. B Increased intracellular uptake of potassium

Insulin in dextrose is used to drive potassium into the cell thereby reducing the high serum potassium, although not reducing the actual total body potassium. Treatment of the cause of renal failure, in this case likely to be as a result of the addition of an angiotensin-converting enzyme inhibitor, will result in resolution of this potentially life-threatening emergency.

4. E Urethral stenosis

Urinary retention is much less common in women than men. Causes in women include: pelvic prolapse, pelvic masses, poststress incontinence procedures, urethral stenosis, drugs, post operation, S2–S4 injury, pelvic surgery, multiple sclerosis, urinary tract infection and hysteria, the latter in young women. As neurological and clinical examinations of pelvis are normal as is ultrasound of the pelvis and renal tract, the cause of urinary retention in this patient is urethral stenosis. This is cured by urethral dilatation.

5. B High pressure chronic urinary retention

This man is in chronic urinary retention as he has a non-painful bladder, which remains palpable or percussible after passing urine. In association with this, the patient has renal dysfunction which is likely to be caused by high pressure in his bladder causing backpressure onto his kidneys. This is known as high pressure chronic retention as opposed to low pressure chronic retention where there would be normal renal function.

5. B Dehydration

Note the 3-day history of nausea and vomiting. Renal failure can be prerenal, renal or postrenal. The degree of dilatation is not indicative of the degree of obstruction in the collecting system. However, in the presence of bilateral normal kidneys a single obstructed kidney would not normally result in acute renal failure as the other kidney would compensate. A CT of kidneys, ureters and bladder is a noncontrast imaging modality used for the diagnosis of urinary tract calculi, and therefore contrast nephropathy is not possible. With 3 days of nausea and vomiting, dehydration (prerenal failure) is the most likely cause. In the presence of kidney stones, one should also consider infection and nonsteroidal anti-inflammatory drugs as contributing factors.

Chapter 18

Endocrine system

A 16-year-old girl with features of acute appendicitis, including vomiting, is scheduled for surgery the next morning. She has suffered from diabetes mellitus from the age of five and gives herself subcutaneous insulin prior to each meal. Her diabetes has been well-controlled on her present insulin regime for several years.

What is the most appropriate management of this patient?

A   Dextrose–potassium–insulin infusion before surgery
B   Normal saline infusion at anaesthetic induction
C   Perioperative blood sugar should not rise above 5 mmol/L
D   Procedure scheduled at the end of the list to allow stabilisation
E   Usual subcutaneous insulin on the day of operation

A 35-year-old woman with features of Grave's disease is on the waiting list for subtotal thyroidectomy. She has been on antithyroid treatment for 2 months. At her preoperative assessment in the outpatient clinic, she complains of feeling too hot and is found to be sweating, with a sinus tachycardia of 90 beats per minute and an arterial blood pressure of 170/90 mmHg.

Which of the following is the most effective management?

A   Postpone operation for further stabilisation
B   Referral to a cardiologist for management of hypertension
C   Reiterate that antithyroid drugs and surgery are the way forward
D   Turn down the thermostat in the outpatient department
E   Urgent treatment for early atrial fibrillation

A 75-year-old man is undergoing emergency closure of a perforated duodenal ulcer. There was difficulty in obtaining a detailed history of his previous condition due to a degree of memory loss and confusion. He mentioned having taken tablets for pains in his hands, which showed features of rheumatoid arthritis. Relatively early in the operation his blood pressure begins to drop despite apparently adequate fluid administration. Several pressor agents are tried without benefit. His pressure becomes satisfactory again after an intravenous injection of hydrocortisone.

Which of the following is most likely to have caused this condition?

A   Nonspecific age-related effects
B   Preoperative paracetamol affecting clotting factors in the bone marrow
C   Preoperative paracetamol affecting clotting factors in the liver

D   Preoperative steroids interfering with adrenocortical function
E   Preoperative steroids interfering with the immune system

4.   A 62-year-old woman has recently been diagnosed with lung cancer and has been admitted for pneumonectomy. She was noted to be somewhat vague about her symptoms when the booking was made and in the subsequent 10 days she has become more confused and drowsy, complaining of vague headache. Arterial blood results for carbon dioxide, oxygen and pH are within the normal range, but serum sodium, chloride and potassium are below normal.

Which of the following is the most appropriate investigation to do next?

A   Blood grouping and cross matching with a view to urgent surgery
B   Brain scan to check for cerebral secondaries
C   Liver function tests to check for hepatic secondaries.
D   Repeat arterial blood gases to determine type of respiratory failure
E   Serum osmolality to establish whether a low osmolality is present

5.   A 25-year-old man on insulin injections for diabetes mellitus (present since childhood) has had total colectomy with ileoanal pouch procedure for familial adenomatous polyposis. Postoperative progress has been satisfactory, and he is now receiving oral nutrition and fluids. Several days after surgery a nurse reports that he is behaving out of character – he became rather unpleasant when she arrived to take his observations and would not allow these to proceed. He is sweating and his hand is shaking when you take his pulse rate. His pulse rate is 90 beats per minute and his blood pressure is 160/70 mmHg.

Which of the following is the most effective management?

A   Cool patient down with a bedside fan
B   Determine blood glucose measurement and give oral glucose
C   Immediate injection of the due dose of insulin
D   Immediate intravenous infusion of 5% dextrose
E   Prescribe a mild oral sedative

6.   A 40-year-old man presents following repeated episodes of renal colic and is being investigated for an underlying cause. His only other complaint is of vague abdominal discomfort. Investigations show no evidence of underlying renal disease. Blood tests reveal an increased calcium level and a reduced phosphate level, his plasma proteins are normal.

Which of the following is the most likely diagnosis?

A   Hyperthyroidism
B   Hypoparathyroidism
C   Hypothyroidism
D   Primary hyperparathyroidism
E   Subclinical hepatic failure

Answers

A Dextrose–potassium–insulin infusion before surgery

The objective is to maintain intracellular glucose levels by means of the insulin and to avoid hypoglycaemia and hypokalaemia by means of the dextrose (10%) and potassium (10 mmol/L). Monitoring the blood glucose is required, with adjustment, when necessary, by varying the insulin administered. This is done by substituting a new dextrose–potassium–insulin bag with the new level of insulin, higher if the blood glucose is too high and lower if it is too low. The aim is to have the patient's blood glucose around 10 mmol/L. This relatively high glucose level is much safer in these circumstances than the normal fasting level of 5 mmol/L (B). Thus, her usual daily doses (C) of insulin would not be inappropriate. She should be scheduled for first thing in the morning, rather than towards the end (E), to minimise the danger of prolonged starvation. A major danger during anaesthesia and surgery is development of hypoglycaemia when the usual clinical signs of hypoglycaemia (confusion, sweating, bounding pulse, and tremor) are masked by the anaesthetic. Saline alone (A) is inappropriate. Overall, the most severe risk is of permanent brain damage due to severe hypoglycaemia.

C Reiterate that antithyroid drugs and surgery are the way forward

This woman still has marked features of hyperthyroidism. They are caused by increased activity in mitochondria whereby energy production is increased and heat production is relatively even more increased. The overall basal metabolic rate is raised and the associated increased heat production mean that she much prefers a cool environment and even mild exertion leads to an increase in the uncomfortable feeling of being too hot. Body temperature starts to rise and this leads to reflex stimulation of sweat glands. Cardiac activity increases, partly from a direct action of excess thyroid hormones, and partly due to reflex activity to increase peripheral blood flow and dissipate the excess heat. Since the adverse effects stem from excessive thyroid activity, antithyroid drugs and sub-total thyroidectomy should eventually control the unpleasant symptoms.

The woman herself is the source of the excess heat, so turning down the thermostat (A) might gradually make her more comfortable, but the other patients are likely to complain of the cold! Typically hyperthyroid patients sit near an open window and hypothyroid patients cover up and go for a source of heat. The tachycardia and hyperdynamic pulse are due to her disorder and do not suggest cardiac disease (B). With sinus tachycardia this patient has no atrial fibrillation to treat (D); hyperthyroidism is a risk factor for atrial fibrillation, but mainly in older patients. Blood pressure readings are likely to return to normal with control of the hyperthyroidism (E).

3. D Preoperative steroids interfering with adrenocortical function

This man developed hypotension which was not responsive to adequate fluid administration and pressor agents. This is the picture seen with an inadequate cortisol response to the stress of major surgery. The prompt response to intravenous hydrocortisone confirms the previous deficiency of the adrenal glucocorticoid, cortisol (hydrocortisone is also a potent glucocorticoid). Long-term glucocorticoid therapy (e.g. prednisone) suppresses by negative feedback the anterior pituitary secretion of adrenocorticotrophic hormone and hence the adrenal secretion of cortisol. The cells forming these two hormones suffer disuse atrophy and so cannot respond in the life-threatening emergency of major surgery. Without adequate cortisol replacement treatment until recovery from the acute stress, death is quite likely.

Although steroids also suppress the immune system, this would not account for the hypotensive crisis observed (B). Clotting is not an issue in this case, and the usual doses of paracetamol would be unlikely to suppress production of clotting factors in the liver or platelets in the red bone marrow (C, D). Neither do nonspecific age-related effects (E) provide an explanation.

4. E Serum osmolality to establish whether a low osmolality is present

Abnormally low results for sodium, potassium and chloride would give a low estimated serum osmolality as together they account for most of the total osmolality. Symptoms of cerebral dysfunction with headache, suggest retention of excess water leading to swelling of the brain with raised intracranial pressure. The lung tumour may be secreting vasopressin (neoplasia can activate latent genetic abilities of tumour cells to secrete hormones, causing para-neoplastic syndromes). Secretion by tumour cells can lead to excessive (inappropriate) levels of the hormone vasopressin, normally released from the posterior pituitary. The antidiuretic action of this excessive vasopressin causes excessive reabsorption of water in the collecting ducts of the kidneys and hence an increase in total body water, including brain intracellular volume. Compression of the brain in the non-expandable skull leads to serious deterioration of brain function. This must be assessed and controlled prior to surgery. Confirming a low osmolality is the first step.

Although respiratory failure can cause confusion and headaches there is no evidence of diffuse lung disease (D). Other tests (A, B, C) are of less urgency than dealing with the serious risk of advancing cerebral dysfunction due to excess body water.

5. B Determine blood glucose measurement and give oral glucose

Episodes of hypoglycaemia are relatively common in diabetic patients on insulin, especially during restabilization after surgery. An early sign of brain function being impaired by lack of its necessary glucose substrate is unreasonable, out of character behaviour. Increasing drowsiness and impairment of consciousness develop as the blood sugar falls appreciably below the 5 mmol/L level and a severe fall can lead to coma and death. The brain has no energy stores and relies on uptake of glucose from a normal extracellular level (insulin does not influence this uptake). This man was still relatively cooperative (allowed his pulse and blood pressure to be taken) so it should not be difficult to persuade him to take a glucose rich drink or sweet snack. It is important to take a prior sample of blood for glucose measurement to establish the diagnosis; the sample can then be sent off after the patient has been resuscitated by oral glucose or sucrose, both of which are absorbed quite rapidly.

His sweating is not due to excessive heat (A) but is part of a reflex sympathetic response which also causes the tremor and hyperdynamic circulation (tachycardia with high pulse pressure, twice the normal in his case). Sympathetic activity helps to combat hyperglycaemia, adrenaline being particularly effective with its β-adrenoceptor action. Intravenous glucose (D) is not necessary when oral glucose or sucrose can be taken; if the patient is unconscious, intravenous 50% glucose must be given immediately after blood is taken for glucose measurement. Sedation (C) is inappropriate and an injection of insulin (B) could be fatal.

D Primary hyperparathyroidism

It is a physical law that when the solubility product of the calcium and phosphate ions exceeds its maximum, solid calcium phosphate is deposited. This law explains two features of this man's situation, in relation to his extracellular fluid, and in relation to his urine. Firstly, the major role of parathyroid hormone is to maintain the extracellular calcium ion level. This is important because interstitial extracellular fluid bathes nerves, muscles, bones, and also the (normally four) parathyroid glands (interstitial fluid and plasma exchange freely their calcium ions). If extracellular calcium ion level falls, nerves and muscles become hyperexcitable leading to tetany. However, a fall in calcium ions stimulates release of parathyroid hormone; this increases phosphate excretion into the urine, lowering extracellular phosphate. The solubility product for calcium and phosphate then falls, favouring release into solution of calcium ions in bone. Parathyroid hormone also favours activation of vitamin D, thereby getting more calcium into the body from the gut.

Secondly, in the urine, the level of phosphate rises because more is being excreted as mentioned above. In addition, because plasma calcium has increased, more filters into the urine. Thus, the calcium and phosphate ions in urine increase; when the maximal solubility product increases, solid calcium phosphate is deposited and grows into renal stones. Treatment of the hyperparathyroidism is the answer to this man's problems. Vague abdominal pains are a feature of hypercalcaemia, which hyperparathyroidism induces.

The other explanations are inappropriate. While hyperthyroidism (B) can erode the protein matrix of bone (to feed its hypermetabolic state), there is no significant erosion of the calcium salts in bone. Hypoparathyroidism (C) by the reversal of the mechanisms in the above paragraphs lowers excretion of calcium and phosphate. Hypothyroidism (D) does not affect calcium and phosphate excretion significantly.

The role of the liver is of interest in that albumin is a major carrier of bound calcium ions. If albumin in the blood falls, it carries less calcium and the total calcium level (as measured in hospital labs) falls, even though the critical physiologically significant calcium ion level may be normal. The reverse holds too. Thus, it is necessary to correct for abnormalities of plasma proteins in order to know the critical calcium level. In this case plasma protein levels were normal so correction is not needed (E).

Chapter 19

The liver

. A 45-year-old man suffering from chronic liver failure presents with bilateral ankle swelling and ascites.

Which of the following is most likely to have caused both these conditions?

A   A low circulating albumin level
B   A low circulating fibrinogen level
C   A raised albumin/globulin level in the circulation
D   Hepatic encephalopathy
E   Portosystemic anastomoses

. A 64-year-old woman with obstructive jaundice is being evaluated for non-urgent surgery within the next few weeks. Her coagulation screening shows an INR of 1.8 with normal values for fibrinogen and platelets.

What is the most appropriate management of this patient?

A   Arrange surgery as soon as possible
B   Commence regular injections of vitamin C
C   Commence regular injections of vitamin K
D   Give factor VIII intravenously over the perioperative period
E   Infuse fresh frozen plasma over the perioperative period

. A 66-year-old man has been admitted with severe vomiting of fresh blood and has required rapid transfusion of six units of blood. He is known to have long-standing hepatic cirrhosis with evidence of liver failure and ascites.

What is most likely source of the bleeding?

A   A duodenal ulcer related to coagulation problems
B   Oesophageal varices related to deficiency of vitamin B_{12}
C   Oesophageal varices related to gastric acid reflux
D   Oesophageal varices related to portal venous hypertension
E   Stress-related gastric ulcers

. A 35-year-old woman with jaundice presents with a raised bilirubin level in which both conjugated and unconjugated forms are above normal. The blood urea and creatinine are both increased, and haemoglobin is decreased. The patient also has several (asymptomatic) gallstones in the gallbladder.

What is the most appropriate management of this patient?

A   Commence vitamin B_{12} injections to treat the anaemia
B   Ignore the raised urea and creatinine because liver failure may be present

C   Investigate a possible haemolytic anaemia
D   Investigate a possible hepatic failure of bilirubin conjugation
E   Proceed to removal of the gallstones

5. A 45-year-old man presents with mild abdominal discomfort and is subsequently found to have several small gallstones. He is otherwise well.

What is the most appropriate management of this patient?

A   Consider elective cholecystectomy after full informed consent
B   Investigate for impaired absorption of bile salts and bile pigments
C   Scan his liver for hepatic secondary tumours
D   Treat the gallstones medically with bile pigments
E   Treat the gallstones medically with bile acids

6. A 55-year-old man with recurrent episodes of liver failure has been admitted with moderate impairment of consciousness (Glasgow coma scale 12) and shows coarse tremor of the outstretched arms.

Which of the following is most likely to have caused this condition?

A   A recent episode of severe jaundice
B   A recent high carbohydrate meal
C   A recent high fat meal
D   A recent high protein meal
E   Vitamin B_{12} deficiency

Answers

1. A A low circulating albumin level

Synthesis of circulating albumin is a major liver function. A low albumin level (together with a low albumin/globulin ratio, C) is a major indicator of liver failure. Since albumin is the major contributor to plasma oncotic pressure which retains fluid in the circulation, deficiency increases fluid filtration from the capillaries. Thus, the low albumin leads to dependent oedema – manifested in the ankles in the upright posture and around the sacrum in those confined to bed. Ascites is related to a combination of increased filtration pressure in the peritoneal capillaries due to portal hypertension (often found in liver failure) and decreased opposing oncotic pressure. Thus both his conditions are strongly related to the low circulating albumin level.

While a low fibrinogen level (B) is often found in liver failure, it does not contribute to portal hypertension or dependent oedema. Neither do hepatic encephalopathy (D) nor portosystemic anastomoses (E). Hepatic encephalopathy is impaired brain function related to toxins accumulating in liver failure and portosystemic anastomoses are enlarged venous channels which, in the oesophagus can rupture, causing sudden severe haemorrhage.

2. C Commence regular injections of vitamin K

With obstructive jaundice, bile is not reaching the gut. Absence of bile salts in the gut impairs absorption of fat and fat-soluble vitamins. Of these vitamin K is essential for formation of prothrombin in the liver. Prothrombin deficiency increases clotting time so INR (patient's clotting time divided by standard normal value) is elevated to 1.8 and there is a clear danger of excessive haemorrhage at operation due to impaired clotting. The vitamin K deficiency can be reversed by injections of the vitamin, bypassing the gut. Advancing the time of non-urgent surgery (A) would increase risks inappropriately. Deficiency of vitamin C is not a problem in obstructive jaundice, so (B) is unhelpful. Factor VIII (D) is used during surgery in patients with haemophilia, and fresh frozen plasma (E) is used when there are multiple or uncertain abnormalities of clotting.

3. D Oesophageal varices related to portal venous hypertension

Hepatic cirrhosis by the scarring it causes often impedes flow of portal blood through the liver, hence causing portal venous hypertension. The presence of ascites supports the diagnosis of portal hypertension, as does the severity of the bleeding. Increased pressure in the portal veins leads to diversion of blood through distended, weak-walled portosystemic anastomoses. These are common in the lower oesophagus and are prone to catastrophic bleeding.

Deficiency of vitamin B_{12} and gastric acid reflux are not significant contributory factors (B, C). Duodenal or gastric ulcers (A, E) are much lower on the list of possible diagnoses. However, coagulation problems may play a part in the severity of bleeding in patients with liver failure coexisting with portal hypertension.

4. C Investigate a possible haemolytic anaemia

With both unconjugated and conjugated bilirubin raised a haemolytic anaemia is suggested. The liver is conjugating more bilirubin than usual and yet is not keeping pace with the build-up of freshly released unconjugated bilirubin from broken-down red cells. The haemolytic anaemia needs to be investigated and treated before dealing with asymptomatic gallstones (E), which in this case may be pigment stones from the increased biliary content of conjugated bilirubin.

There is no suggestion of liver failure in this case and even if present it would not explain the raised urea and creatinine (B) which also need investigation (urea is normally formed in the liver, so its value may fall slightly in liver failure). Equally there is no suggestion of vitamin B_{12} deficiency (A). A raised conjugated bilirubin level suggests good liver function, particularly in excreting bilirubin (D).

5. A Consider elective cholecystectomy after full informed consent

This is a young patient with gallstones who is otherwise well. Although he has minimal symptoms, as he is young, cholecystectomy should be considered after full informed consent. Although a case can be made to leave things alone, he may develop complications later in life when he might have developed co-morbid disease. Laparoscopic cholecystectomy is one of the safest operations in good hands and eliminates the dreadful possibility, although rare, of cancer of the gallbladder which carries a dismal prognosis.

Investigating the patient for impaired absorption of bile salts and bile pigments (B) and hepatic secondaries (C) is not necessary as he remains otherwise well. Bile pigments are not a method of treatment (D). Medical treatment with bile acids (E) is a long-term treatment, hardly ever used. It will require regular monitoring of the size of the stones and after dissolution needs continued prophylaxis to prevent recurrence.

6. D A recent high protein meal

Dealing with the toxic products of protein digestion and bacterial action on protein products is a major function of the liver, which maintains normal consciousness in people with unimpaired liver function. A high protein meal in someone with liver failure can mimic the effects of alcoholic intoxication and may even lead to coma. In a patient with liver failure and portal hypertension, there may be bleeding in the gut from oesophageal varices. Absorption of this blood from the gut may have the same effect as a high protein meal causing impaired consciousness.

Carbohydrate (B) and fat (C) meals are processed in the liver, but absorption of large amounts of glucose or fat do not normally impair consciousness. Bilirubin (A) is harmful to infant brains, but adult brains are protected from it by the blood-brain barrier. While vitamin B_{12} is normally stored in the liver there is no reason to suspect that this man does not have adequate dietary vitamin B_{12} to avoid the nervous system problems of severe B_{12} deficiency (E).

Chapter 20

Inflammation

A 40-year-old woman is admitted for surgery having been diagnosed with autoimmune thyroid (Grave's) disease. Damage to the thyroid causing diffuse hyperplasia and high vascularity is caused by mechanisms similar to a type II hypersensitivity reaction.

What is the most likely mechanism for this reaction?

A   Activated T cells sensitised to nickel compounds
B   Antibody binding to antigens
C   Antigens becoming trapped inside macrophages
D   Bacterial infection in the gland
E   Circulating immune complexes deposit in the gland

A 55-year-old man presents with severe respiratory problems after elective cardiac surgery. He is diagnosed with acute respiratory distress syndrome triggered by endotoxin liberation.

What are the most likely immunological effects of endotoxin liberation?

A   Activation of CD8+ cytotoxic T cells
B   Decreased vascular permeability and prevention of vasodilation
C   Induction of B cells and the antibody response.
D   Macrophage activation and initiation of the cytokine cascade
E   Sensitisation of mast cells by antigen specific IgG

A 43-year-old man has received a renal transplant after kidney failure. Three weeks after his transplant, he starts showing symptoms of acute rejection.

What is the most likely immunological mechanism involved in acute rejection?

A   Alloreactive T cells infiltrate the graft
B   Immune complexes producing an inflammatory response
C   Immunosuppressive drug related toxicities
D   Pre-existing antibodies to major histocompatibility class I or ABO antigens
E   Reoccurrence of the original disease.

A 65-year-old man, recently retired, has taken up bee-keeping. After being stung several times, his most recent sting causes him to collapse with anaphylactic shock. His symptoms were very similar to the anaphylactoid reactions he had occasionally seen previously when handling the bees.

What is the most likely difference in mechanism between the anaphylactic and the anaphylactoid reaction?

    A   Anaphylactoid reactions are allergic reactions to milk proteins

    B   Anaphylactoid reactions are caused by direct activation of mast cells and are not immune mediated.

    C   Anaphylactoid reactions require high circulating levels of immunoglobulin E

    D   Anaphylactoid reactions require primary sensitisation of mast cells by the immune response

    E   There is no difference – they are both the same

5. A 45-year-old man presents with a wound infection for investigation. The wound contains high levels of phagocytic (pus) cells. Elimination of infection by phagocytic cells is a major mechanism in the prevention of sepsis and inflammation.

What is their most likely mechanism of action?

    A   Provide the main defence against virus infected cells

    B   Inhibit complement activation

    C   Ingest and kill invading bacteria

    D   Provide 'help' for B-cells in primary adaptive immune response

    E   Secrete antibodies during the immune response

6. A 36-year-old woman with systemic lupus erythematosus is admitted for a kidney transplant after her own organ has ceased to function.

What is the most likely immunological mechanism that initiated the damage to her kidney?

    A   Activation of the alternative complement pathway

    B   Antibody binds to antigens immobilised on kidney cells and tissues

    C   Antigen binds directly to proximal tubule cells causing cell sensitisation

    D   Circulating immune complexes deposit in the tissues

    E   Damage to the tissues is caused by activated T cells

7. A 30-year-old woman sustained a leg injury while gardening and was admitted to hospital. Dirt and soil in the wound caused an infection, initiating an acute inflammatory response. Activation of the alternative complement pathway is central to this process.

What is the most likely mechanism of complement activation by this pathway?

    A   Complement attaches to IgE antibody on mast cells

    B   Complement attaches to immune complexes bound to phagocytic cells

    C   Complement coated bacteria bind directly to CD8+ cytotoxic T cells

    D   Complement components in blood are activated by bacteria

    E   T lymphocytes bind to bacterial peptides complexed with MHC class II molecules

Answers

. B Antibody binding to antigens

The inflammatory response is a normal, necessary part of the immune response (**Figure 20.1**). Hypersensitivity reactions occur when an antigenic stimulus cannot be removed (e.g. chronic infection, autoimmune disease). In type II reactions, antibody is formed against antigen on the surface of cells in individual organs (**Table 20.1**). When the antigen is a cell receptor, antibody binding can either initiate or inhibit stimulation by the natural ligand. In Grave's disease autoantibody binds to the thyroid stimulating hormone receptor on the thyroid gland, permanently stimulating the production of thyroxine. Normally this is controlled by feedback regulation when high levels of thyroxine inhibit release of thyroid-stimulating hormone from the pituitary gland, but will have no effect on autoantibody production.

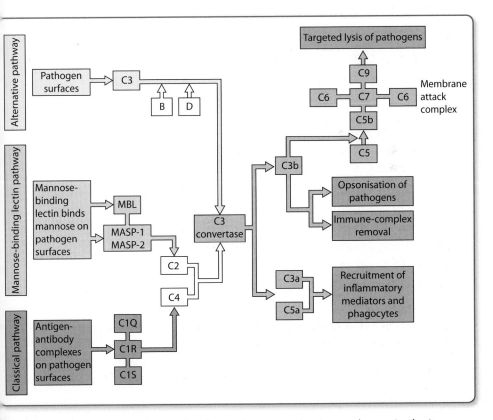

Figure 20.1 An overview of the role of complement activation pathways in the immune response.

Table 20.1	
Hypersensitivity reaction	**Mediated by**
Type I (immediate)	Allergen-specific IgE bound to mast cells is cross-linked by initiating allergen leading to mast cell degranulation
Type II	Antigen-specific IgG or IgM antibody binds to antigen on tissues and organs
Type III	Antigen-specific IgG or IgM antibody forms complexes with circulating antigen which then deposit in a range of tissues
Type IV (delayed)	Three variants: contact, tuberculin, granulomatous mediated by T lymphocytes

Table 20.1 Comparison of the immune mechanisms which lead to the initiation of the four types of hypersensitivity reaction.

2. D Macrophage activation and initiation of the cytokine cascade

Endotoxins are structural components of Gram-negative bacterial cell walls made up of polysaccharides and lipids called bacterial lipopolysaccharides. Their active component, responsible for most toxic effects, is lipid A. Picogram quantities of lipopolysaccharides entering the circulation will rapidly stimulate macrophages (through TLR4 receptors) to release tumour necrosis factor-α. This initiates an inflammatory cascade through release of IL-1, IL-6, platelet activating factor and eicosanoids. Neutrophils activate, aggregate and adhere to endothelial cells. Endotoxins also directly activate coagulation, fibrinolytic and contact dependant pathways. Classical and alternative complement pathways are also activated (**Figure 20.1**). This results in vasodilation, hypotension and poor organ perfusion.

3. A Alloreactive T-cells infiltrate the graft

Major histocompatibility (MHC) molecules on the cell surface have a major role in immune recognition, presenting antigen to either CD8+ T cells (MHC class I) or CD4+ T cells (MHC class II). Most of the rejection response is to these molecules which show wide genetic variability between individuals. Rejection involves different immune effector mechanisms and timing is important in determining which is occurring. Acute rejection occurs in days to weeks and is initiated when donor dendritic cells (passenger leucocytes) migrate out of the transplanted kidney to recipient lymph nodes and stimulate a primary allogeneic response. Activated T-cells return to the kidney where they generate cytotoxic T-cells and induce delayed type hypersensitivity reactions (type IV (**Table 20.1**). Both CD4+ and CD8+ T cells can cause graft rejection.

4. B Anaphylactoid reactions are caused by direct activation of mast cells and are not immune mediated

In type I hypersensitivity reactions, adjacent allergen-specific IgE molecules on mast cells, cross-linked by their specific allergen, activate the mast cell to release its pharmacological mediators (**Table 20.1**). Pollen, house dust mite, animal dander elicit local responses, but food, bee stings, drugs can cause a systemic response (anaphylactic shock) when all the mast cells release their pharmacological mediators at the same time. Anaphylactoid reactions are also caused by systemic release of mast cell mediators but here there is no immune involvement, no sensitisation phase and no IgE production. The agent acts directly on the mast cells or by activating the alternative complement pathway (**Figure 20.1**). Nonsteroidal anti-inflammatory drugs, radio-opaque organic iodines and intravenous anaesthetic induction agents may do this.

5. C Ingest and kill invading bacteria

Phagocytic cells (macrophages and neutrophils) are the main immune mechanism for removal of invading microbes, and act by ingesting and killing them. Toll-like receptors, C-type lectins and 'scavenger receptors' have been identified as pathogen-associated molecular patterns (PAMPs) recognised by phagocytes on microbial surfaces. Intracellular PAMPs such as unmethylated guanosine cytosine (CpG) sequences of bacterial DNA and double-stranded RNA from RNA viruses also act in this way. The organism is phagocytosed into a vacuole which fuses with cytoplasmic granules which release their contents to kill and digest the organism by oxygen-dependent and independent mechanisms. Uptake by the phagocyte is significantly enhanced by coating the organism (opsonisation) with complement, antibody or both (**Figure 20.1**).

6. D Circulating immune complexes deposit in the tissues

Systemic lupus erythematosus is the classic systemic or non-organ-specific autoimmune disease and is characterised by chronic production of large numbers of small immune complexes which overwhelm normal disposal mechanisms (**Table 20.1**). They deposit in the walls of small blood vessels in the renal glomerulus, joints and other organs leading to complement fixation by the classical pathway and migration of inflammatory cells to the site (type III hypersensitivity reaction) (**Figure 20.1**). The consequent tissue damage causes more immune complexes to form and the inflammation induced can cause sufficient damage for the organ to cease functioning and require transplantation.

7. D Complement components in blood are activated by bacteria

Microorganisms activate the alternative complement pathway (**Figure 20.1**). Once activated, C3b binds to the surface of the organism opsonising it for phagocytosis. C3a and C5a act on mast cells to release mediators that affect vascular permeability and also neutrophil chemotactic factors. Their combined effects allow fluid and plasma components including more complement to move to the site of infection. Upregulation of adhesion molecules allows neutrophils (which have a C3b receptor) to adhere to capillary walls (margination), move along a chemotactic gradient to the infection site and phagocytose the C3b coated bacteria which started the process. This is the acute inflammatory response, an important mechanism in innate immunity. Macrophages can also initiate this response independently of mast cells through activation by endotoxin, C5a, and C3b coated bacteria.

Chapter 21

Cellular injury and infection

A 25-year-old man has suffered multiple injuries in a road traffic accident. There are open fractures to both knees. He has a major intra-abdominal injury and there is a clear intracranial injury associated with significant bruising of his neck.

Which of the organs below are made up of cells capable of responding to injury by starting to divide rapidly?

A   Articular cartilage
B   Bowel mucosa
C   Brain
D   Liver
E   Salivary glands

A 28-year-old woman is concerned that her breasts fluctuate in size according to the stage of her menstrual cycle. It is explained to her that this is in response to changes in the hormone levels in her body causing the cells of her breast tissue to proliferate and regress each month.

What is the name given to the process whereby cells proliferate and regress under hormonal influence?

A   Atrophy
B   Apoptosis
C   Avascular necrosis
D   Degeneration
E   Dysplasia

A 35-year-old woman is informed that the result of her cervical smear test shows dysplastic changes of the cervical epithelium.

Which description most accurately describes dysplasia?

A   All different types of cells mixed together
B   Cells showing changes which look malignant
C   Cells which are failing to become fully mature
D   Cells which are looking primitive and not differentiated
E   Cells with lightly coloured large nuclei

4. A 75-year-old man presents with increasing generalised weakness due to neuropathy. A muscle biopsy shows small widely dispersed muscle fibres.

    Which term most accurately describes the findings?

    A   Atrophy of muscle
    B   Fibrous infiltration
    C   Hypoplasia of muscles
    D   Metaplasia
    E   Myopathy

5. A 55-year-old woman has developed the clinical and biochemical features of chronic renal failure. A CT guided renal biopsy shows signs of swelling with clear vacuoles appearing in the cytoplasm. There are also some fatty globules in the cytoplasm.

    Which process is most likely to explain these microscopic changes?

    A   Defence against viral infection
    B   High intracellular potassium levels
    C   Permanent cell damage
    D   Rapid repair and division of cells
    E   Reversible cell injury

6. A 25-year-old man, an intravenous drug user, has died of a fulminating chest infection. At postmortem the lungs look like a piece of cheese when viewed macroscopically. Microscopically they show fragmented pieces of cells enclosed within a clear inflammatory border.

    What is the underlying pathology?

    A   Abscess formation
    B   A carbuncle
    C   Caseous necrosis
    D   Coagulative necrosis
    E   Liquefactive necrosis

7. A 60-year-old man underwent a femoropopliteal bypass using an artificial graft. Postoperatively the wound becomes infected and the graft is found to be infected with *Staphylococcus epidermidis*.

    What special mechanism is this organism using to protect itself from attack?

    A   Ability to produce collagenase
    B   Absorption of plasmids from other resistant bacteria
    C   Developing a glycoprotein biofilm in which it can lie dormant
    D   Lying dormant inside erythrocytes for part of its life cycle
    E   Rapid mutation to give it antibiotic resistance

8. A 35-year-old woman on a surgical ward is found to have a methicillin-resistant *Staphylococcus* urinary tract infection three days after a urinary catheter was inserted. During the following week, swabs taken from wounds on two other

patients on the ward, one with a leg ulcer and the other with a bed sore, are found to culture the same organism with a similar pattern of resistance.

What is the most likely cause of this outbreak?

A   Beds too close together
B   Dirty floors
C   Inadequate hand cleaning by doctors and nurses when moving between patients
D   Inadequate ventilation of the ward
E   Medical outlier patients transferred into surgical beds owing to a shortage of medical beds

Answers

1. D Liver

Liver cells are normally non-dividing. However, when the liver is injured by trauma or by toxins then the cells start dividing to replace those which have been damaged. This is the definition of a quiescent cell.

The cells making up other organs cannot do this. Once the brain has finished growing, then brain cells do not divide further even when the brain is damaged (C). The same applies to the cells which form articular cartilage (A). They are defined as non-dividing. At the other extreme some organs are made up of cells which are dividing continuously throughout the life of the organism. Examples of these are bowel mucosa (B) and salivary glands (E). The cells which make up an organ can therefore be defined by their behaviour into three categories:

- Non-dividing cells
- Quiescent cells
- Continuously dividing cells

2. B Apoptosis

The natural process of cell death which occurs in embryological development and in adult humans under the influence of hormone changes is called apoptosis. Unlike necrosis (C), which is a result of external or pathological agents, there is usually very little inflammation and no other tissues are involved. Apoptosis is a normal not a pathological part of the anatomy and physiology of the human body. Atrophy (A) denotes reduction in the size of cells or decreased function which is not the case here. Similarly, degeneration (D) is not the process here as it signifies change of tissue to a lesser functionally active form. Dysplasia (E) signifies abnormality of development in pathology and is precancerous and so is not the process here.

3. C Cells which are failing to become fully mature

Cells showing rapid division but failing to become fully mature are dysplastic. It is a response by cells to stress. The cells start to divide more rapidly and fail to mature into their fully differentiated state. They have a higher nuclear to cytoplasmic ratio. They also lose the normal architecture of the nucleus. They are not malignant cells, but in some cases, such as the cervix, the dysplastic changes can indicate that malignant change is likely to occur in future. The other possibilities (A, B, D, E) are not the changes occuring here – A shows mixed cellularity, B shows malignancy, D denotes undifferentiated cells and E are just cells with hyperchromatic nuclei.

4. A Atrophy of muscle

The muscle fibres are showing atrophy. The reduction in function is primarily a result of decrease in cell size and reduction in cell numbers but is not primarily a result of cell death. The atrophying organ may not actually decrease in size because the space created is replaced by adipose tissue. There is no fibrous tissue formation and hence B is not a possibility. Hypoplasia (C) is defined as inadequate or underdevelopment and is not happening here. Metaplasia (D) is a response to chronic injury and occurs in glandular epithelium. Myopathy (E) can be of autoimmune inflammatory origin and pathology would show muscle injury.

. E Reversible cell injury

Swelling is a cardinal sign of temporary cell injury. In those injured cells, which normally metabolise actively, this may be accompanied by the accumulation of triglycerides because these cells are not able to metabolise fatty acids properly. In irreversibly damaged cells, there will also be coagulation of proteins and disruption of cell membranes. The nucleus becomes small and dense (pyknotic) and may even start to fragment.

. C Caseous necrosis

The features in the history here point to tuberculosis. *Mycobacterium tuberculosis* which produces a very characteristic necrotic lesion with contents the consistency of cheese. Liquefactive necrosis (E) would be more characteristic of a staphylococcal infection, which produces an abscess. Coagulative necrosis (D) is characteristic of non-infective causes of death such as ischaemia. A carbuncle (B) is a subcutaneous collection of pus so it is not found in the lung.

. C Developing a glycoprotein biofilm in which it can lie dormant

Staphylococcus epidermidis is a normal skin commensal and so it is not normally a pathogen. However, it has an unexpected ability to form a glycoprotein biofilm on the surface of implants which is impervious to antibodies and antibiotics. So long as it remains dormant in the matrix of this biofilm, it can survive in the human and wait for an opportunity to break out. Other pathogenic organisms employ a variety of methods to protect themselves from their host. Many bacteria especially *Escherichia coli* gain resistance to antibiotics by rapidly mutating to new strains which have resistance (E). Some of these bacteria can transfer resistance to antibiotics to other species of bacteria by the direct transfer of naked DNA in plasmids. Again *Escherichia coli* is commonly implicated. Collagenase (A) destroys collagen and is implicated in the rapid spread of *Clostridium* through tissues. Plasmodium spends part of its life cycle within the erythrocyte (D).

. C Inadequate hand cleaning by doctors and nurses when moving between patients

Methicillin-resistant *Staphylococcus aureus* (MRSA) infection is most common in hospitals (nosocomial) and is much more rarely seen in the community. The resistant organisms seem to arise as a result of heavy use of antibiotics and thrive in an environment where a significant number of patients are immunocompromised. However, the spread of infection seems to be directly related to the failure of staff to adhere properly to universal precautions, especially proper hand cleaning between patients. The spread is not usually air-borne, so poor ventilation is not likely to be the cause of this problem (D). Outlying patients may have introduced the infection into the ward but will not have been responsible for its spread (E).

Chapter 22

Wounds and wound healing

A 20-year-old healthy female college student is caught in a bomb blast and sustains an injury to her right leg. There is skin loss with abrasions, and a wood splinter hidden deep beneath a laceration on the outside of her thigh.

What is the most likely cause for the delay in wound healing?

A   Diabetes mellitus
B   Foreign body
C   Malnutrition
D   Site of wound
E   Smoking

A 36-year-old man underwent an emergency conventional open appendicectomy for acute appendicitis and was discharged after 48 hours. He presented to the emergency department 3 days later with a high swinging pyrexia and severe pain in the stitch line. There were signs of inflammation and a yellowish discharge from the wound.

Which of the following is the most appropriate management of this patient?

A   CT scan of the abdomen
B   Open the wound on the ward
C   Re-exploration in operating theatre
D   Start antibiotics
E   Start intravenous fluids and antipyretics

A 45-year-old woman presents with bouts of right upper abdominal pain associated with fatty meals. She is diagnosed as has having multiple gallstones with chronic cholecystitis and undergoes an elective laparoscopic cholecystectomy with a conventional four-port approach.

Which of the following terms best describes the wounds created for the ports?

A   Clean
B   Clean contaminated
C   Contaminated
D   Dirty
E   Dirty infected

4. A 55-year-old man, who is a smoker and an alcoholic, presents to the emergency
    department with acute upper abdominal pain and shock. He is diagnosed as
    having peritonitis with free gas under the dome of diaphragm. He undergoes
    emergency laparotomy with repair of a duodenal ulcer perforation and thorough
    peritoneal lavage. The abdominal fascia is closed with polypropylene but the skin
    is left open due to extensive contamination of the wound during surgery. The
    wound is dressed daily and the skin is closed after 72 hours.

    Which of the following best describes the procedure carried out above?

    A   Primary closure (healing by first intention)
    B   Secondary closure (healing by secondary intention)
    C   Delayed primary closure
    D   Delayed secondary closure
    E   Tertiary closure

5. A 35-year-old man was admitted with a sebaceous cyst on the front of the
    sternum which was excised and the incision was closed primarily. The patient
    presents 6 months later with local itchiness and nodular swelling at the incision
    site. The swelling is firm in consistency and extended into the adjoining skin
    beyond the incision. Intralesional triamcinolone therapy improved the lesion
    symptomatically.

    Which of the following is the most likely diagnosis?

    A   Cylindroma
    B   Fibroma
    C   Hypertrophic scar
    D   Keloid
    E   Recurrent sebaceous cyst

6. A 66-year-old diabetic man sustained an unstable pelvic fracture after a fall from
    height. He was initially treated with several weeks of bed rest. Upon transfer to a
    tertiary care centre, examination of the sacral region revealed a 10 × 12 cm area of
    full thickness skin loss with exposed sacral bone.

    Which of the following stages of pressure bed sore best describes the above
    ulcerated wound?

    A   Stage 1
    B   Stage 2
    C   Stage 3
    D   Stage 4
    E   Stage 5

Answers

. B Foreign body

Wound healing depends on local and systemic factors. Some important local factors which can hinder healing are the presence of a foreign body, blood clot or dead/devitalised tissue in the wound, infection, tissue hypoxia, and vascular compromise, e.g. due to poor blood supply/vascular insufficiency or tight sutures in a wound. The vascularity in the wound may be reduced from previous irradiation or diabetes leading to microangiopathy or atherosclerosis. The presence of any foreign body in the wound leads to the persistence of infection and should be suspected as a cause of delayed healing when other local or systemic factors are absent. Systemic factors include advancing age, insufficiency of vitamins A and/or C, zinc and proteins, systemic malignancy, chemotherapy, radiotherapy, immunosuppressive illness, venous oedema, diabetes, malignancy, uraemia, obesity and peripheral vascular disease.

. B Open the wound on the ward

Signs suggestive of surgical site infection are increasing local pain at the surgical site with signs of inflammation (redness, shiny skin, a discharge, induration of the surrounding tissue and tenderness to palpation). This is usually accompanied by a swinging pyrexia. The most appropriate management is to open the wound and collect any discharge for gram stain, culture and sensitivity. The wound should then be washed out and a non-stick, absorbent dressing applied. Starting antibiotics alone would convert the wound abscess into an antibioma, prolong the illness, postpone local wound healing and increase the risk of septicaemia. Any collection of pus needs to be found and drained. If there had been signs of peritonitis (abdominal distension, bowel ileus, widespread tenderness and rebound tenderness beyond the midline) or an intra-abdominal collection visible on ultrasound or CT scan, then formal exploration in the operating theatre would be more appropriate.

. B Clean contaminated

One classification of wounds is based on the extent or degree of contamination. According to this, there are the following classes of wounds:

- **Class I or clean wound:** This refers to all elective surgical wounds which are uninfected and where the respiratory, gastrointestinal, hepatobiliary or genitourinary systems are not entered. These wounds are closed at the end of the surgery and may involve the use of drains or foreign body like mesh, etc. Operations involving the parotid, thyroid, breast, hernia or vascular system, e.g. varicose vein removal fall into this category.

- **Class II or clean contaminated wound:** This refers to a surgical wound created when the respiratory, gastrointestinal, hepatobiliary or genitourinary systems are entered under controlled conditions and without any significant contamination. Procedures such as cholecystectomy, oral surgery, interval appendicectomy and gynaecological operations fall into this category.
- **Class III or contaminated wound:** Wounds involving significant contamination from the gastrointestinal tract or a major breach in the sterile technique are included in this category. Thus, operations on the colon or rectum with spillage or cases of trauma to the gastrointestinal tract treated early would come under this classification.
- **Class IV or dirty/infected wound:** Contamination of the wound with purulent material from an existing source of infection like perforation of a hollow viscus, severe inflammation like peritonitis, gangrenous appendicitis or acute diverticulitis or old traumatic infected wounds would be classified in this category.

The above classification is valuable in deciding on whether to use antibiotics and for how long. Prophylactic antibiotics are given either as a single dose at induction or three doses over the first 24 hours and are used for Class I and II wounds. Therapeutic antibiotics are given to patients with Class III and IV wounds and may need to be continued for 5 or more days. Class III and Class IV wounds include those with significant contamination or pre-existing bacterial organisms which warrant the use of therapeutic antibiotics for up to 5 days.

4. C Delayed primary closure

Class I and Class II category wounds which have been created in elective surgery, such as those after an incised traumatic wound with little or no contamination, or after elective surgical procedures as described in Question 3, may be closed by primary closure. This leads to primary healing or 'healing by first intention'. It is now a standard practice to irrigate the wound with saline before approximating the skin with sutures or staples. Closure of the subcutaneous tissue separately is no longer thought to be necessary. However, presence of infection at the surgical site or significant contamination of the wound to pus, intestinal contents or faecal matter is best managed by leaving the wound open with daily return to the operating theatre for cleaning and redressing. Once the wound is clean (2–5 days later) it is closed by delayed primary closure. In cases where there is heavy contamination or presence of dead tissue requiring daily debridement or extensive tissue destruction, the wound is allowed to heal by granulation. Such a wound progressively contracts with the maturation of collagen and undergoes epithelialisation from the edges. It closes by the formation of a scar over several weeks or months. Such a form of healing is referred to as secondary healing or 'healing by secondary intention' and produces a scar which is usually wide and thick. It is possible to tell by simple inspection whether the wound has been managed by primary intention or left to heal by secondary intention.

5. D Keloid

All wound heals by scarring and no matter how fine the incision or the type of procedure; a scar is an inevitable result of the process of healing. Excessive healing creates a wider and thicker scarring and is described by some as a hypertrophic scar and by others as keloid. There is a delicate difference between the two conditions which needs to be made if appropriate treatment is to be given.

Hypertrophic scars are usually raised above the skin level but stay within the confines of the original wound and may actually decrease in size over the passage of time. They usually stop growing within 1 year and are more frequently seen when scars cross areas of tension or are located on flexor surfaces crossing the joints. Hypertrophic scars initially appear erythematous and raised and gradually with time become paler and flatter in appearance. Histologically, the scars have collagen bundles that are placed more randomly are flatter with the collagen fibres appearing in a wavy pattern. In contrast to keloid scarring there is no site, racial or sex predilection for their formation. Hypertrophic scars are particularly prone to occur after extensive burns which have healed by scarring. Hypertrophic scars can be prevented by meticulous approximation of skin edges without tension, combined with the use of compression garments and stockings especially in burn patients.

In contrast to hypertrophic scars, keloid scars are almost always raised above the skin level and also tend to invade the normal skin surrounding the initial scar. They continue to grow even after the first year and have a predilection for certain anatomical sites such as the ear lobe, the pre-sternal region, the back and the deltoid region. There is an autosomal dominant trait in inheritance of the tendency to form keloids; both males and females are equally affected. They are commoner in peoples with darker skins. The lesions may vary from small nodules to broad swellings which are occasionally pedunculated, and which may appear firm or hard in consistency on palpation. Histologically, the collagen fibres are larger and thicker than normal. They lack their normal arrangement in bundles and are loosely packed. They are also found to be connected haphazardly and randomly with respect to the epithelial surface. Dark-pigmented skin patients undergoing surgical procedures need careful examination for any previous lesions, and should be warned of the increased risk of keloid formation. The first-line treatment of keloid is non-surgical with the use of intralesional injection of steroids like triamcinolone . This helps in softening the lesion and relieves itching and pain. Radiation, pressure garments and the topical application of silicone sheets may also be useful. Surgery combined with radiotherapy is the last option and is valuable for debulking very large lesions.

6. D Stage 4

Bed sores are pressure sores, defined as skin ulceration accompanied with tissue necrosis as a result of prolonged pressure. These are not uncommon in patients who are debilitated and on prolonged bed rest, immobilised for trauma or due to paraplegia. Elderly and immunocompromised people are particularly vulnerable. A pressure sore passes through the following stages:

Stage 1: non-blanching erythema or redness of the skin in the absence of any breach in the continuity of the overlying skin

Stage 2: partial thickness loss of skin involving the epidermis and dermis

Stage 3: full thickness skin loss with exposed subcutaneous tissue but intact fascia

Stage 4: the same as above but extending into deeper tissues like muscle, tendons, bones or joints

Figure 22.1 illustrates a typical Stage 4 bed sore. **Figure 22.2** shows the various stages in the formation of a bed sore. **Table 22.1** summarises the pathology and management of a bed sore.

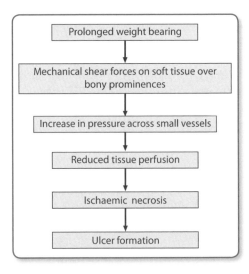

Figure 22.1 Stage 4 type of pressure bed sore with exposed sacral bone and deep muscles. Note the sloping type of edges consistent with healing ulcer. Such a patient needs to be nursed in the lateral position if possible and needs the help of a plastic surgeon to plan an appropriate wound cover.

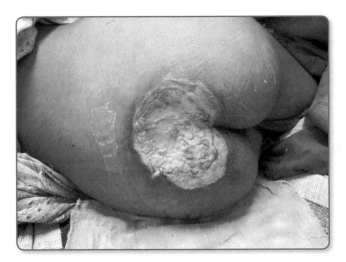

Prolonged weight bearing

Mechanical shear forces on soft tissue over bony prominences

Increase in pressure across small vessels

Reduced tissue perfusion

Ischaemic necrosis

Ulcer formation

Figure 22.2 Stages in the formation of a bed sore.

Table 22.1	
Definition	A chronic wound following tissue necrosis from pressure
Aetiology	Paraplegia
	Peripheral vascular disease
	Unconscious and confused bed-bound patients
Sites	Any bony prominences:
	• Sacrum
	• Ischium
	• Trochanter
	• Heel
Treatment	*Supportive*
	Improve tissue perfusion, oxygenation, correct anaemia and malnutrition, relieve pressure
	Surgery
	Consider only after careful and detailed assessment
	Prevention
	Multidisciplinary approach is necessary

Table 22.1 Summary of pathology and management of bed sore.

Chapter 23

Disorders of growth and differentiation

A 72-year-old man presents with symptoms of bladder outflow obstruction. Ultrasound of the bladder shows a bladder diverticulum.

Which of the following is most likely to have caused the formation of the diverticulum?

A   Apoptosis of prostatic cells
B   Hyperplasia of bladder musculature
C   Hypertrophy of bladder musculature
D   Inflammatory response in bladder neck
E   Regeneration of transitional bladder epithelium

A 55-year-old woman has suffered from chronic renal failure for 10 years and has been on haemodialysis over the same period. During this 10-year period, she has developed renal osteodystrophy from secondary hyperparathyroidism.

Which of the following is most likely to have caused the hyperparathyroidism?

A   Carcinoma of parathyroid glands
B   Combined pattern growth of parathyroid glands
C   Hyperplasia of parathyroid glands
D   Hypertrophy of one parathyroid gland
E   Multiplicative growth of parathyroid glands

A 52-year-old man presents following emergency left hemicolectomy surgery for an annular carcinoma of the upper descending colon. The resected specimen showed huge dilatation and thickening of the bowel proximal to the growth.

Which of the following is most likely to have caused this change in the macroscopic appearance of the proximal large bowel?

A   Hyperplasia of the bowel musculature
B   Hypertrophy of the bowel musculature
C   Inflammatory response from the carcinoma
D   Pseudomalignant epithelial hyperplasia
E   Regeneration of columnar intestinal epithelium

A 45-year-old woman complained of a breast lump. After formal triple assessment, she underwent surgical removal of the lump. Histology showed no malignancy with fibrocystic changes.

Which of the following is most likely to have caused these changes?

    A Apoptosis
    B Breast duct hypertrophy
    C Dystrophic calcification
    D Hyperplasia of breast epithelium
    E Granulomatous mastitis

5.　A 50-year-old man, a heavy smoker, suffers from long-standing gastro-oesophageal reflux disease. Histology of the lower one-third of the oesophagus shows a Barrett oesophagus with an associated mucosal abnormality.

　　Which of the following is the most likely abnormality?

    A Accretionary growth
    B Differentiation
    C Dysplasia
    D Heterotopia
    E Metaplasia

6.　A 30-year-old man recently arrived from North Africa to the UK presents with haematuria. Cystoscopy reveals the presence of bilharzial nodules with papillomas. Histology does not show a carcinoma but does show a mucosal abnormality.

　　Which of the following is the most likely abnormality in the mucosa?

    A Dysplasia
    B Granuloma
    C Metaplasia
    D Multiplicative growth
    E Pseudotubercles

7.　A 65-year-old woman, on medical treatment for ulcerative colitis for 10 years, has been on annual colonoscopic surveillance. This is combined with random colonic biopsies.

　　Which of the following changes is the pathologist looking for in the biopsies?

    A Auxetic growth
    B Dysplasia
    C Hyperplasia
    D Metaplasia
    E Regeneration

8.　A 40-year-old woman sustained a blunt injury to her breast as a result of a road traffic accident where the steering wheel struck her chest wall. Two weeks later presents to a surgeon with a breast lump at the site of the injury.

　　Which of the following is the most likely diagnosis?

    A Apoptosis
    B Caseous necrosis
    C Coagulative necrosis
    D Colliquative necrosis
    E Fat necrosis

Answers

. C Hypertrophy of bladder musculature

In this patient, there is hypertrophy of the urinary bladder musculature causing it to be thickened. The stimulus to this change is mechanical. Because of bladder outflow obstruction, most commonly from an enlarged prostate, there is increased workload on the bladder to empty. The stimulus to enlarge to overcome the obstruction results in increased cellular size without cell replication. The bladder muscle thus hypertrophies. With continued obstruction, the intravesical pressure increases causing trabeculation. When the obstruction is not relieved, it results in sacculation which is herniation of the mucosa through the trabeculated musculature of the bladder. Ultimately sacculation leads to formation of a diverticulum. The commonest site of a diverticulum is next to the ureteric orifice as it is the site of maximum weakness. This common pathological outcome in bladder outflow obstruction can be summarised as:

Bladder outflow obstruction → hypertrophy of bladder musculature → trabeculation → sacculation → diverticulum formation (**Figure 23.1**).

Hypertrophy is produced by certain mechanisms or signals such as growth factor stimulation, neuroendocrine stimulation, calcium channel activity, chemical mediators such as nitric oxide and angiotensin II and angiogenesis.

Apoptosis is programmed cell death, which is not the process that occurs in the prostate; it is benign prostatic hyperplasia. Hypertrophy and not inflammatory response is also a feature that may occur in the bladder neck resulting in bladder outflow obstruction. Chronic inflammation may cause hyperplasia of the transitional epithelium seen as whitish plaques.

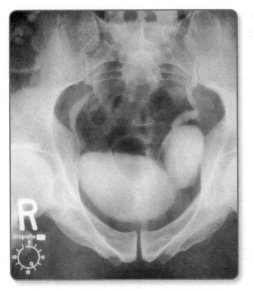

Figure 23.1 Intravenous urogram showing bladder diverticulum.

2. C Hyperplasia of parathyroid glands

This patient has parathyroid hyperplasia where all four parathyroid glands are enlarged. The increase in size of the glands is due to proliferation of the chief cells (specialised parathyroid C-cells) in response to the renal failure, causing low serum calcium and high serum phosphate. This clinical situation is called secondary hyperparathyroidism, where there is an increased demand for function resulting in multiplication of the number of cells, and also resulting in diffuse enlargement of the glands. Rarely, one of the glands may become hyperplastic when it is called an adenoma. Such a clinical scenario is referred to as tertiary hyperparathyroidism. Microscopically the normal glandular adipose tissue is replaced by sheets and trabeculae of hyperplastic chief cells.

The stimulus here is chemical and hormonal and hence the cause of enlarged gland is hyperplasia; when the stimulus is mechanical such as obstruction, the outcome is hypertrophy.

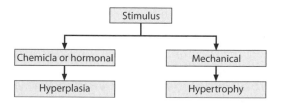

Parathyroid carcinoma (A) shows trabecular pattern with marked mitotic activity and capsular and vascular invasion; it is extremely rare and does not occur in secondary hyperparathyroidism. Combined pattern growth (B), a combination of multiplicative auxetic and accretionary types of growth is seen in embryological development. When a single gland is involved it is always an adenoma, a benign neoplasm. Microscopically there are sheets of neoplastic chief cells. Hypertrophy is not the underlying growth disorder. Multiplicative growth where there is increase in the number of cells by mitosis (E) occurs during embryogenesis.

3. B Hypertrophy of bowel musculature (Figure 23.2)

The growth disorder here is classical hypertrophy of the proximal large bowel. The stimulus here is mechanical, caused by prolonged obstruction from the annular colonic carcinoma. As a result of the functional demand to overcome the obstruction, changes occur to adapt to the pathology in an attempt for the solid faecal matter to negotiate the narrowed lumen. This leads to increased cellular size. In organs made of terminally differentiated cells (e.g. heart, skeletal muscle, intestinal muscle) such adaptive response is accomplished by increase in cell size, i.e hypertrophy.

Hyperplasia (A), an increase in the number of cells, does not occur here. Inflammatory response from the carcinoma (C) does not play a part in this process. Pseudomalignant epithelial hyperplasia (D) is a condition seen in the skin, an example of which is keratoacanthoma and hence is not the process happening here. Regeneration is the renewal of a damaged tissue, which is not the feature here (E).

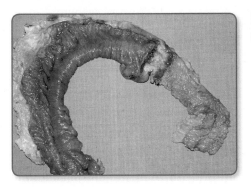

Figure 23.2 Carcinoma of the left colon.

4. D Hyperplasia of breast epithelium

The underlying pathology here is hyperplasia of the breast epithelium, aptly called epithelial hyperplasia (epitheliosis). There is proliferation of epithelial cells which occurs in the interlobular and intralobular ducts and the acini resulting in a mass obliterating the lumina, which is filled by hyperplastic epithelium. Sometimes there is atypical hyperplasia, a sinister finding. Here there is disordered orientation of cells: nuclear pleomorphism with occasional mitotic cells. This is termed atypical ductal or lobular hyperplasia which has a 4 to 5-fold increased risk of developing invasive cancer, a risk that is further enhanced by a strong family history. In fibrocystic disease, there is a combination of cystic dilatation of terminal ducts, increase in fibrous stroma and proliferation of duct epithelium.

Apoptosis (A) which is programmed cell death occurs in normal breasts at the end of a menstrual cycle and is not the cause of the disorder here. Hypertrophy (B) is not the problem here; it occurs in women with abnormally high hormonal levels as seen in functioning ovarian, adrenal or pituitary tumours (C). Dystrophic calcification occurs in tissue already affected by disease. In the breast it may occur in tuberculosis or in a carcinoma when it may show up on mammography. Granulomatous mastitis (E) is a rare inflammatory condition produced by insertion of foreign material such as in breast enhancement.

5. C Dysplasia

The abnormality here is dysplasia, a pre-malignant change occurring in the presence of Barrett's oesophagus. Barrett's oesophagus occurs as a result of metaplasia from long-standing chronic gastro-oesophageal reflux disease. The condition is usually confined to the lower one-third of oesophagus but may extend higher. The squamous epithelium is replaced by a 'specialised epithelium' which consists of a mixture of intestine-like epithelium of well-formed goblet cells, gastric foveolar cells and Paneth cells. In dysplasia this specialised epithelium is altered by variation in size and shape of the cells, nuclear enlargement, irregularity, hyperchromatism, larger nucleus-to-cytoplasm ratio and disorderly arrangement. The dysplasia may be mild, moderate or severe, the latter being considered by some as carcinoma in situ. The risk of cancer in such a situation is 25 times higher than in the general population, which is further enhanced by the increased length of the involved oesophagus.

Accretionary growth (A) is a disorder where there is an increase in intercellular tissue components as occurs in bone and cartilage. Differentiation (B) occurs when the cell develops a different specialised function to its parent cell. Neither of these occurs here. Heterotopia (D) is where mature tissue from one organ is found in another, e.g. gastric mucosa in a Meckel's diverticulum. Metaplasia (E) is a reversible change where there is transformation of one type of differentiated cell into another type of fully differentiated cell. This change is reversible if the cause is removed. If the stimulus continues, it undergoes transformation into dysplasia and then on to cancer, as in this scenario.

6. C Metaplasia

This patient has metaplasia of the bladder from long-standing bilharzial infestation with *Schistosoma haematobium*. Presence of ova in the bladder submucosa results in cystitis glandularis and cystitis cystica. In due course pseudotubercles form, which coalesce to form nodules. In long-standing cases, areas of transitional cell epithelium transform into squamous metaplasia which is also called leucoplakia. This will ultimately give rise to squamous cell carcinoma which is not the usual type of bladder cancer (transitional cell carcinoma) and has a poor prognosis. A similar type of change may occur anywhere in the urinary tract infested with this parasite with an equally sinister outcome.

Dysplasia (A) is not a result of bilharzial infestation. Granulomas (B) may occur from aggregation of nodules. Histologically they are a collection of epithelioid histiocytes; this is a feature of some specific chronic infective or inflammatory conditions. Multiplicative growth (D), which is an increase in cell numbers from mitosis, occurs during embryogenesis. 'Sandy patches' (E) seen in this condition are not mucosal changes but are the result of calcified dead ova with degenerated overlying epithelium.

7. B Dysplasia

In this instance, dysplasia is the change that the pathologist is particularly looking for. Ulcerative colitis is a diffuse mucosal disease with acute and chronic inflammatory cells. Crypt abscesses are a typical feature where aggregates of polymorphs are seen within distended crypts. There is lack of mucin in the epithelium with mucosal atrophy. In long-standing cases, there is epithelial dysplasia which is precancerous. Microscopically, there is alteration in mucosal architecture and epithelial abnormalities showing hypercellularity with variation in the size, shape and staining qualities of the nuclei. High-grade dysplasia will soon result in colorectal cancer which may occur in more than one site (synchronous cancer). Therefore, this is an indication for colectomy. The longer the duration of the disease, the greater is the chance of developing cancer. Hence, all patients with the disease longer than 10 years should be on annual colonoscopic surveillance.

Auxetic growth (A) is an increase in size of individual cells as seen in growing skeletal muscle. Hyperplasia (C) is an increase in the number of cells. Neither of these happens in this situation. Metaplasia (D) is conversion of one differentiated cell type to another and is an after-effect of chronic injury. Regeneration (E) is where cells destroyed by injury or disease/are replaced by identical cells.

3. E Fat necrosis

This woman classically has developed fat necrosis, a condition that can easily be confused with breast carcinoma. The condition results from direct trauma to adipose tissue resulting in extracellular liberation of fat. Here the release of intracellular fat produces a brisk inflammatory response with phagocytosis by polymorphs and macrophages, ultimately leading to fibrosis. This results in a palpable mass in the breast as in this patient.

The condition can also occur in acute pancreatitis due to the release of pancreatic lipase. The lipase acts on the fat cells to split the fat into fatty acids which combine with calcium to form irregular whitish plaques on the pancreas as calcium soap, a process called saponification.

Apoptosis (A) is the phenomenon of programmed cell death. This can occur as a method of physiological growth control which helps in maintaining organ size. Reduced apoptosis causes neoplasia while increased apoptosis results in atrophy. In caseous necrosis (B), the necrotic cells do not retain their cellular outline and lack structure. The debris is greyish-white, soft, friable and resembling cheese, hence the name. This is typical in tuberculosis although may be seen in other conditions. Coagulative necrosis (C) is the most common form of necrosis which follows ischaemia. Here the cells retain their outline as their proteins coagulate ceasing any function. Colliquative necrosis (D) is where the necrotic material becomes softened and liquefied as in the brain. None of these conditions cause the disorder in this patient.

Chapter 24

Neoplasia

1. A 35-year-old woman presents with a lump in the region of her right femoral triangle. This has gradually been growing in size over 2 years. It is neither painful nor tender, 8 cm in diameter, easily mobile and slips under the finger.

   What is the most likely diagnosis?

   A   Aneurysm of femoral artery
   B   Angioma
   C   Lipoma
   D   Lymphoma
   E   Soft tissue sarcoma

2. A 70-year-old man undergoes an anterior resection for rectal cancer. The histology, from a biopsy taken during surgery, is reported as Dukes' stage B cancer.

   Which statement describes the degree of spread?

   A   Confined to the bowel wall
   B   Metastasised to liver
   C   Metastasised to regional lymph nodes
   D   Penetrating mucosa
   E   Spread to perirectal (extra rectal) tissues

3. A 60-year-old man undergoes a total gastrectomy for carcinoma of the stomach. The histology of the surgical specimen shows a well-differentiated carcinoma.

   Which of the following does this pathological feature indicate?

   A   Anaplastic growth
   B   Fibrous infiltration
   C   Increased mitosis
   D   Marked nuclear pleomorphism
   E   Original intestinal type epithelium

4. A 16-year-old boy has recently arrived in the UK for treatment of a Burkitt's lymphoma which is affecting the jaws.

   Which of the following is most likely to have precipitated this condition?

   A   Aromatic amines
   B   Bacteria
   C   Genetically inherited

    D   Ultraviolet radiation

    E   Virus

5. A 60-year-old man, who had a malignant tumour excised some 5 years before, presents with a painful pulsatile lump in the middle of his upper thigh. An X-ray of his femur shows a solitary lytic lesion on the upper shaft of the femur.

    Which of the following is the most likely malignant tumour that was resected 5 years ago?

    A   Colorectal carcinoma

    B   Gastric carcinoma

    C   Prostatic carcinoma

    D   Renal cell carcinoma

    E   Testicular teratoma

6. A 56-year-old man, who has tested positive for AIDS, presents with a slightly painful, non-itchy, reddish-brown ulcerative skin lesion, 4 cm in diameter, on the dorsum of his left foot. This has been gradually increasing in size over 6 months. There is marked swelling of the foot and distal leg.

    What is the most likely diagnosis?

    A   Angiosarcoma

    B   Kaposi's sarcoma

    C   Lymphangiosarcoma

    D   Secondary skin metastasis

    E   Soft tissue sarcoma

7. A 3-year-old boy is brought to the emergency department by his mother, who says that while bathing her son she noticed asymmetry of her child's abdomen, with the right side looking much larger. He also had three episodes of haematuria over the previous 4 months. On examination, there is a mass in the right side of the abdomen and loin. The right iris is absent.

    What is the most likely diagnosis?

    A   Ganglioneuroma

    B   Hepatoblastoma

    C   Neuroblastoma

    D   Rhabdomyosarcoma of the urinary bladder

    E   Wilms' tumour (nephroblastoma)

Answers

1. C Lipoma

This patient has a lipoma on the front of her thigh, a benign tumour arising from the subcutaneous fat. The classical clinical features of the condition are: a slow-growing painless lump, non-tender, mobile and easily slips under the finger referred to as the 'slipping' sign (**Figure 24.1**).

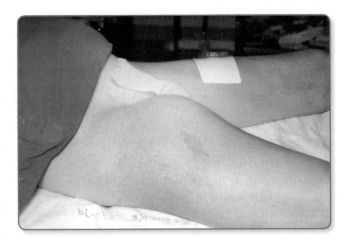

Figure 24.1 A fatty swelling that slips easily under the finger tip: lipoma.

A neoplasm, also called a tumour, is a lesion that results from the autonomous growth of cells which persist after the initiating cause has ceased. According to their biological behaviour, neoplasms are classified as benign and malignant. The latter can be a carcinoma arising from epithelial tissues or sarcoma arising from connective tissues. Any tumour, benign or malignant is named by its cell or tissue of origin with the suffix '-oma'. A benign tumour replicates the parent cell of origin, is slow-growing and remains localised (non-invasive) and well-circumscribed by a surrounding capsule; it never spreads to distant organs (metastasis). Benign tumours cause clinical problems because of cosmesis, pressure on neighbouring structures as in the brain or by producing a hormone as in the thyroid gland.

An aneurysm of the femoral artery (A) will exhibit expansile pulsation. An angioma (B) usually occurs in children, is compressible and containing large, dilated thin-walled blood vessels. A lymphoma (D) is a primary malignant tumour arising from the lymph nodes and may have evidence of the disease elsewhere in the reticuloendothelial system. A soft tissue sarcoma (E) is a rapidly growing, fixed malignant tumour.

2. E Growth spread to perirectal (extra rectal) tissues

Dukes' stage B denotes the spread of cancer to perirectal tissues beyond the rectal wall. In 1932 Cuthbert Dukes (1890–1977), a pathologist from St Mark's Hospital in London, described the post-operative staging of rectal carcinoma in three stages (A to C) according to the spread. In stage A, the cancer is confined to the rectal wall, i.e. involving mucosa, submucosa and muscle; in stage B, the cancer has gone beyond the muscle into the perirectal tissues without lymph node involvement; when there is lymph node metastasis, it is stage C. In some quarters stage C is subdivided into C1 and C2, the latter denoting involvement of the apical lymph node at the origin of the inferior mesenteric artery. Later, a 4th stage (stage D) was added to a growth that had spread to the liver. At the time of resection, 15% belong to stage A, 35% to stage B and the remaining 50% to stage C.

The significance of Dukes' staging is twofold: to decide upon postoperative treatment and to get an idea of the prognosis. Lymph node positive patients (stage C) should be given post-operative chemotherapy. The younger and high-risk patients of stage B should be offered chemotherapy. The approximate 5 year survival figures are: 90% in stage A, 70% in stage B, 30–40% in stage C and 15% in stage D.

3. E Original intestinal type epithelium

When a carcinoma is reported as being well-differentiated, it signifies that the cells have a strong resemblance to the parent structure. Differentiation is a term used to mean the degree to which the tumour histologically resembles its cell of origin; the more the cancer cell is akin to its original cell, the better differentiated the tumour is, and therefore the prognosis is better. Thus, tumors may be graded as well-differentiated (good prognosis), moderately differentiated (intermediate prognosis) and poorly differentiated (bad prognosis).

In the case of the stomach, intestinal type gastric cancers originate from sites of intestinal metaplasia which are typically well-differentiated adenocarcinoma. Biologically, these types of gastric cancers, referred to as early gastric cancer, behave in a more benign manner with a much better prognosis than advanced gastric cancer.

An anaplastic growth (A) is poorly differentiated with cellular atypia. The changes are nuclear pleomorphism (D) (variation in the size and shape of cells and nuclei), enlarged hyperchromatic (darkly stained) nuclei, atypical and abundant mitoses (C) – all histological features accounting for a poor outcome.

4. E Viruses as carcinogen

The carcinogen in Burkitt's lymphoma is a virus discovered in 1964 by Michael Epstein, a pathologist, and Yvonne Barr, a virologist, from Bristol and hence called Epstein–Barr virus (EBV). The tumour is named after Denis Burkitt who first brought attention to this condition in Uganda in 1958. Epstein–Barr virus is a human herpesvirus which is so common all over the world that the vast majority of adults have antibodies to it. Epstein–Barr virus was the first virus to be confirmed as a causal agent for a human malignant tumour. Burkitt's lymphoma is a B-cell tumour in which EBV is within the DNA of the lymphocytes. Normally suppressor T cells keep the B-cell proliferation under control. However, in chronic malaria, there is a lack of T cell response. This results in uncontrolled B-cell proliferation going on to formation of the lymphoma. Nasopharyngeal carcinoma is another tumour caused by EBV.

Bacteria (B) can also produce cancer, e.g. *Helicobacter pylori* can cause gastric cancer and *Aspergillus flavus* produces aflatoxin, the causative agent in hepatocellular carcinoma. The chemical carcinogen β-naphthylamine is an aromatic amine that causes urinary bladder cancer (A). Examples of genetically inherited tumours (C) are retinoblastoma and Wilms' tumour. Ultraviolet light (D) is a physical carcinogen which gives rise to skin malignancies such as basal cell carcinoma, squamous cell carcinoma and malignant melanoma, particularly in fair-skinned people.

D Renal cell carcinoma

The primary tumour would have been a renal cell carcinoma It is also known as Grawitz tumour, hypernephroma or clear cell carcinoma. Renal cell carcinoma most often metastasises via the blood stream to the lungs and bones, particularly long bones. Secondary bone cancer is typically very vascular, hence the pulsatile lump in the thigh. This bone secondary is lytic, and therefore eventually, a pathological fracture will result. If a fracture is imminent then surgical stabilisation with an intramedullary nail should be planned as soon as the vascularity of the tumour has been reduced with arterial embolisation. Histologically, the bone secondary replicates the clear cell cancer of the kidney.

Bone secondaries from colorectal (A) or gastric (B) cancers are extremely rare; if they do occur, vascularity is not a feature and therefore they are not pulsatile. Bone secondaries from prostatic cancer (C) are sclerotic and mostly occur in the axial skeleton – pelvis, vertebrae and ribs. Testicular teratoma (E) is highly unlikely because these tumours occur in the third decade.

B Kaposi's sarcoma

As this patient is known to have AIDS, a vascular, ulcerative skin lesion in a limb is a Kaposi's sarcoma. It was described in 1872 by Moritz Kaposi, a Viennese dermatologist. This is a malignant proliferative tumour arising from vascular endothelial cells. It occurs in immunocompromised patients. The lesion commences as a reddish-brown or purple cutaneous nodule that ulcerates and may be solitary or multiple. Lymphatic obstruction may give rise to swelling of the limb from lymphoedema. Histologically there is granulation tissue with proliferation of vessels with poorly differentiated, spindle-shaped, neoplastic endothelial cells and extravasation of red blood cells and inflammatory cells.

Angiosarcoma and lymphangiosarcoma are highly malignant tumours of blood vessels or lymphatics. They are rare and arise at irradiated sites or chronically oedematous limbs as in postmastectomy patients. Histologically there may be difficulty in separating malignant blood vessel tumours from their lymphatic counterparts because of intimate anastomosis between both sets of vessels. A fibrosarcoma is a tumour of mesenchymal origin arising from fibroblasts which make up the majority of soft tissue sarcomas.

7. E Wilms' tumour (nephroblastoma)

This child has a right Wilms' tumour, the commonest abdominal solid tumour in children. Haematuria, a rare symptom, denotes that the growth has invaded the renal pelvis and is therefore at a locally advanced stage. Both aniridia and hemi-hypertrophy of the body are associated with this condition. An intravenous urogram may show a soft tissue shadow with irregular pelvicalyceal pattern (**Figure 24.2a**). Macroscopically the tumour is a soft solid mass of whitish tissue with cystic cavities, haemorrhage and necrosis (**Figure 24.2b**). Histologically the tumour consists of normal fetal tissue of primitive mesenchyme cells of embryonic nephrogenic blastema. Hence there are highly cellular areas of undifferentiated mesenchymal cells, immature tubules, striated muscle fibres, cartilage and bone.

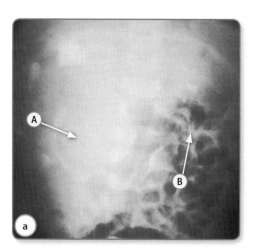
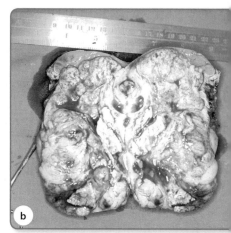

Figure 24.2 (a) Nephrotomography showing: huge soft tissue shadow on the right (A) with normal excretion on the left (B). (b) Cut section of Wilms' tumour.

Ganglioneuroma and neuroblastoma may have similar physical findings; the former arises from retroperitoneal ganglia, the latter from the adrenal medulla. Hepatoblastoma is a rare tumour arising from the liver. It usually attains a large size destroying much of the liver. Rhabdomyosarcoma of the urinary bladder causes urinary frequency, recurrent urinary infection or acute retention. Haematuria is rare as the tumour is sub-epithelial.

Malignant tumours in infancy and childhood are embryonic tumours derived from immature tissues which have undergone malignant change during development. The component cells are poorly differentiated and immature because they retain their embryonic characteristic and not because they have become anaplastic.

Chapter 25

Surgical immunology

A 17-year-old man is admitted to hospital following a road accident. His spleen is removed because it is ruptured.

What role of the spleen will be lost with its removal, that may affect the patient's future health?

A   Deletion of immature autoreactive T cells
B   Major site of insulin producing cells
C   Primary lymphoid organ where immature lymphocytes arise
D   Removal of encapsulated bacteria by phagocytic mechanisms
E   Responds to the pituitary gland to produce thyroxine

A 55-year-old man scheduled for surgery was found to be HIV positive at pre-assessment.

What is the most likely effect of this infection on his immune response to infection?

A   Ability to phagocytose and kill bacteria will be lost
B   Activation of an effective adaptive immune response will be impaired
C   Activation of the alternative complement pathway will be prevented
D   None. HIV infection does not affect the immune response
E   Innate immune defences will be impaired

A 60-year-old man with septicaemia due to an antibiotic resistant infection was admitted to hospital. In septicaemia, uncontrolled activation of inflammatory cytokines can lead to acute respiratory distress syndrome and multiorgan failure.

What are cytokines?

A   Antigen-specific molecules produced by B lymphocytes
B   Part of an enzyme cascade activated by immune complexes
C   Small signalling proteins that regulate immune activation
D   Subtype of cytotoxic T cells
E   Ultracellular enzymes which kill bacteria within phagocytic cells

A 70-year-old woman is admitted for hip replacement. She had suffered for many years from chronic rheumatoid arthritis, an autoimmune disease with progressive joint destruction.

What is the most likely mechanism causing autoimmune disease?

A   Body mounts an immune response against itself

B   Chronic activation of allergen specific IgE sensitised mast cells initiates the disease

C   Deficient immune response due to the action of an external agent

D   Genetic defect causing a deranged immune response

E   T cell activation is inhibited

5. A 21-year-old woman is admitted to hospital for removal of wisdom teeth. Investigations reveal that she has high levels of circulating IgM antibody.

What statement below best describes IgM antibodies?

A   Antibodies that can survive on mucosal surfaces

B   Antibodies which bind to mast cells during allergic reactions

C   Antibodies which can confer protection to newborn infants

D   Long-lived antibodies that provide long-term protection against infection

E   Short-lived antibodies produced during the early stages of ongoing infection

6. A 30-year-old man is going to work in Uganda for 6 months. As a precaution he has a Heaf (six-needle) test, and this gives a positive reaction.

What is the most likely immunological significance of this result?

A   Determines exposure to Lyme disease

B   Determines protective antibody responses to vector-borne infections

C   Determines T cell responses to the tubercle bacillus

D   Measures allergic responses to grass and flower pollens

E   No immunological significance

7. A 70-year-old woman, admitted for a corneal graft, will not require immunosuppressive therapy after surgery because the anterior chamber of the eye is considered to be 'immunologically privileged'.

What is the most likely immunological mechanism involved?

A   Adaptive immune responses do not occur there.

B   All immune cells are destroyed immediately upon arrival

C   Beneficial responses are promoted while damaging ones are suppressed.

D   Immune cells arrive but are prevented from entering

E   Immune cells become functionally inactive on entering the site

Answers

1. D Removal of encapsulated bacteria by phagocytic mechanisms

The spleen is a secondary lymphoid organ composed of red pulp and white pulp and a marginal zone. In white pulp, lymphoid tissue forms a periarteriolar sheath composed of B cell follicles and a T cell area. B cell germinal centres (stimulated follicles) also contain follicular dendritic cells and phagocytic macrophages. Aged platelets and red cells are destroyed in the red pulp. Various antigen-presenting cell types and a distinct subset of long-lived B cells are present in the marginal zone. The spleen filters foreign antigens present in the blood and provides a site where antigen presentation and activation of lymphocytes can take place. It has a unique role in the phagocytic removal of encapsulated bacteria.

2. B Activation of an effective adaptive immune response will be impaired

Human immunodeficiency virus (HIV) selectively targets and kills CD4+ T lymphocytes. Activated CD4+ T cells provide help to CD8+ cytotoxic T cells and B cells in activating an adaptive immune response (see Figure 20.1). Repeated cycles of infection eventually eliminate all the CD4+ T cells and their bone marrow precursors. AIDS is defined by a CD4+ T cell count of less than 200 cells/μL and takes an average of 10 years to develop.

3. C Small signalling proteins that regulate immune activation

Cytokines are small soluble signalling molecules that enable all immune cells to regulate themselves, each other and any cell that expresses the requisite cytokine receptor. Chemokines are a cytokine subset that orchestrates immune cell movement to the optimal anatomical site to carry out their function (see Figure 20.1). Once cytokine activation occurs, a cascade of inflammatory and regulatory cytokines is initiated which serves to self-regulate the system. In septicaemia, the cytokine tumour necrosis factor alpha (TNFα) synergising with other cytokines such as IL-1 and interferon gamma can override these regulatory mechanisms.

4. A Body mounts an immune response against itself

Autoimmune disease occurs when a genetically susceptible individual comes in contact with an environmental trigger. Immune tolerance mechanisms, which prevent recognition of self proteins by the immune system, are bypassed by a number of mechanisms and an autoimmune response occurs. Diseases form a spectrum from organ-specific (e.g. Graves' disease) at one end to non-organ-specific or systemic (e.g. systemic lupus erythematosus) at the other end. Rheumatoid arthritis lies towards the systemic end of the spectrum and damage to the joints is caused by deposition of immune complexes in the joints (type III hypersensitivity reaction) leading to complement activation by the classical pathway and inflammation (see Figure 20.1).

5. E Short-lived antibodies produced during the early stages of ongoing infection

Five classes of antibody are produced by activated B cells (See Figure 20.1) namely IgG (a monomer of the basic structure); IgM (a pentamer of the basic structure); IgA (a dimer of the basic unit); IgE (which circulates bound to mast cells) and IgD (monomeric surface receptor on B cells). IgM is the first antibody produced during the primary immune response. It is short-lived and eventually replaced by IgG. At second and subsequent exposure, the main antibody class produced is IgG which is long-lived and confers long-term protection against subsequent exposure to the same infection. High circulating IgM levels are indicative of an ongoing current infection.

6. C The Heaf test determines T cell responses to tubercle bacillus

Type IV delayed type hypersensitivity reactions come in three variants – contact, tuberculin and granulomatous all mediated by T cells. The heaf test employs the tuberculin reaction and can be used to determine previous exposure to mycobacterium tuberculosis and efficacy of vaccination. On first exposure, either to the natural infection or vaccine, primary sensitisation of the adaptive immune response occurs and memory T cells are formed. On second contact, when small amounts of organism are injected into subcutaneous tissue, memory cells are activated, and CD4+ T helper 1 lymphocytes move to the site of inoculation (see Table 20.1). The response evolves over 24 or 48 hours.

7. C Beneficial responses are promoted while damaging ones are suppressed.

'Privileged sites' were thought to be locations where immune responses did not occur. More extensive tests have revealed that these sites are not immunologically impaired but have differences in their self-regenerative capacity. The eye is poorly regenerative and can be completely destroyed by a pro-inflammatory cell-mediated adaptive response (see Figure 20.1). It therefore promotes beneficial responses while suppressing those that would cause local damage. Anterior chamber epithelial cells express Fas ligand which preferentially leads to destruction of Th1 lymphocytes but allows Th2 responses. Tumour growth factor-β present in the fluid limits T cell proliferation and induces Th2 and T regulatory cells thus inflammatory responses are prevented.

Chapter 26

Surgical microbiology

. A 70-year-old man, who is an insulin-dependent diabetic and a smoker, is due to undergo a below-knee amputation for gangrene of his foot that cannot be re-vascularised. He is not allergic to any antibiotic.

What is the most appropriate antibiotic prophylaxis for this patient?

A   Benzylpenicillin
B   Cefuroxime
C   Erythromycin
D   Tetracycline
E   Vancomycin

. A 50-year-old man with severe acute pancreatitis is in the intensive treatment unit. A contrast-enhanced CT showed pancreatic necrosis.

What is the most appropriate next step in his management?

A   Antibiotic treatment
B   Fine needle aspiration cytology (FNAC) of the pancreatic necrosis
C   Intravenous nutrition
D   Laparotomy
E   Observe with daily ultrasound

. A 15-year-old girl underwent an emergency splenectomy for trauma. She is now at increased risk of infection.

Which one of the following organisms is most likely to be the causative agent?

A   Clostridia
B   Encapsulated bacteria
C   *Klebsiella*
D   *Pseudomonas aeruginosa*
E   *Staphylococcus aureus*

. A 45-year-old man underwent emergency surgery 2 weeks ago for severe soft tissue injury around an open comminuted fracture of his tibia and fibula. An external fixator was applied. He has now developed osteomyelitis of his tibia.

Which of the following is the most likely organism causing his osteomyelitis?

A   *Clostridium tetani*
B   *Escherichia coli*
C   *Pseudomonas aeruginosa*

    D   *Staphylococcus aureus*
    E   *Streptococcus*

5. A 72-year-old man underwent aortobifemoral bypass graft. Following this he spent 2 days in the intensive treatment unit because he had medical complications. The right groin wound became infected on the 8th postoperative day. The swab report came back as methicillin-resistant *Staphylococcus aureus*. He had received the usual antibiotic prophylaxis according to the unit's protocol.

Which of the following is the most appropriate antibiotic to be started?

    A   Aminoglycoside
    B   Carbapenems
    C   Cephalosporins
    D   Glycopeptides
    E   Imidazoles

6. A 75-year-old woman underwent an emergency sigmoid resection and Hartmann procedure for perforated diverticulitis. Postoperatively she is in the intensive treatment unit. On the 2nd day her readings are as follows:
- Temperature: 39.8°C
- Heart rate: 98 beats per minute
- Respiratory rate: 28 breaths per minute
- White cell count: 3×10^9 with immature neutrophils

Which of the following is she most likely to have?

    A   Infection
    B   Multiple organ dysfunction syndrome
    C   Sepsis
    D   Severe sepsis
    E   Systemic inflammatory response syndrome

7. A 45-year-old man, an insulin-dependent diabetic for 20 years, presents as an emergency with painful scrotal oedema, sloughing of a part of scrotal skin and a perianal abscess. A clinical diagnosis of Fournier's gangrene was made.

Which organism is most likely to have caused this condition?

    A   *Clostridium difficile*
    B   *Clostridium perfringens*
    C   Combination of organisms
    D   Gonococci
    E   Tubercle bacillus

8. A 52-year-old man underwent small bowel resection 4 weeks ago for Crohn's disease, this being his fourth resection in as many years. He has been left with only a few feet of small bowel. Therefore, it was felt necessary to give him parenteral nutrition for which he has a right subclavian tunnelled central venous line inserted. For almost a week he has been pyrexial with a temperature ranging from 38°C to 39°C.

What is the most likely cause of his pyrexia?

A Central line catheter
B Deep wound infection
C Pneumonia
D Subphrenic abscess
E Urinary tract infection

Answers

1. A Benzylpenicillin

Benzylpenicillin is the prophylactic antibiotic of choice as this patient has no history of drug allergy. 1.2 g is given intravenously during induction of anaesthetic and every 6 hours for the next 48 hours. This prophylaxis is against *Clostridia perfringens* to avoid gas gangrene. Bactericidal prophylaxis prevents intraoperative microbial contamination. All hospitals have a local policy which is followed except in exceptional cases of drug allergy.

Cefuroxime, a cephalosporin, is used when the patient is allergic to benzylpenicillin. Vancomycin is reserved for methicillin-resistant *Staphylococcus aureus*.

2. B Fine-needle aspiration cytology (FNAC) of the pancreatic necrosis

FNAC should be carried out by the radiologist at the time of contrast-enhanced CT. If cytology confirms that the necrosis is infected, then the appropriate antibiotic is started after culture and sensitivities are obtained. More importantly in case of infected necrosis, the patient should undergo a laparotomy for thorough necrosectomy and lavage of the lesser sac under broad spectrum antibiotic cover. At the same time a feeding jejunostomy is performed. The abdomen is closed by a laparostomy as second-look procedures are not uncommon. If the necrosed tissue is sterile, close observation is continued by repeated ultrasound or CT scan.

In some units, the presence of necrosed tissue in the lesser sac is an indication to start prophylactic antibiotics although this is controversial. Intravenous nutrition is not yet indicated because in the first instance a feeding jejunostomy should be inserted when the patient next requires a laparotomy (**Figure 26.1**).

3. A Encapsulated bacteria

Patients who have undergone splenectomy are in danger of developing septicaemia from encapsulated organisms such as *Streptococcus pneumoniae, Neisseria meningitidis* and *Haemophilus influenzae*. The risk is enhanced in the child, the immunosuppressed, and in those undergoing splenectomy for haematological disorders. Such infections are referred to as opportunist post-splenectomy infection (OPSI). This risk is highest during the first 3 years after splenectomy. In elective splenectomy, patients should have prophylactic vaccination 2 weeks prior to surgery (repeated every 5 to 10 years) against these organisms, or in emergency splenectomy immediately after the operation. Annual influenza vaccination is recommended for all asplenic patients.

After splenectomy antibiotic prophylaxis should be given to all in the first 3 years, and then continued in children up to the age of 16 years and in immunocompromised patients. Prophylaxis should consist of twice daily penicillin in doses of 500 mg for

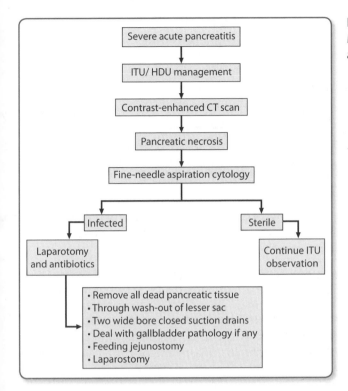

Figure 26.1
Management of severe acute pancreatitis.

adults, 250 mg for and then continued in children up to the age of 16 years and in 125 mg for those below 2 years. Patients allergic to penicillin should be protected by erythromycin or chloramphenicol.

The other organisms in the list do not contribute towards OPSI although *Escherichia coli* may sometimes be the offending organism. On discharge, the splenectomised patient should carry a card containing details of their condition, vaccination status and medication. They should be advised to see a doctor at the slightest suspicion of signs of any infection or starting on an antibiotic until seen by a doctor. The risk of death from OPSI is 600 times greater than in the general population.

4. D *Staphylococcus aureus*

The most likely organism is *Staphylococcus aureus* which is the causative pathogen in more than 90% of patients. In children and neonates rarely *Haemophilus influenzae*, *E. coli* and group B streptococci and in those with sickle-cell disease *Salmonella* may be the causative organism; very rarely gram-negative bacilli such as *Pseudomonas* may be responsible. *Clostridium tetani* which would result in severe constitutional symptoms is almost unknown nowadays.

The cause in this patient is post-traumatic. There are no bone changes in the first 2 weeks. Therefore, an X-ray will only act as a baseline for future reference. Ultrasound-guided fluid aspiration and blood cultures will confirm the organism so that the appropriate antibiotic can be used. Until the causative organism has been isolated and sensitivities established, 'best-guess' intravenous antibiotics are started. Monitoring is carried out by clinical parameters and haematological blood results including inflammatory markers. Prompt recognition and treatment prevents long-term complications of chronic osteomyelitis which may be seen in about 5%. In chronic osteomyelitis, there may be formation of dead bone (sequestrum) surrounded by normal bone (involucrum). The involucrum may have perforations (cloaca) through which parts of sequestrum may exude out as a sinus.

5. D Glycopeptides

This patient has a methicillin-resistant *Staphylococcus aureus*. He should be started on a glycopeptide, such as vancomycin or teicoplanin. Vancomycin is the initial drug of choice, but some strains are developing resistance to it and in that case teicoplanin is the next choice. These drugs act by inhibiting peptidoglycan synthesis in the bacterial cell wall. MRSA is a type of nosocomial infection, a term used to signify infection acquired within the hospital.

The condition is easily transmissible and once acquired can be very difficult to eradicate. Hence prevention is of the utmost importance. Prevention strategies must be in place in all hospitals. They are: meticulous hand-washing, patient screening before high risk major surgery, isolation of infected patients and postponement of elective surgery in carriers. Serum levels need to be carefully monitored as the therapeutic range is narrow and nephrotoxicity and ototoxicity are well described in patients who receive too high a dose. The other group of drugs, particularly the carbapenems, although they have a broad spectrum, are not effective against MRSA.

6. E Systemic inflammatory response syndrome

This patient has the typical parameters of systemic inflammatory response syndrome (SIRS). The term is used to describe the widely disseminated inflammatory reaction that can complicate a range of disorders such as severe acute pancreatitis, major trauma, burns and major emergency surgical procedures. SIRS is a hypermetabolic state where there is an exaggerated and generalised manifestation of a local immune and inflammatory reaction. This massive inflammatory reaction with cell damage, results from systemic release of cytokines such as tumour necrosis factor-alpha (TNF-α), interleukin-1 (IL-1), IL-6 and platelet activating factor.

Several pathophysiological changes occur. These are loss of microvascular integrity, increased vascular permeability, systemic vasodilatation, decreased myocardial contractility and poor oxygen delivery to tissues that suffer from oxygen debt. The condition is associated with organ system dysfunction. In the intensive treatment unit, prompt management consists of controlling the source of infection by surgery or interventional radiology, prevention of tissue hypoxia (this may require ventilation), metabolic support by total parenteral nutrition and prevention of nosocomial infections by appropriate antibiotics. Unsuccessful management will lead to sepsis, then severe sepsis, multiple organ dysfunction syndrome and finally to multiorgan failure and death (**Figure 26.2**).

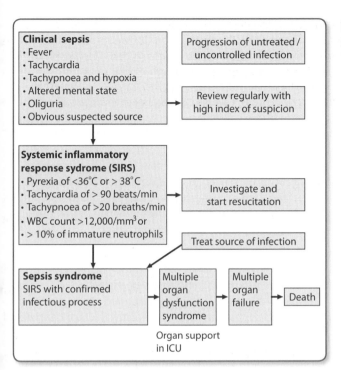

Figure 26.2 Steps in sepsis.

C Combination of various organisms

This condition is caused by a mixed group of organisms which are coliforms, staphylococci, *Bacteroides,* Clostridia and anaerobic streptococci. Gonococci and tubercle bacillus do not play a part. There is synergistic action between these organisms. The underlying pathology is necrotising fasciitis with spreading dermal gangrene. This may develop in devitalised tissues within areas of trauma. It is known to occur after relatively minor trauma. Similar infection in the anterior abdominal wall is called Meleney's synergistic gangrene. Patients, usually immunocompromised, are systemically ill and their pain is very severe, out of proportion to the clinical picture where signs may be minimal. Crepitus may be felt from underlying gas. This may be confirmed by ultrasound or CT scanning.

The key to successful management is early diagnosis, vigorous resuscitation by circulatory support and aggressive intravenous antibiotic therapy combined with radical surgical debridement. Regular review under a general anaesthetic will be needed to ensure that all necrotic tissue is removed. Hyperbaric oxygen, not widely available, may have a role. In the long-term extensive plastic surgery will be required to cover the defects.

8. A Central line catheter

This patient's pyrexia is from central line catheter unless proven otherwise. Central line catheter infection occurs more commonly in lines used for parenteral nutrition The responsible pathogens are skin commensals such as coagulase-negative *Staphylococcus*, *Staphylococcus aureus*, *Candida*, enterococci and *Klebsiella*. Infectio results from initial colonisation of the catheter hub from the hands of the carers; organisms establish themselves in the fibrin sheath of the intravascular part of the catheter thus gaining access to the bloodstream and cardiac valves. Lines with multiple lumens are particularly prone to catheter sepsis. Subclavian lines and peripherally inserted central catheters placed in the antecubital fossa have a low risk of infection. Routine flushing with an anticoagulant and strict catheter handlin protocols and a dedicated nursing team will reduce the incidence of this septic complication which carries a significant mortality and morbidity.

The diagnosis is confirmed by isolating the organism in blood withdrawn from the central line in numbers greater than those isolated from peripheral blood culture. I proven catheter infection, the line is removed and a new one inserted at a different site. If the diagnosis is in doubt, the catheter may be exchanged over a guide wire. The tip of the removed catheter is sent for culture and sensitivity. Once central and peripheral blood cultures have been taken, antibiotic treatment should be started.

The other causes on the list can be excluded on clinical grounds combined with th relevant investigations such as abdominal ultrasound and cultures.

Chapter 27

Surgical haematology

A 35-year-old woman is having preoperative screening before laparoscopic cholecystectomy. She has had four children in the last 10 years, during which time she suffered from heavy periods. For many years she has been on oral iron preparations intermittently. A full blood count shows haemoglobin of 105 g/L, mean cell volume is low, reticulocyte count is normal, red blood cells are pale.

What is the most likely diagnosis?

A   Macrocytic anaemia due to failure of DNA replication
B   Macrocytic anaemia due to iron deficiency
C   Microcytic anaemia due to failure of DNA replication
D   Microcytic anaemia due to iron deficiency
E   Normocytic anaemia due to bone marrow failure

A 74-year-old woman complains of gradually increasing tiredness over the last 6–12 months. She is anaemic, with a haemoglobin level of 105 g/L. Mean red cell volume is above the normal range. The reticulocyte count is around the lower limit of normal.

What is the most likely diagnosis?

A   Macrocytic anaemia due to deficiency of vitamin B_2
B   Macrocytic anaemia due to deficiency of vitamin B_{12}
C   Microcytic anaemia due to deficiency of vitamin B_{12}
D   Normocytic anaemia due to chronic liver failure
E   Normocytic anaemia due to chronic renal failure

A 32-year-old man is being treated by peritoneal dialysis for chronic renal failure. His haemoglobin level is 105 g/L. His mean cell volume is normal and the red cells look normal microscopically.

Which of the following is the most effective management of his anaemia?

A   Erythropoietin to stimulate his bone marrow
B   Oral iron plus vitamin B_{12} to stimulate his bone marrow
C   Oral iron to stimulate his bone marrow
D   Parenteral iron and B_{12} to stimulate his bone marrow
E   Regular transfusions of red cells

4. A 6-year-old girl is awaiting surgery for cyanotic heart disease. Her cyanosis is central. Her haemoglobin is 165 g/L.

    Which of the following is most likely to have caused her polycythaemia?

    A   Decreased circulating erythropoietin
    B   Direct stimulation of her red bone marrow by hypoxia
    C   Direct stimulation of her red bone marrow by a raised carbon dioxide level
    D   Frequent blood transfusions
    E   Increased circulating erythropoietin

5. A 60-year-old man is being managed as an outpatient on a chemotherapy regimen for non-Hodgkin lymphoma. He has developed a painful throat with irregular ulceration on his pharynx.

    Which one of the following is most likely to have caused his throat problem?

    A   Acute depression of bone marrow function
    B   Acute lymphatic leukaemia
    C   Exacerbation of chronic myeloid leukaemia
    D   Throat infection with *Clostridium difficile* organisms
    E   Throat infection with MRSA organisms

6. A 27-year-old man has been brought to hospital unconscious, with many superficial cuts and abrasions. Blood loss from these is much more extensive and persistent than would be expected. His personal details, previous medical history and possible medication are unknown at this stage.

    Which of the following is the most likely cause of this man's excessive bleeding?

    A   He completed, two weeks previously, a course of low molecular weight heparin to prevent deep venous thrombosis
    B   He is on warfarin treatment and his INR is 1.2
    C   He is on warfarin treatment and his INR is 0.8
    D   His factor VIII level is about 20% of the normal average
    E   His platelet count is slightly below the lower limit of the normal range

Answers

. D Microcytic anaemia due to iron deficiency

The history strongly suggests chronic iron deficiency due to increased loss of iron in her heavy periods; blood loss at the time of delivery would add to this. Iron deficiency is the major cause of microcytic anaemia. There is no problem with DNA replication and cell division (A, C), but the cells are small and pale because of inadequate iron content. Normal red cells are in essence cellular bags filled with haemoglobin. In this case the anaemia should be corrected with oral iron before major surgery. A rising reticulocyte count during treatment with iron would confirm increased bone marrow activity and a response to the iron. The more active the bone marrow the greater is the percentage of circulating red cells showing the reticular pattern, which is lost during final maturation in the first day or so in the circulation.

In macrocytic anaemia (B), the cells are large because cell division in the red bone marrow is slowed. In normocytic anaemia (E), the cells are normal but the bone marrow is not able to maintain the required rate of production.

. B Macrocytic anaemia due to deficiency of vitamin B$_{12}$

Deficiency of vitamin B$_{12}$ is a major cause of macrocytic anaemia particularly in elderly women. The B$_{12}$ deficiency slows DNA formation and hence cell division, so too few red cells are produced. Unless there is coexisting iron deficiency, there is plenty of haemoglobin to fill the cells, so they are large, well filled with haemoglobin, and not pale. However, the number of cells is so small that the total haemoglobin level is reduced. Other rapidly multiplying cells which require much DNA replication can be affected too, so there may be a shortage of platelets and white cells, and the tongue epithelium may be affected, becoming painful and red. Production of myelin may also be impaired and this can ultimately impair brain and peripheral nerve function. Adequate replacement of vitamin B$_{12}$ should reverse all these effects.

. A Erythropoietin to stimulate his bone marrow

The anaemia of renal failure is due to failure of the diseased kidneys to produce the hormone erythropoietin. This hormone is normally released by renal tubular cells in response to hypoxia, which in turn is caused by anaemia (anaemic hypoxia) as the red cell count falls. Thus, the erythropoietin level normally rises in anaemia and stimulates the red bone marrow to restore the haemoglobin level to normal. In renal failure the bone marrow can restore the haemoglobin to normal if exogenous erythropoietin is administered (produced pharmaceutically by bacteria with appropriate DNA modification) – or if renal transplantation occurs. In this patient's case, increased amounts of iron and vitamins will not stimulate the bone marrow (B, C, D) and blood transfusion is not appropriate (E). The erythropoietin administered should be adjusted to produce moderate relief of the anaemia, but bringing the level to or above the normal level can produce complications, such as increased risk of thrombosis.

4. E Increased circulating erythropoietin

This girl has central cyanosis, so her arterial oxygen level is seriously reduced (by desaturated blood bypassing the lungs). The hypoxia is detected by renal tubular cells which are genetically programmed to produce increased erythropoietin when they are hypoxic (these cells are metabolically very active, so hypoxia is readily detected). The increased circulating erythropoietin then acts in the usual way on he red bone marrow (more widely distributed in children than in adults) to raise the haemoglobin level above normal (secondary polycythaemia). Hopefully, with relief of her cardiac abnormality, the hypoxia, cyanosis and secondary polycythaemia will be abolished.

The renal cells respond to hypoxia only, not to increased carbon dioxide (C). Abnormal blood gases do not stimulate the red bone marrow (B, C). There is no reason why she would be treated by regular blood transfusions (D). Decreased circulating erythropoietin (A) of course leads to anaemia.

5. A Acute depression of bone marrow function

This man has a painful ulcerated throat. The most likely cause in his case is that some chemical in his body, such as one of his cytotoxic drugs has caused an idiosyncratic reaction which has depressed his bone marrow. This has resulted in aplastic anaemia as a result of reduction in the number of stem cells and early progenitor cells. The throat is the main portal of entry of pathogens. Normally the lymphoid ring around the pharynx (Waldeyer's ring) intercepts such organisms, leading to defence mechanisms such as antibody formation and accumulation of neutrophils. Pus consists of dead neutrophils, slain in the battle with the bacteria. Bone marrow depression can interfere with production of red and white cells and platelets, but deficient neutrophils – neutropenia – is a common presenting feature as in this case

The other options can produce some of the features in this case, but there is nothing in the details given to support the diagnoses, B–E.

6. D His factor VIII level is about 20% of the normal average

Excessive bleeding can be due to a wide range of haematological disorders, but there must be a severe abnormality (as in this case) before problems arise. Thus for Factor VIII values around 90–110% of the average normal would not cause problem As the value for Factor VIII falls below around 75% of the normal average, problems can be expected with major injury or surgery. More serious problems emerge (and with less injury such as tooth extraction) around 50%, and at the severely low level of 20% there is risk of severely increased bleeding. There may also be spontaneous bleeding into brain or joints, when no injury is apparent.

In testing for prothrombin deficiency, INR values around 0.8 to 1.2 (B, C) represent the normal range and should not cause problems. Values of 1.5 and above indicate a risk for surgery – the higher the value, the greater the risk. Above 3–4 there is a seriously increased risk of spontaneous bleeding. Platelet counts just below the lower limit of normal (E) do not usually cause problems; the count would have fallen to around 25% of the lower limit of normal for serious problems. Low molecular weight heparin (A) does not require haematological monitoring as the risks of bleeding are small, and they would be negligible two weeks after the end of a course.

Chapter 28

Surgical biochemistry

A 50-year-old woman requires total parenteral feeding.

Which of the following is the most appropriate management to meet her 24-hour energy requirements?

A   5% dextrose and 10% amino acid solution
B   20% dextrose and 10% lipid
C   5% dextrose as the sole provider of energy
D   50% dextrose as the sole provider of energy
E   20% lipid as the sole provider of energy

A 60-year-old man with a long history of duodenal ulcer has the typical clinical features of gastric outlet obstruction with incessant non-bilious vomiting, visible gastric peristalsis and succussion splash. He has Chvostek's sign (tapping in front of the ear causes spasm of the facial muscles).

Which of the following is most likely to have caused his spasm?

A   Acidotic tetany from respiratory acidosis
B   Acidotic tetany from respiratory alkalosis
C   Alkalotic tetany from metabolic alkalosis
D   Alkalotic tetany from respiratory acidosis
E   Alkalotic tetany from respiratory alkalosis

A 25-year-old woman, who does not look after her type 1 diabetes well, has been brought into the emergency department with diabetic ketoacidosis. She has a high anion gap acidosis.

Which of the following is most likely to have caused the acidosis?

A   A decrease in bicarbonate concentration
B   A decrease in chloride concentration
C   An increase in potassium concentration
D   An increase in sodium concentration
E   Combined increase in sodium and decrease in chloride

A 50-year-old man with cancer of the pyloric antrum is severely malnourished with hypoalbuminaemia due to gastric outlet obstruction. He is to have parenteral feeding prior to radical gastrectomy.

Which of the following is the most effective feeding regimen?

A   Amino acids, derived from animal and vegetable proteins
B   Amino acids including essential amino acids

    C   Dextran

    D   Mixture of dextrose, intralipid and amino acids

    E   Mixture of dextrose, intralipid and dextran

5. A 20-year-old man has been admitted with multiple injuries after his car crashed. Several days after admission, he has to be taken to theatre for debridement of his wounds. A preoperative screen shows that he has developed a dangerously low circulating fibrinogen level.

Which of the following is most likely to have caused this condition?

    A   Congenital hypofibrinogenaemia

    B   Liver damage either pre-existing or due to the crash

    C   Loss of fibrinogen with the blood he lost

    D   Normal clotting to limit blood loss

    E   Widespread activation of clotting in regions of injury

6. A 60-year-old woman is being investigated prior to possible hip replacement for osteoarthritis. She has fairly well-controlled multiple myeloma, although she has increased circulating myeloma proteins. During her assessment she appears very tense, is hyperventilating and then develops carpopedal spasm. However, a plasma calcium measurement taken at this time is normal.

Which of the following is the most likely to have caused her spasms?

    A   Non-specific muscle cramps

    B   Respiratory acidosis combined with hyperproteinaemia

    C   Respiratory acidosis combined with hypoproteinaemia

    D   Respiratory alkalosis combined with hyperproteinaemia

    E   Respiratory alkalosis combined with hypoproteinaemia

Answers

. B 20% dextrose and 10% lipid

As in normal life, this woman requires a blend of carbohydrate and lipid for daily energy. Carbohydrate is required for efficient functioning of the Krebs cycle in the mitochondria. However, lipid has the advantage of a high energy content (around 9 kcal per gram) compared with carbohydrate (and protein) which each delivers around 4 kcal per gram. However, lipid alone (E) cannot be metabolised in the Krebs cycle efficiently and leads to increasing ketoacidosis. A litre of 5% dextrose (C) provides only 200 kcal of energy – just about one-tenth of the daily need. The higher the concentration of dextrose, the more energy it provides but the more irritant it is (hence the need to deliver into a large central vein for dilution). One litre each of 20% dextrose and 10% lipid provides 800 + 900 = 1700 kcal. Together with energy derived from the necessary amino acid infusion, this makes a reasonable contribution to her daily energy needs, and can be adjusted in relation to individual needs. Lipids are also vehicles for delivery of fat-soluble vitamins. Clearly the woman also requires appropriate amounts of minerals and other micronutrients.

Solution A provides inadequate energy, and Solution D is highly irritant.

. C Alkalotic tetany from metabolic alkalosis

This man has alkalotic tetany due to incessant vomiting. The vomiting is non-bilious, consistent with gastric outlet obstruction. Thus, he is losing large amounts of gastric hydrochloric acid. The acid is produced in the parietal cells. These generate hydrogen ions in a process that involves combination of water and carbon dioxide:

$H_2O + CO_2$ combine to form $H^+ + HCO_3^-$

The parietal cells secrete the hydrogen ions (together with chloride ions) into the gastric lumen and the bicarbonate ions pass into the circulation. Normally the hydrogen ions are reabsorbed in the small intestine, but in this case they are lost to the body in the vomit, so the bicarbonate level rapidly soars to give a metabolic alkalosis. An alkalosis, either respiratory or metabolic, alters the properties of the plasma proteins, so that they bind more of the circulating calcium ions, giving rise to a critical reduction in free calcium ions; this causes the tetany.

Acidosis protects against tetany, so A and C are wrong. There is no respiratory alkalosis in this case (D) and a respiratory acidosis cannot cause alkalotic tetany (E).

. A A decrease in bicarbonate concentration

In diabetic ketoacidosis, the deficiency of glucose in cells causes them to rely on excessive lipid metabolism for energy. This generates ketoacids which liberate huge amounts of hydrogen ions. These swamp all the compensatory mechanisms and in the process reduce the bicarbonate level which can fall to half or less of the normal value. The anion gap is a simple calculation of the combined sodium and potassium (ionic) blood levels, minus the combined chloride and bicarbonate levels, all in mmol/L. The normal gap is thus around $(140 + 5) - (105 + 25) = 15$. In severe cases of ketoacidosis the bicarbonate can slump to 10, doubling the gap in this case to 30. Other causes of a high anion gap acidosis are lactic acidosis and salicylate poisoning where the bicarbonate is again depleted by buffering.

Changes in the other ions mentioned in B–E have little effect on the gap in this case.

4. D Mixture of dextrose, intralipid and amino acids

The aim is to improve this man's nutrition, and particularly his albumin level, promptly prior to urgent surgery. He requires a high energy diet to maintain his metabolism and allow some restoration of lost weight, so amino acids alone would be inappropriate (C, D, E). In addition to a blend of carbohydrate and fat to provide energy, he requires an appropriate mix of essential amino acids to build up his circulating and muscle proteins. Essential amino acids are those which the body cannot synthesise. An appropriate mix of amino acids would be similar to those in plasma albumin. Dextran (B) is used to temporarily expand the blood volume but is of no nutritional value.

This man's survival and recovery from major surgery depend on an adequate stress response, which in turns depends on adequate reserves of energy and protein.

5. E Widespread activation of clotting in regions of injury

This young man has developed a low fibrinogen which must be corrected before surgery. The condition is consumptive coagulopathy due to disseminated intravascular coagulation. Extrinsic factors generated by widespread tissue damage initiate the widespread laying down of fibrin clot within blood vessels, depleting body levels of fibrinogen and other clotting factors. This is a relatively rare complication (C, D) and there is no evidence given in the question for options A and B.

6. D Respiratory alkalosis combined with hyperproteinaemia

This woman has two causes for hypocalcaemic tetany rather than non-specific muscle cramps (A) – her hyperventilation and her hyperproteinaemia (myeloma proteins adding to normal plasma proteins – E). Hyperventilation (due to stress) leads to a respiratory alkalosis (B, C). The mechanism of the alkalosis is lowering of the body's carbon dioxide level by increased excretion. This moves the equation below to the right, mopping up hydrogen ions:

$$H^+ + HCO_3^- \text{ combine to form } H_2O + CO_2$$

With body fluids somewhat depleted of hydrogen ions, circulating proteins subtly alter their properties and mop up more free calcium ions in the plasma. We need to bear in mind that biochemistry laboratories measure total plasma calcium whereas it is the free calcium ions that determine whether or not there is tetany. Thus, we would expect her total serum calcium to be normal in alkalotic tetany and the ionized calcium to be low. Furthermore, in a patient with raised plasma proteins, the level of bound calcium ions will also sustain a compensatory rise.

A fall in free calcium ions changes the properties of proteins in excitable tissue membranes so that muscle spasms occur. Thus, her total plasma calcium can be normal while the free ions are seriously reduced and the bound calcium is correspondingly elevated. A 'corrected' calcium level can be calculated by a formula involving plasma protein measurements.

Chapter 29

Central nervous system

A 25-year-old male roofing contractor fell off a ladder onto a concrete floor and hit his temporal region. He was talking coherently as he came into the emergency department but rapidly became unconscious. He is found to have a dilated pupil reacting to light and a Glasgow coma score of 8.

What is the most likely diagnosis?

A   Acute subdural haematoma
B   Brainstem injury
C   Cerebral concussion
D   Extradural haematoma
E   Subarachnoid haemorrhage

A 65-year-old man, a heavy smoker, is being treated with radiotherapy for an inoperable bronchogenic carcinoma. He has attended with an intense headache for 1 week which is associated with vomiting and loss of visual acuity.

What is the most likely diagnosis?

A   Acoustic neuroma arising from the 8th cranial nerve
B   Cerebral metastasis
C   Medulloblastoma
D   Meningioma
E   Pituitary adenoma

A 57-year-old man is admitted complaining of a sudden onset of intense occipital headache, which he describes as a 'hammer blow' to the back of his head. As he is giving this history he lapses into unconsciousness.

What is the most likely diagnosis?

A   Acute subdural haematoma
B   Bleeding into a meningioma
C   Extradural haemorrhage
D   Ruptured berry aneurysm causing subarachnoid haemorrhage
E   Transient ischaemic attack from internal carotid artery stenosis

A 45-year-old man presents complaining of a 6-week history of a throbbing headache with vomiting every morning when he wakes. Recently he has noticed that he has lost lateral vision on both sides and his vision is blurred.

What is the most likely diagnosis?

    A   Bilateral optic neuritis
    B   Glioma in the frontal lobe
    C   Haemangioblastoma of cerebellum
    D   Migraine
    E   Pituitary adenoma

5. A 75-year-old woman on the medical ward has cognitive impairment with episodes when she is sleepy. Her medication includes dipyridamole and warfarin. One week ago she accidentally fell out of bed, striking her head. At no time after this has her Glasgow coma score fallen below 14.

What is the most likely diagnosis?

    A   Acute subdural haematoma
    B   Cerebral infarction
    C   Chronic subdural haematoma
    D   Dementia
    E   Reversible intermittent neurological deficit from carotid artery stenosis

Answers

1. D Extradural haematoma

This patient has extradural haematoma. Having had a head injury he has had a lucid interval followed by a deteriorating Glasgow coma score and a dilated pupil. This classical pattern is only seen in one-third of the patients with this condition. Extradural haematoma is caused by rupture of the middle meningeal artery where it lies under the squamous part of the temporal bone, the thinnest part of the skull. As the haematoma enlarges in the confined space of the cranium, features of raised intracranial pressure develop. The enlarging haematoma displaces the medial part of the temporal lobe against the midbrain which is displaced downward through the tentorial opening. This transtentorial herniation pushes the uncus against the 3rd cranial nerve which is compressed by the sharp edge of the tentorium causing pupillary dilatation.

Before this event occurs a protective response, called the Cushing reflex, sets in to improve cerebral circulation and oxygenation. The heart rate slows to increase ventricular filling. This, combined with enhanced myocardial contraction, leads to a rise in systolic pressure. If the bleeding continues the dilated pupil becomes fixed (unresponsive to light) and irreversible brain damage occurs once the haematoma has reached 50–60 mL.

2. B Cerebral metastasis

Metastatic tumours are the most common intracranial neoplasms. They spread to the brain by the bloodstream. In order of frequency, the tumours most likely to spread to the brain are: lung, breast, melanoma, kidney and colon. Overall 25% of cancer sufferers will develop cerebral secondaries. In almost 15% of cerebral secondaries, the primary remains undetected.

In contrast to a glioma, a metastasis has a discrete appearance, round in shape with a surrounding halo of oedema. It is the pressure effects of the oedema that can be palliated by steroids.

If you exclude metastases, gliomas account for 60% of primary brain tumours and meningiomas for a further 20%. The rest are made up of pituitary tumours, acoustic neuromas and a miscellaneous group including ependymomas. Clinically intracranial tumours present with features of raised intracranial pressure – early morning headache associated with nausea and vomiting and visual disturbances due to papilloedema. Primary tumours will exhibit focal neurological deficits depending upon the anatomical site of origin or as an emergency with seizures.

3. D Ruptured berry aneurysm causing subarachnoid haemorrhage

Berry (saccular) aneurysms are responsible for 75% of subarachnoid haemorrhages. They appear to occur during development as a result of a defect in the circular muscle layer at the bifurcation of an artery, and this is where 90% are found. The turbulence of blood flow at this point causes fragmentation of the internal elastic membrane. This leads to expansion of an aneurysm shaped like a berry, which is covered only in adventitia.

They occur with equal incidence at the junction of the anterior cerebral and anterior communicating arteries, the internal carotid complex (internal carotid–anterior communicating–anterior cerebral) and the trifurcation of the middle cerebral artery; in 20% they are multiple. Silent aneurysms are seen in 25% of people over the age of 55. Aneurysms in the region of the basilar artery account for 5% of cerebral aneurysms. The commonest presentation is subarachnoid haemorrhage as an emergency. This may be preceded by severe cervical and occipital headaches.

4. E Pituitary adenoma

This patient has all the clinical features of raised intracranial pressure. In addition he has bitemporal haemianopia, caused by pressure from the tumour on the optic chiasma. This is the characteristic presentation of a pituitary tumour, but in the case of large tumours the 3rd, 4th and 6th cranial nerves may also be involved. Some tumours may produce endocrine dysfunction, and rarely a pituitary tumour may be a part of multiple endocrine neoplasia type 1 (MEN-1 syndrome or Wermer's syndrome). This is a hereditary condition where there is pituitary adenoma, parathyroid adenoma, pancreaticoduodenal endocrine tumours.

Pituitary adenomas can be classified into three types: acidophil adenomas produce excessive quantities of growth hormone; basophil adenomas overproduce adrenocorticotrophic hormone. Chromophobe adenomas have no endocrine properties. Tumours under 10 mm are called microadenomas. They are only symptomatic if they produce a hormone; tumours over 10 mm are called macroadenomas. They can produce symptoms from pressure effects and from hormone overproduction.

5. C Chronic subdural haematoma

This patient has chronic subdural haematoma, a condition most common in the elderly. There is a typical history of minor head injury in the recent or distant past. Those on anticoagulants and antiplatelet drugs are particularly prone to bleeding after minor trauma. The cerebral hemispheres float in the cerebrospinal fluid being loosely fixed by blood vessels and cranial nerves. When the cerebral hemispheres strike the inside of the skull, the force of displacement causes the dura to move with the skull and the arachnoid to move with the cerebrum. This shearing effect causes the bridging and cortical veins in the subdural space to rupture and the haematoma to spread in the subdural space and hence is frequently bilateral.

Clinical features are variable: headaches, focal signs, seizures and cognitive impairment. A CT scan shows a hyperdense lesion which is diffuse and concave in appearance. The treatment is surgical evacuation.

Chapter 30

Cardiovascular system

1. A 70-year-old man, a heavy smoker, complains of cramp-like pain in both his calves after walking 400 metres when he has to stop. He can continue for a similar distance after a 10 minute rest.

   What is the most likely diagnosis?

   A   Bilateral varicose veins
   B   Intermittent claudication
   C   Morton's metatarsalgia
   D   Osteoarthritis of both knees
   E   Prolapsed intervertebral disc

2. A 35-year-old woman presents to her general practitioner with headaches and general feelings of tiredness and lethargy. The general practitioner did not find anything untoward except for a blood pressure of 140/90 mmHg. The general practitioner heard a systolic bruit over the renal area.

   What is the most likely diagnosis?

   A   Malignant hypertension
   B   Nephrotic syndrome
   C   Pheochromocytoma
   D   Renal artery stenosis
   E   Renal cell carcinoma

3. A 33-year-old man returns home to the UK after a 6-week trekking holiday in the Amazon rainforests in Brazil. Twenty-four hours later he develops gross swelling of his entire left lower limb from the groin distally; and the limb felt heavy and painful. He has a temperature of 38°C.

   What is the most likely diagnosis?

   A   Deep vein thrombosis
   B   Femoral artery embolism
   C   Filariasis
   D   Lymphangitis
   E   Acute thrombophlebitis

4. A 65-year-old man presents to his general practitioner complaining of throbbing lower backache for a fortnight, which has kept him awake at night. The general practitioner could find no abnormality in his musculoskeletal system, but felt a pulsating mass in his epigastrium and a blood pressure of 160/90 mmHg.

What is the most likely diagnosis?

A   Abdominal aortic aneurysm (AAA)
B   Dissecting abdominal aortic aneurysm
C   Leaking abdominal aortic aneurysm
D   Carcinoma of stomach
E   Horseshoe kidney

5. A 50-year-old man is admitted with increasing recurrent angina and severe
    dyspnoea. Six months ago, he had a fairly severe myocardial infarct of the left
    anterior descending and circumflex arteries. His present ECG shows persistent ST
    segment elevation and abnormal Q waves.

    What is the most likely diagnosis?

    A   Cor pulmonale
    B   Dressler's syndrome
    C   Ischaemic cardiomyopathy
    D   Myocardial rupture
    E   Left ventricular aneurysm

nswers

B Intermittent claudication

This patient has intermittent claudication which is the result of atherosclerosis. The condition affects the aorta and medium-sized arteries and develops slowly over several decades. Risk factors are male sex, obesity, increasing age, family history, hypertension, diabetes, increased C-reactive protein, smoking and the use of the contraceptive pill; environmental and genetic factors also play a part. An increased level of low-density lipoprotein cholesterol and a decreased level of high-density lipoprotein predisposes to atheroma formation. Infection with *Chlamydia pneumonia* has been incriminated as a cause of atherosclerosis.

The typical lesion in atherosclerosis is a fibroinflammatory lipid plaque which progressively enlarges to obstruct the vessel lumen. The plaques grow into and involve the tunica media. In coronary and cerebral arteries, the plaque is eccentric so that it obstructs only a part of the lumen. Over the following years complications arise. These include thrombus formation, plaque rupture and stenosis (frequently a problem in the carotids). Aneurysmal dilatation can also occur, especially in the aorta (**Figure 30.1**).

Arteriosclerosis is a condition that affects the smaller arteries and arterioles as a result of the ageing process. There is increase in the thickness of the arterial wall due to smooth muscle hypertrophy with extra layers of collagen giving an 'onion-skin' appearance. The condition results in mild chronic hypertension.

If symptoms merit intervention, the optimal investigation is a digital subtraction angiogram. This will accurately define the site and extent of the obstruction.

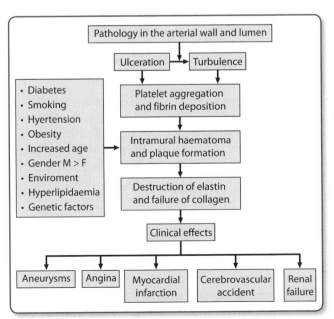

Figure 30.1 Pathogenesis of atherosclerosis, the process of chronic inflammation mediated by monocytes and macrophages.

2. D Renal artery stenosis

This patient has renal artery stenosis causing renovascular hypertension. The commonest cause is atherosclerosis, but in younger patients, especially women of child bearing age, it may be fibromuscular hyperplasia (dysplasia). This leads to thickening of the walls of medium sized arteries, such as the renal, splanchnic, vertebral and internal carotid. Unlike atherosclerosis, the proximal part of the artery is less involved than the distal part where the tunica media causes stenosis. Macroscopically fibrous and muscular ridges project into the lumen where smooth muscle is replaced by fibrous tissue; intimal hyperplasia may also occur with connective tissue encircling the adventitia. When the condition is due to atherosclerosis, the entire vascular system will be affected with involvement of the origin of the artery from the aorta.

Clinically patients present with hypertension and a systolic bruit over the renal artery. A renal angiogram shows smooth localised narrowing of the artery away from its origin. The treatment is percutaneous transluminal angioplasty, with or without stenting. If left untreated, it may result in deterioration of renal function.

3. A Deep vein thrombosis

Following a long flight from South America to the UK, this man has developed iliofemoral deep vein thrombosis (DVT; sometimes referred to as 'economy class syndrome'). Venous thrombosis results from any condition that predisposes to impaired venous return and stasis. The risk factors for DVT are prolonged immobility (as in this patient), pregnancy, oral contraceptives, long major surgical procedures, malignancy, haematological disorders and multiple traumas. More than 90% occur in deep veins of the legs beginning in the calf. The causative factors are endothelial injury, stasis and a hypercoagulable state. A thrombus in the vein may result in thrombophlebitis in which there is inflammation superimposed on bacterial infection. Here the clot is adherent to the vein wall and is unlikely to get dislodged. In phlebothrombosis, on the other hand, there is no underlying inflammation or infection; the clot can get dislodged and cause pulmonary embolism. The term deep venous thrombosis encompasses both thrombophlebitis and phlebothrombosis. Large venous thrombi that propagate proximally into the iliofemoral veins will be a significant hazard for dislodgement producing fatal pulmonary embolus.

It is believed that only large venous thrombi which extend proximally into the iliofemoral veins are liable to break off and produce a clinically significant pulmonary embolus. The diagnosis can be confirmed by a duplex scan, supplemented if necessary by a venogram. If a significant clot is present the patient should initially be fully heparinised then converted to long-term anticoagulation. In patients where there is a large iliofemoral thrombus, the insertion of an inferior vena caval filter may prevent fatal pulmonary embolism.

4. A Abdominal aortic aneurysm (AAA)

A patient with a pulsating epigastric mass has an AAA until otherwise proven. It should be clinically confirmed that the mass shows expansile pulsation. The throbbing backache is because the aneurysm causes pressure on and erosion of the lumbar vertebral bodies.

The vast majority (95%) of AAAs are infrarenal. The definition of a significant aneurism is a permanent localised dilation of the aorta by more than 50% of normal. They are usually fusiform but can be saccular, and are symptomatic once their diameter exceeds 5–6 cm. Occasionally, they may involve the common iliac arteries. The aneurysm wall is lined by raised, ulcerated, calcified atherosclerotic lesions with the lumen occupied by a mural thrombus. Dislodgement of a part of the mural thrombus may result in distal embolisation. The thrombus may obstruct the origin of the inferior mesenteric artery; however, in the majority this does not cause ischaemic symptoms because of the formation of collateral circulation. Microscopically there is destruction of the arterial wall which is replaced by fibrous tissue. Small islands of normal media may be seen with the plaques extending to variable depths. The adventitia is thickened (**Figure 30.2**). This patient requires an abdominal ultrasound, a CT scan and an operation after thorough assessment.

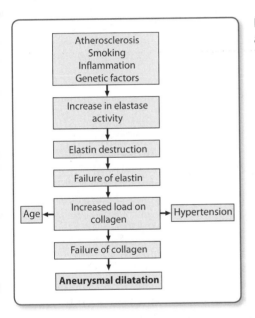

Figure 30.2 Pathogenesis of abdominal aortic aneurysm.

The most common emergency presentation is a retroperitoneal leak of the aneurysm (**Figure 30.3**). This requires immediate resuscitation and operation. However, one-fifth rupture directly into the peritoneal cavity. This event is invariably fatal.

. E Left ventricular aneurysm

This patient has a ventricular aneurysm, a delayed complication of left ventricular transmural myocardial infarct. It occurs in 10–15% of cases. A transmural infarct involves the full thickness of the ventricular wall while a subendocardial infarct involves one-third to one half of the ventricular muscle. After thrombosis of the left circumflex and left anterior descending branches of the left coronary artery, the left ventricular muscle infarcts. The damaged area is later replaced by dense fibrosis, which then becomes solid mature scar tissue. The characteristic ECG changes are of persistent ST elevation. The scar tissue goes on to form an aneurysm which can be true or false.

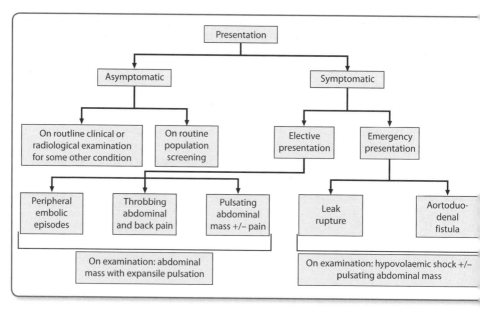

Figure 30.3 Presentation of abdominal aortic aneurysm.

A true aneurysm, much more common, is caused by the weakened and intact left ventricular wall. A false aneurysm results when there is a rupture of a portion of the ventricular wall that is contained externally by adherent pericardium. Thus a true aneurysm is lined with a ventricular wall (**Figure 30.4a**), scar tissue and pericardium while a false aneurysm has only scar tissue and pericardium (**Figure 30.4b**). Confirmation is by an echocardiogram. Treatment is medical with surgical treatment reserved for selected cases. **Figure 30.5** shows the pathogenesis of ventricular aneurysm.

The aneurysm wall consists of a thin layer of necrotic ventricular muscle and collagen. As the aneurysm becomes more fibrotic, it dilates increasing the workload of the heart causing ventricular tachycardia. A mural thrombus develops within the

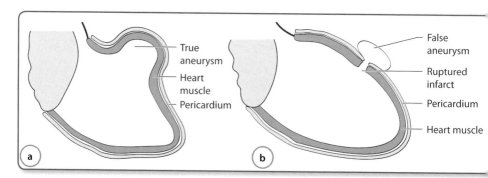

Figure 30.4 (a) Left ventricular true aneurysm. (b) Left ventricular false aneurysm. The true aneurysm contains heart muscle and pericardium. The mouth of a false aneurysm is much narrower than that of a true aneurysm. It is contained only by pericardium, and is therefore more liable to rupture.

aneurysmal sac; a part of the thrombus can get dislodged resulting in a peripheral embolus, yet another complication in a patient recovering from a myocardial infarction (**Figures 30.6** and **30.7**).

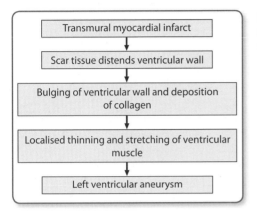

Figure 30.5 Pathophysiology of left ventricular aneurysm, which occurs in 10–15% of myocardial infarctions.

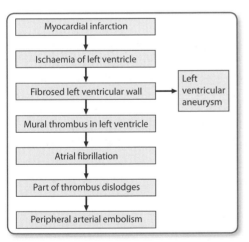

Figure 30.6 Pathogenesis of arterial embolism. An embolus is a mass (e.g. blood clot, foreign body) that is transported by the bloodstream (arterial or venous) and lodges at a site away from its origin.

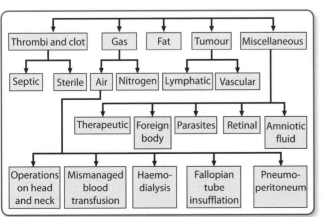

Figure: 30.7 Types of embolus.

Chapter 31

Respiratory system

A 60-year-old man had a right hemicolectomy. On the first postoperative day he has developed a temperature of 39°C, is very short of breath and looks slightly cyanosed; his oxygen saturation is 92%.

What is the most likely diagnosis?

A   Acute respiratory distress syndrome
B   Aspiration pneumonia
C   Atelectasis
D   Lobar pneumonia
E   Pulmonary embolus

A 28-year-old man, 1.93 m (6′4″) tall, presents to the emergency department with sudden chest pain and rapid onset of breathlessness. A short time after admission, his pain improves although he continues to be breathless. Since childhood he has suffered from asthma for which he uses inhalers intermittently.

What is the most likely diagnosis?

A   Boerhaave's syndrome
B   Cardiac tamponade
C   Spontaneous pneumothorax
D   Tension pneumothorax
E   Tracheal rupture

A 55-year-old Caucasian man, who has been a smoker for 40 years, complains of recent haemoptysis. He has had a 'smoker's' cough for as long as he can remember. Recently, he has developed pain in his left shoulder and on examination has a left Horner's syndrome.

What is the most likely diagnosis?

A   Carcinoma of the lung
B   Mesothelioma
C   Pulmonary metastasis
D   Pulmonary tuberculosis
E   Thoracic inlet (outlet) syndrome

A 45-year-old man, a non-smoker, complains of increasing shortness of breath for 5 days. He is orthopnoeic. During this period his neck, face and upper limbs have become swollen. The jugular veins are distended as are the veins on the front of his chest.

What is the most likely diagnosis?

A   Acute respiratory distress syndrome
B   Chronic obstructive pulmonary disease
C   Congestive cardiac failure
D   Superior vena cava syndrome
E   Surgical emphysema

5. A 55-year-old man, a non-smoker, presents with haemoptysis and gradual shortness of breath for 2 months. Over the last 4 months or so he has developed a Cushingoid appearance. A chest X-ray showed a smooth shadow in the right lung with lower lobe collapse. At the age of 25 he had right orchidectomy for a testicular teratoma.

What is the most likely diagnosis?

A   Bronchiectasis
B   Bronchial carcinoid tumour
C   Pulmonary hamartoma
D   Pulmonary secondary
E   Small cell lung carcinoma

Answers

. C Atelectasis

This patient has atelectasis. Examination will reveal poor basal air entry, bronchial breathing and dullness on percussion. Atelectasis is a collapse of lung tissue. This may affect part or all of one lung. The condition prevents normal oxygenation of tissues.

It is seen as a postoperative complication after major abdominal surgery. It results from mucus obstruction of a bronchus, the effect being exacerbated by reduced movement of the chest wall due to splinting of the respiratory muscles from pain. Postoperative atelectasis can be prevented and the risks reduced by: preoperative cessation of smoking for 6 to 8 weeks, physiotherapy and weight reduction, postoperative physiotherapy, adequate analgesia in the form of patient-controlled epidural to help coughing and deep breathing. Patients with fractured ribs, particularly flail chest, are also prone to this condition. The absence of surfactant will also lead to atelectasis. A surfactant is an insoluble lipoprotein consisting of dipalmitoyl lecithin secreted by type 2 cells of the alveoli. This forms a thin layer at the air-fluid interface which reduces surface tension of pulmonary fluids thus contributing to the elastic properties of the lungs. The surface-tension-lowering effect of the surfactant can be improved by increasing the surface area of the alveoli by deep breathing exercises.

Treatment is prompt and vigorous physiotherapy with humidified oxygen. If secondary infection supervenes, appropriate antibiotic treatment is instituted.

. C Spontaneous pneumothorax

This young man has a spontaneous pneumothorax. It usually occurs in tall young men during exercise and in asthmatics. It presents with acute chest pain and shortness of breath. Pneumothorax is defined as air in the pleural cavity. It may be 'spontaneous' or 'tension', the latter being life-threatening. The cause of spontaneous pneumothorax is rupture of a pulmonary bulla produced by a defect in the connective tissue of the alveolar cells. There may also be underlying chronic obstructive pulmonary disease. It presents with shallow painful breathing, as the sensitive parietal pleura rubs on the lung surface. Paradoxically mild cases are more painful while complete collapse causes less pain but more dyspnoea. Small pneumothoraces may be left to resolve spontaneously. Larger ones may be aspirated. But if they reform or are causing respiratory distress a chest drain may be required. If they recur a pleurodesis may be required.

In tension pneumothorax a valvular mechanism causes air to be sucked into the pleural space during inspiration but not expelled by expiration; this causes air to be trapped causing a rise in the intrapleural pressure (which is normally negative). With every breath the positive intrapleural pressure increases with collapse of the lung, shift of the mediastinum to the opposite side and decrease in the venous return with cardiac compromise – an emergency situation that requires immediate intervention. This should be a needle thoracostomy in the 2nd intercostal space in the mid-clavicular line followed by a formal insertion of an intercostal drain in the triangle of safety.

3. A Carcinoma of the lung

This patient, a long-term smoker, with haemoptysis has a primary lung cancer. His symptoms and signs suggest that the cancer is arising from the upper lobe. Horner's syndrome is due to involvement of the cervical sympathetic chain and shoulder. Pain is from infiltration of the upper ribs and the lower cords of the brachial plexus. Involvement of the phrenic nerve can cause paralysis of the ipsilateral dome of the diaphragm (see Figure 4.3); recurrent laryngeal nerve involvement will cause hoarseness of voice. A lung cancer that arises from the upper lobe is called a Pancoast's tumour.

Carcinoma of the lung is the most common cause of cancer death in the world. More than 85% occur in cigarette smokers. There are two main types; non-small cell lung cancer (NSCLC) and small cell lung carcinoma (SCLC) which is also called oat cell carcinoma. The latter makes up 20% of lung cancers, is highly malignant, and is considered by some to be a systemic disease. It metastasises early through the lymphatics and the blood stream but responds well to chemotherapy. They can also produce paraneoplastic syndromes such as diabetes insipidus and ectopic adrenocorticotrophic syndrome. The NSCLC group consists of adenocarcinoma, squamous cell carcinoma and bronchoalveolar carcinoma. Adenocarcinoma is the most common type in women, arises from the peripheral part of the lung as irregular masses, and is associated with pulmonary fibrosis and scarring. Squamous cell carcinoma, most common amongst smokers, is usually hilar in origin and is prone to necrosis and cavitation. Bronchoalveolar carcinoma is a variant of adenocarcinoma.

4. D Superior vena cava syndrome

This patient has superior vena cava syndrome. He is very short of breath with facial and neck swelling brought on by external compression and obstruction of the superior vena cava. As a result, he has distended jugular veins with collateral venous circulation on the chest wall. In advanced cases there may be suffusion, brawny facial oedema of the upper arms, conjunctival oedema, visual disturbances, cyanosis and dysphagia – a symptom complex caused by gross mediastinal lymphadenopathy; in the younger age group this arises from primary malignancy of the lymph nodes such as a lymphoma. In the older age group it is more likely due to secondary metastases from a lung cancer.

In order to make a diagnosis an X-ray and CT of the chest may need to be followed by biopsy (CT guided or excision) of the enlarged lymph nodes. On rare occasions emergency radiotherapy may need to be started before investigation. Histology can then be obtained once the swelling has been reduced. Treatment is radiotherapy and/or chemotherapy. In some instances stenting of the inferior vena cava gives good palliation.

. B Bronchial carcinoid tumour

This patient has bronchial carcinoid tumour. The unusual combination of pulmonary symptoms of haemoptysis and shortness of breath associated with the endocrine disturbance of a Cushingoid appearance gives away the diagnosis. The chest X-ray shows a lung shadow with post-obstructive collapse from obstruction of the bronchus by the tumour. These features are typical of a bronchial carcinoid which account for 2% of primary lung cancers. These are neuroendocrine tumours that arise from neuroendocrine cells of the bronchial epithelium. There are two types: a majority that have no endocrine manifestations and a group that has endocrine features such as Cushing syndrome where the tumour cells produce adrenocorticotrophic hormone.

True carcinoid syndrome is manifested in only 1% of cases when there are liver metastases. This produces an excess of serotonin which leads to the protean manifestations of the syndrome. Confirmation is by finding an excess of urinary 5-hydroxyindoleacetic acid, which is a derivative of 5-hydroxyindoleacetaldehyde.

One-third of the tumours originate in the central bronchus, one-third is peripheral and one-third is in the middle of the lung. The tumour is a fleshy smooth polypoid mass that projects into the bronchus causing haemoptysis and if large enough causes obstruction with distal lobar collapse as in this patient. The 5-year survival after surgery is 60–90% depending upon the histological nature of the tumour.

Chapter 32

Gastrointestinal system

A 65-year-old woman complains of left iliac fossa pain associated with passage of dark red blood per rectum. She is habitually constipated and takes regular laxatives for a satisfactory bowel action. She is overweight and is tender in the left iliac fossa.

What is the most likely diagnosis?

A   Colorectal carcinoma
B   Crohn's disease
C   Diverticular disease
D   Ischaemic colitis
E   Ulcerative colitis

A 70-year-old man complains of waking in the morning and having to rush to the lavatory to have a motion. He then finds that he only passes mucous, blood and watery stool. He has tenesmus and a continuous feeling of insufficient evacuation. Recently he has lost some weight.

What is the most likely diagnosis?

A   Acute fissure-in-ano
B   Fistula-in-ano
C   Prolapse of rectum
D   Rectal carcinoma
E   Thrombosed piles

A 46-year-old man presents with a 6-month history of dyspeptic symptoms despite regular use of pantoprazole. On upper gastrointestinal endoscopy and biopsy and a rapid urease test, he is found to have a *Helicobacter pylori* infection.

Which one of the following conditions is most likely to develop if left untreated?

A   Acute oesophageal ulcer
B   Oesophageal carcinoma
C   Acute gastric ulcer
D   Gastric lymphoma
E   Duodenal adenoma

A 55-year-old man is investigated for persistent gastro-oesophageal reflux disease symptoms. He undergoes an oesophagogastroduodenoscopy. Biopsies taken from his distal oesophagus suggest the presence of intestinal metaplasia.

Which condition is the patient most likely to develop?

    A   Oesophageal adenocarcinoma
    B   Oesophageal squamous cell carcinoma
    C   Oesophageal oat cell carcinoma
    D   Gastric adenocarcinoma
    E   Gastric squamous cell carcinoma

5. A 19-year-old male student is admitted with a 2-day history of right sided abdominal pain and raised inflammatory markers. Following a clinical diagnosis of acute appendicits, he is laparoscoped prior to his proposed appendicectomy. At laparoscopy, a 5 cm segment of the proximal transverse colon appears red, inflamed and thickened.

What is the most likely diagnosis?

    A   Crohn's disease
    B   Diverticulitis
    C   Infective colitis
    D   Ischaemic colitis
    E   Ulcerative colitis

nswers

C Diverticular disease

The diagnosis here is diverticular disease. The symptoms are produced by diverticula, which are small mucosal herniations through the gut wall. They can be congenital or acquired. A congenital diverticulm is one where there is herniation of all the layers of the bowel wall (mucosa, muscle and serosa); an acquired diverticulum is herniation of mucosa covered only by serosa. The term usually refers to acquired diverticula in the sigmoid colon, where faecal contents are solid and high colonic pressures can be found. These are a consequence of a low-fibre diet, constipation, high intraluminal pressure, disordered motility, segmentation and ageing (changes in collagen and elastin). Chronic high-pressure contractions lead to hypertrophy and thickening of the colonic muscle. Diverticula tend to occur at the taenia coli, where arterial vasa recta penetrate the inner muscle layer, the point of maximum weakness.

One-fifth of patients with diverticula are symptomatic – left iliac fossa cramps, bloating, pellet-like stools and the passage of mucus. Rupture of a peridiverticular submucosal blood vessel may result in severe colonic haemorrhage. Inflammation results in acute diverticulitis. Untreated this will progress to a paracolic abscess which may perforate causing purulent peritonitis; perforation of the inflamed diverticula itself results in faecal peritonitis. The inflamed segment of diverticulitis may penetrate into adjacent structures causing a fistula – colo-vesical, colo-vaginal, colo-cutaneous, colo-enetric. Patients with recurrent diverticulitis and subsequent healing end up with scarring, fibrosis and luminal narrowing with resultant stricture formation (see Figures 48.16 and 48.17). Figure 48.18 summarises the various presentations of diverticular disease.

D Rectal carcinoma

The most likely diagnosis is a rectal carcinoma. Colorectal cancers are the second most common cause of cancer death in the United Kingdom; rectal cancers accounting for more than a third of them. The macroscopic types of rectal cancers are ulcerating (see Figure 48.9), polypoid, tubular and annular (see Figure 48.10), the latter two causing stenosing lesions. Polypoid cancers are more common in the right colon where the capacious lumen allows unimpeded growth; left colonic growths are more often annular or tubular. The vast majority are adenocarcinomas. A minority of them secrete mucin and hence are referred to as mucinous adenocarcinoma; they carry a poorer prognosis which is also influenced by the degree of differentiation; the greater the differentiation the better the prognosis.

These cancers extend in a circumferential manner and then outward to penetrate through the rectal wall and into adjacent structures, sometimes resulting in fistulation. They also spread via the lymphatics to regional lymph nodes and by bloodstream to distant organs (34% liver, 22% lung). They are staged according to Dukes' classification (**Table 32.1**) and TNM staging.

Table 32.1

Stage	Description	5-year survival (%)
A	Beneath muscularis propria	90
B	Through muscularis propria	65
C	Spread to regional lymph nodes	35
D	Distant spread	10

Table 32.1 Dukes' classification

Rectal cancers tend to cause local symptoms, particularly early morning spurious diarrhoea. Stenosing cancers however, may present with constipation and symptoms of partial obstruction. Patients may also present with general effects of malignant disease (weight loss, anorexia) and metastatic spread such as a seconda hepatomegaly.

3. D Gastric lymphoma

This patient might develop a gastric lymphoma if left untreated. Gastric mucosa-associated lymphoid tumour (MALToma) occurs in long-standing *Helicobacter pylor* chronic gastritis which provides the immunological stimulus for β cell proliferation There are several causes of gastritis (see Figure 46.5) of which *H. pylori* is one. Gastrointestinal lymphomas account for 10 to 15% of all primary lymphomas; stomach is the commonest site for a gastrointestinal lymphoma, and these make up 3–6% of all gastric malignancies. The tumour takes the form of a diffuse mucosa thickening, not unlike linitis plastica; ulceration may be present. The antrum and th pylorus are most commonly affected.

Diagnosis is confirmed by deep biopsies on oesophagogastroduodenoscopy. Primary gastric lymphoma is different from generalised lymphoma that happens to involve the stomach, the latter situation being more common. In order to be able to distinguish the two conditions, proper staging is carried out by full blood picture, CT scan of the chest and abdomen and bone marrow biopsy. The histology in the vast majority is a diffuse large non-Hodgkin's β-cell tumour. Perforation and haemorrhage are the usual complications, which may sometimes be the initial presenting feature. Lymphatic spread to the regional lymph nodes is late.

The clinical presentation is similar to that of carcinoma, the common symptoms being abdominal pain, anaemia, anorexia, asthenia and weight loss. *H. pylori* is causally associated with gastritis, duodenitis, chronic peptic ulceration (10–20% ris gastric cancer (1–2% lifetime risk), gastric lymphoma and intestinal metaplasia.

4. A Oesophageal adenocarcinoma

The most likely diagnosis is an oesophageal adenocarcinoma. The oesophagus is normally lined by a stratified squamous non-keratinised epithelium up to the gastro-oesophageal junction. Chronic reflux oesophagitis leads to a metaplastic change of the epithelium of the distal oesophagus to a columnar type epithelium, which may be gastric, intestinal or mixed in composition (upward migration of the squamo-columnar junction). This condition is called Barrett's oesophagus and is visible endoscopically because it appears salmon-pink in colour. The length of the affected segment is variable with contiguous or patchy changes. In patients with long-standing Barrett's oesophagus, the columnar epithelium may become dysplastic . There is then a 40-fold increase in the risk of adenocarcinoma developing. This risk is directly proportional to the length of oesophagus involved and the degree of dysplasia.

Histologically the epithelium contains goblet cells with gastric foveolar cells. It shows a villiform architecture and may progress to dysplastic glands with hyperchromatic nuclei. Traditionally dysplastic changes are classified microscopically as negative, indefinite, low-grade or high-grade. In some quarters, high-grade dysplasia is regarded as carcinoma in situ and an indication for oesophageal resection. Once a patient has been diagnosed with dysplasia he should undergo regular endoscopic surveillance with four-quadrant biopsies as follow-up.

. A Crohn's disease

The most likely cause of this appearance is Crohn's disease also called regional enteritis. The condition is a chronic transmural inflammatory disease that can affect any part of the gastrointestinal tract. The ileocaecal region is affected in about 40% of patients, small bowel disease in 30%, while in 20% the disease is confined to the large bowel with the right side more often affected than the left. Only 5% of patients have disease limited to the anal or perianal region.

A characteristic feature of the disease is the patchy distribution of inflammation, with diseased segments interspersed between normal bowel, a situation referred to as 'skip lesions'. Typically, all the layers of the bowel wall are involved giving rise to a strictured lumen. The mesentery is oedematous and thickened with typical fat-wrapping on the bowel surface (see Figure 48.6). Macroscopically the bowel lumen exhibits oedema with shallow, discrete aphthoid ulcers and serpinginous fissures. The intervening mucosa acquires a coarsely textured, cobblestone appearance with pseudopolyps which are isolated islands of bulging normal mucosa. The condition is associated with the following complications (see Figures 48.5a and b).

Microscopically, every layer of the bowel wall is involved. The features are lymphoid aggregates, patchy inflammation, crypt abscesses, ulceration and scattered granulomas. Non-caseating granulomas (see Figure 48.4) so often described as typical of Crohn's disease, are seen in less than 70% of patients. They occur more frequently in younger patients and those with more distal disease. Foreign body giant cells are another important feature.

Chapter 33

Genitourinary system

. A 64-year-old man has had a transurethral resection of the prostate (TURP). Immediately following his surgery, he has stress incontinence which does not resolve with conservative measures. On subsequent cystoscopy his verumontanum cannot be visualised.

Which structure is most likely to have been damaged during this patient's TURP?

A   Internal urethral sphincter
B   Pelvic floor muscles
C   External urethral sphincter
D   Ureteric orifices
E   Penile urethra

. A 66-year-old man attends the urology outpatient clinic with progressive voiding lower urinary tract symptoms (hesitancy, poor flow and incomplete emptying). As part of his clinical examination he has a digital rectal examination, which reveals an enlarged, smooth and non-tender prostate, consistent with benign prostatic hyperplasia.

In which zone of the prostate does benign prostatic hyperplasia largely develop?

A   Peripheral zone
B   Fibromuscular stroma
C   Anterior zone
D   Central zone
E   Transitional zone

. A 65-year-old man presents to his general practitioner with fever, sweats, frequency of micturition, suprapubic pain and dysuria. On further questioning the man has had voiding lower urinary tract symptoms of poor urinary stream, hesitancy, and incomplete emptying for several months.

What is the most likely underlying cause of this patient's urinary tract infection?

A   Benign prostatic hyperplasia
B   Bladder cancer
C   Renal stone
D   Colovesical fistula
E   Ureteric reflux

4. A 73-year-old man presents to the urology department with 2 weeks of visible haematuria. He is investigated with a flexible cystoscopy and CT urogram. The cystoscopy reveals a 1 cm papillary growth on the posterior wall of the bladder. Which is excised.

In the Western world, what is the most likely histological subtype of this bladder tumour?

A Adenocarcinoma
B Melanoma
C Sarcoma
D Squamous cell carcinoma
E Transitional cell carcinoma

5. A 40-year-old man presents with a 3-week history of left testicular swelling. He has no systemic upset and no history of trauma. He does have a history of bilateral orchidopexy when aged 2 years. On examination he has a hard craggy mass arising from his left testicular parenchyma and ultrasound confirms this as a likely testicular tumour. Tumour markers are given in the table.

Tumour marker	Result	Reference range
α-Fetoprotein	4 kU/L	26–kU/L
Human chorionic gonadotrophin	2 IU/L	<9 IU/L
Lactate dehydrogenase	250 U/L	208–460 U/L

What is the most likely diagnosis?

A Leydig cell tumour
B Non-seminomatous germ cell tumour
C Rhabdomyosarcoma
D Seminoma
E Sertoli tumour

6. A 45-year-old woman presents with a first episode of right renal colic and on CT scan is found to have a 3 mm calculus in her distal right ureter with no hydronephrosis. She is comfortable following analgesia, her renal function is normal and there is no sign of infection.

What is the most appropriate treatment option?

A Conservative management
B Cystoscopy
C Open ureterolithotomy
D Percutaneous nephrolithotomy
E Shockwave lithotripsy

A 12-year-old boy attends with a 4-hour history of sudden onset of right testicular pain and nausea. The right testis is high riding and transverse. Testicular torsion is suspected.

What is the most appropriate initial management?

A   Immediate scrotal exploration
B   Observation
C   Scrotal exploration that day
D   Scrotal ultrasound scan
E   Two week course of antibiotics

A 55-year-old man complains of pain in his right loin which has been present for 3 months. This pain occasionally radiates to the ipsilateral groin. This is also associated with haematuria, where the blood is in the form of worm-like clots. He has a firm lump in the right loin which moves with respiration, bimanually palpable and ballotable.

What is the most likely diagnosis?

A   Hydronephrosis
B   Medullary sponge kidney
C   Renal calculus
D   Renal cell carcinoma
E   Renal pelvis carcinoma

Answers

1. C External urethral sphincter

Continence in men is mainly controlled by the external urethral sphincter. The internal sphincter does not add much to the control of urine. During a transurethral resection of the prostate (TURP) the internal sphincter is resected together with the prostatic urethra and the prostate adenoma. The position of the external urethral sphincter is approximately marked by the verumontanum where the ejaculatory ducts enter the prostatic urethra. As such, during a TURP the operator must be aware at all times where the verumontanum is situated in relation to the resection loop. If the verumontanum is damaged the external urethral sphincter may be damaged or resected completely. Pelvic floor muscle training may help some return to continence but if not further evaluation is required and surgery in the form of an artificial urinary sphincter or a male urethral sling may be necessary for cure.

2. E Transitional zone

Benign prostatic hyperplasia develops in the transitional zone of the prostate. This makes possible resection of a benign enlarged prostate transurethrally. However, 75% of prostatic cancer occurs in the peripheral zone where it can easily be palpated by digital rectal exam.

3. A Benign prostatic hyperplasia

Benign prostatic hyperplasia (BPH) causes a range of symptoms in men as they grow old. There are two main classes of symptoms: voiding symptoms (hesitancy, poor flow, abdominal straining and incomplete emptying) and storage symptoms (frequency, nocturia and incontinence). In this case, the patient has voiding symptoms due to bladder outlet obstruction, most likely due to BPH. He will retain urine and have the feeling of incomplete emptying of urine. The urine will stagnate and be prone to urinary tract infection.

4. E Transitional cell carcinoma

90% of bladder tumours in the Western world are transitional cell cancer. Squamous cell cancers are common (75%) where schistosomiasis is endemic (e.g. Egypt), it is caused by the ova of *Schistosoma haematobium*. Squamous cell cancers are also caused by chronic inflammatory states such as long-term catheterisation. Adenocarcinoma is rare; one-third will originate in the urachus. Sarcoma and melanoma both occur very rarely in the bladder.

5. D Seminoma

Non-seminoma germ cell tumour (NSGCT) and seminoma (germ cell tumours) are the most common forms of testicular tumours. The others are rare. Cryptorchidism is a significant risk factor for both. NSGCT are more common in those aged 20–35 years, while seminoma is more common in those aged 35–45 years. Both α-fetoprotein and human chorionic gonadotrophin are more likely to be raised in NSGCT. Lactate dehydrogenase levels are raised in 10–20% of seminomas and can indicate the extent of disease but the test is not specific.

. A Conservative management

In the absence of ureteric obstruction, renal impairment and infection it is safe to adopt a conservative approach to small ureteric calculi, if pain is controlled easily with simple analgesics. Stones <5 mm in size have approximately 90% spontaneous passage rate and this can be improved with the addition of medical expulsion therapy, such as an alpha-blocker (e.g. tamsulosin). This relaxes the distal ureter and aids stone passage as well as reducing analgesic requirements. Stones 5–9 mm in size have an approximate 50% spontaneous passage rate while those greater than 10 mm have <10% spontaneous passage rate.

. A Immediate scrotal exploration

This is a typical history of torsion and the examination findings suggest a 'bell-clapper' deformity, which is the result of a high insertion of the tunica vaginalis and is a risk factor for torsion due to the increased ability for rotation of the testis on its axis. Immediate surgical intervention is important to save the testis and should not be delayed for investigations such as ultrasound. Surgical intervention includes de-torsion and bilateral fixation of the testes to prevent recurrence.

. D Renal cell carcinoma

This 55-year-old man has the typical features of a renal cell carcinoma (hypernephroma, Grawitz tumour), which are the triad of loin pain, haematuria and lump. The blood clots are also the typical shape of those arising from the kidney as they have the shape of the ureter being worm-like. The pain is that of clot colic. Pathologically, the tumours are yellowish in colour, with cystic spaces and haemorrhage separated by septa (see Figure 44.1). Microscopically, it is a clear-cell adenocarcinoma which produces abundant glycogen. The tumour may sometimes grow along the renal vein into the inferior vena cava and then spread to the right atrium. 25% of patients may present with secondaries such as haemoptysis or bone pain in a long bone with a pathological fracture.

Chapter 34

Endocrine system

A 50-year-old man complains of early morning headache associated with occasional projectile vomiting of 2 months duration. Recently, he has noticed that he has double vision and has difficulty seeing objects in the peripheral part of his vision.

What is the most likely diagnosis?

A   Anterior communicating artery aneurysm
B   Cavernous sinus thrombosis
C   Meningioma
D   Optic neuritis
E   Pituitary adenoma

A 70-year-old woman presents with severe explosive diarrhoea with colicky abdominal pain of 3 months duration. She has an enlarged nodular liver, raised jugular venous pressure and features of pulmonary stenosis and tricuspid regurgitation. Eight years ago, she underwent a right hemicolectomy for a tumour arising from the terminal ileum.

What is the most likely diagnosis?

A   Carcinoid syndrome
B   Cor pulmonale
C   Inflammatory bowel disease
D   Irritable bowel syndrome
E   Recurrent small bowel tumour

A 45-year-old woman complains of a central neck lump, present for 8 months, which moves upward with deglutition. Four months later, she developed more lumps on the left side of her neck.

What is the most likely diagnosis?

A   Anaplastic carcinoma of the thyroid
B   Follicular carcinoma of the thyroid
C   Lymphoma of the thyroid
D   Multinodular goitre
E   Papillary carcinoma of the thyroid

A 35-year-old woman complains of episodic attacks of visual disturbances in the form of double and blurred vision associated with sweating, tremor, nausea, palpitations. On a couple of occasions she has lost consciousness. People brought her round by feeding her sugar cubes.

What is the most likely diagnosis?

A   Gastrinoma
B   Glucagonoma
C   Insulinoma
D   Somatostatinoma
E   VIPoma

5. A 35-year-old-woman has put on a considerable amount of weight mostly around her trunk for 4 months. During this period she has been found to be a diabetic with a blood pressure of 160/90 mmHg and noticed hair on her upper lip. She has amenorrhoea.

What is the most likely diagnosis?

A   Conn's syndrome
B   Cushing's syndrome
C   Incidentaloma
D   Phaeochromocytoma
E   Secondary metastasis in the adrenal

6. A 55-year-old man complains of increasing thirst, polyuria, abdominal pain and occasional vomiting for 3 months. He has felt unduly tired with malaise for which he saw his general practitioner. The only abnormality on routine blood tests showed a serum calcium of 3.1 mmol/L.

What is the most likely diagnosis?

A   Diabetes mellitus
B   Disseminated malignant disease
C   Multiple endocrine neoplasia type 1
D   Primary hyperparathyroidism
E   Sarcoidosis

Answers

. E Pituitary adenoma

This patient suffers from a pituitary adenoma. He has symptoms of raised intracranial pressure – early morning headache, projectile vomiting and visual disturbances. The latter symptom specifically is bitemporal hemianopia caused by the space-occupying lesion of the pituitary pressing upon the optic chiasma. Macroadenomas, as they enlarge produce pressure symptoms and may invade the cavernous sinus causing paralysis of the 3rd, 4th and 6th cranial nerves. Microadenomas more often cause endocrine disturbances. This depends upon the hormone secreted: galactorrhoea, amenorrhoea, impotence in a prolactinoma; Cushing's disease in an adrenocorticotrophic hormone producing tumour; acromegaly and gigantism in a growth-hormone secreting tumour. Rarely, pituitary adenomas are a part of multiple endocrine neoplasia syndrome type 1.

They arise from the anterior lobe of the pituitary and macroscopically are of two types: microadenoma when the tumour is less than 1 cm and macroadenoma when larger than 1 cm. They are almost always benign. Microadenomas manifest as endocrine disturbances. Macroadenomas produce pressure symptoms and hormonal disturbances if hormonally active.

Depending upon how the cells stained by haematoxylin and eosin, they were classified as acidophil adenomas associated with overproduction of growth hormone, basophil adenomas producing excess adrenocorticotrophic hormone and chromophobe adenomas which are non-secretory. In 2004, the World Health Organisation classified pituitary adenomas according to the histological, histochemical, immunohistochemical and electron microscopic features. Histologically they comprise of nests and cords of a single cell type. These are in the form of islands supported on a very vascular framework; sometimes there is amyloid deposition and calcification.

2. A Carcinoid syndrome

This patient has carcinoid syndrome. This is due to the effects of excess circulating serotonin (5-hydroxytryptamine). She has an enlarged nodular liver, typical of hepatic secondaries from a carcinoid tumour from the ileum that was removed by right hemicolectomy in the past. Ileal carcinoids are often multiple and more aggressive. These tumours are neuroendocrine tumours that arise from the enterochromaffin cells also called APUD (amine precursor uptake and decarboxylation) cells. They constitute 10% of all small intestine tumours.

Carcinoid syndrome occurs as a result of liver secondaries elaborating the enzyme 5-HT. This occurs in 5% of patients with carcinoid tumours. The classical presentation is explosive diarrhoea (often the most distressing symptom), episodic flushing, bronchospasm and pellagra-like skin lesions of the legs (from niacin deficiency from disturbance in tryptophan metabolism). 5-Hydroxytryptamine is metabolised to

5-hydroxyindoleactaldehyde which is excreted in the urine as 5-hydroxyindoleacetic acid a high level of which in the urine is diagnostic of the condition. The hormone released by the liver has a high concentration in the inferior vena cava and the right side of the heart ultimately causing pulmonary stenosis and tricuspid regurgitation

Macroscopically, the tumour is yellowish-white in colour and arises as a submucous nodule; large tumours may be polypoid or annular with surface ulceration. Microscopically, there are nests, cords and rosettes of small, round cells.

This patient should have the diagnosis confirmed by US and/or CT scan and urinary 5-hydroxyindoleacetic acid. She should be palliated by hepatic artery chemoembolisation.

3. E Papillary carcinoma of the thyroid

This woman has typical papillary carcinoma of the thyroid (PCT), which has a predilection for women in this age group. She has a thyroid nodule with a mass of cervical lymph nodes on the side of the original lesion (**Figure 34.1**). This is the commonest type (seen in 60–70% of all thyroid cancers). The diagnosis is confirmed by fine-needle aspiration cytology. In more than 75% of patients, PCT is multicentric in origin. This feature may represent multifocal origin of the tumour or lymphatic spread within the gland from a solitary tumour. Sometimes the condition may present as a mass of cervical lymphadenopathy without a clinically obvious thyroid lesion. The diagnosis is then made after a biopsy or fine-needle aspiration cytology of the lymph node which shows features of papillary carcinoma. These lesions used to be called 'lateral aberrant thyroid'; now they are referred to as 'incidentalomas'.

Macroscopically, the tumour is yellowish-white, firm and solid with foci of cystic changes and an irregular and infiltrative border. Microscopically branching papillae are lined by neoplastic columnar epithelium with large nuclei with central clear areas giving it a ground glass appearance and hence sometimes termed Orphan Annie-eyed nuclei. Calcospherites (calcified globular body) also called psammoma bodies are diagnostic; there is dense fibrosis. To assess the aggressiveness of the tumour, various scoring systems are available which are used to decide upon the

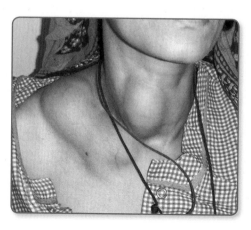

Figure 34.1 Papillary carcinoma of the thyroid.

type of surgical treatment, whether total or hemithyroidectomy. Overall PTC has an excellent prognosis.

4. C Insulinoma

This patient has an insulinoma (β-cell tumour), the commonest pancreatic endocrine tumour. She has the classical clinical symptoms of hypoglycaemia (diplopia and blurred vision) associated with the clinical features of catecholamine release (nausea, tremor, palpitations and sweating); these symptoms may progress to confusion, lethargy and loss of consciousness. This patient's symptoms are referred to as Whipple's triad: the three features are first, typical hypoglycaemic symptoms after fasting or exercise; second, blood glucose levels of <2.8 mmol/L and third, recovery after oral or intravenous glucose. In the vast majority of cases the diagnosis is strongly suspected by the biochemical demonstration of hypoglycaemia with inappropriate and excessive insulin secretion. This tumour occurs sporadically but may be a part of multiple endocrine neoplasia 1 syndrome.

Most insulinomas are solitary and benign; when multiple tumours are present they form a part of multiple endocrine neoplasia 1 syndrome. A small minority are malignant. These tumours are no more than 3 cm in diameter and occasionally smaller and are equally distributed within the gland. Accurate localisation is achieved by endoscopic ultrasound and intraoperative ultrasound. Surgical excision laparoscopically or by laparotomy is the treatment of choice. The tumours are most often well-localised so that they are amenable to enucleation.

Histologically, the tumuor cells resemble normal β-cells seen as nests in trabecular or solid patterns. Tumours larger than 3 cm showing a high mitotic rate and nuclear atypia denote malignancy. Even in these tumours excision should be attempted as they are not as aggressive as the more common adenocarcinoma.

5. B Cushing's syndrome

This woman has the classical features of Cushing's syndrome: recent onset of central obesity, diabetes, hirsutism, pigmentation of skin and menstrual irregularity (**Figure 34.2a**). 85% of cases of this syndrome are ACTH-dependent (adrenocorticotrophic hormone dependent). This sub-group of Cushing's syndrome, caused by excessive secretion of ACTH from a pituitary adenoma are labelled as having Cushing's disease. However, 15% of cases of Cushing's syndrome are actually caused by an adrenocortical adenoma or by ectopic ACTH production, as may occur in paraneoplastic syndrome from a small cell lung cancer. Adrenocortical carcinoma is very rare. In Cushing's disease excessive amount of ACTH is secreted, whereas in Cushing's syndrome the level of ACTH is low.

Diagnosis is made by determining plasma cortisol levels, dexamethasone suppression of 24-hour urinary cortisol excretion and serum ACTH levels. Localisation is by CT scan and MRI of the adrenal glands. Pathologically the adenoma is encapsulated, firm, yellow and lobulated (**Figure 34.2b**) about 5 cm in diameter. The cut surface is yellowish brown with a thin rim of normal compressed gland

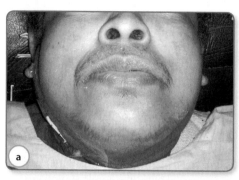

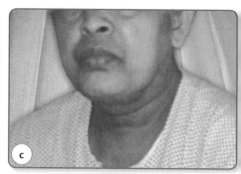

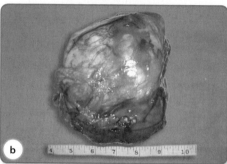

Figure 34.2 Cushing's syndrome. (a) Preoperative appearance. (b) The excised adrenal tumour. (c) The same patient, postoperative.

surrounding it; necrosis and calcification may be present. Microscopically clear, lipid-rich cells are seen arranged in sheets or nests. The distinction between an adenoma and a carcinoma may sometimes be difficult. Large size, multinodularity, heterogenous structure, vascular and capsular invasion are criteria of malignancy. Adrenalectomy is the treatment of choice and gives good results (**Figure 34.2c**). This can be done by the open method or laparoscopically.

6. D Primary hyperparathyroidism

This man has the features of primary hyperparathyroidism, the commonest cause of which is a parathyroid adenoma (80–90%). In a small minority the cause is parathyroid hyperplasia (10–15%) while parathyroid carcinoma as a cause of hypercalcaemia is even rarer (1–5%). Secondary hyperparathyroidism occurs in chronic renal failure, in vitamin D deficiency and intestinal malabsorption; this is due to compensatory parathormone hypersecretion where all the glands are hyperplastic. Rarely, in these situations one of the glands may become an autonomous adenoma, when the condition is called tertiary hyperparathyroidism. In 20% an adenoma may occur as a part of multiple endocrine neoplasia syndrome type 1.

A parathyroid adenoma is a discrete, reddish brown tumour usually no larger than 3 cm in diameter. Haemorrhagic areas are usual while cystic changes are occasional; histologically, sheets of chief cells are seen within a rich capillary network. They have a capsule which distinguishes it from parathyroid hyperplasia.

Chapter 35

Breast disorders

. A 38-year-old woman presents with thick discharge from a single duct in the right breast. Clinical examination of the breast reveals no palpable lump or axillary lymphadenopathy. The nipple and areola are normal.

What is the most appropriate first investigation?

A   Excision of the duct and histopathology
B   Magnetic resonance imaging
C   Mammography
D   Biopsy of the nipple
E   Occult blood test and cytology on nipple discharge

. A 40-year-old woman presents with a 1 cm nodule in the upper outer quadrant of right breast. She undergoes excision biopsy.

Which pathological entity carries the highest risk for development of malignancy?

A   Atypical ductal hyperplasia
B   Duct ectasia
C   Fibroadenoma
D   Florid papillary hyperplasia
E   Sclerosing adenosis

. A 58-year-old woman presents with a 6 cm lump with an ulcer in her left breast with a palpable node in the axilla. Mammography reveals a mass with speculate margins. Core needle biopsy from breast and axilla shows invasive duct carcinoma with metastasis to axilla.

What is the most appropriate treatment?

A   Breast conservation surgery
B   Neoadjuvant chemotherapy
C   Neoadjuvant radiotherapy
D   Modified radical mastectomy
E   Palliative mastectomy

. A 46-year-old woman presents with recurrent episodes of serous discharge from the right breast for 6 months. She noticed a swelling beneath the areola 1 month ago. She recently noted a periareolar discharging sinus. On examination, there is an ill-defined retroareolar mass with a periareolar sinus. Mammography reveals a retroareolar glandular lesion with multiple dilated ducts.

What is the most likely diagnosis?

A   Carcinoma of breast
B   Duct ectasia
C   Paget's disease
D   Ruptured breast cyst
E   Tuberculosis

5. A 34-year-old woman is referred to the breast clinic by her general practitioner. He
paternal aunt had breast cancer. Her father also suffered from breast cancer at the
age of 39 years. Based on the fact that she has had two first-degree relatives with
breast cancer in her family, she appears to be at a higher risk for development of
breast cancer.

What is the most likely gene to be mutated in this family?

A   *APC* gene
B   *BRCA1* gene
C   *BRCA2* gene
D   *CHEK2*
E   *p53* gene

Answers

. E Occult blood test and cytology on nipple discharge

Nipple discharge for occult blood test and cytology is the first line of evaluation. It can exclude carcinoma effectively. Other radiological investigations are indicated if malignancy is suspected. Duct excision is indicated only in patients in whom bloody discharge is confirmed. Many of the discharges from the nipple are physiological, or are caused by benign breast disease and do not require surgery.

Mammography is not the first-line investigation in nipple discharge. In a patient who is 36 years old, mammography is relatively insensitive and ultrasound is better. MRI has very high sensitivity and specificity in breast lesions but is not used as a first line investigation for evaluation of nipple discharge. MRI can distinguish between scar tissue and recurrence. It is the best imaging modality in the presence of implants. Nipple biopsy is indicated in nipple ulcers and excoriations.

. A Atypical ductal hyperplasia

Atypical ductal hyperplasia carries the highest risk (five times) of malignant transformation. It has two varieties, ductal and lobular. Both of them can turn into malignancy. Duct ectasia is a dilatation of breast ducts associated with periductal mastitis. It does not carry any risk of malignancy.

Fibroadenoma arises from hyperplasia of single lobule. They are well-encapsulated and carry minimal risk of malignancy. Florid papillary hyperplasia is a part of the spectrum of benign breast disease and carries no risk of malignant transformation. Sclerosing adenosis is usually asymptomatic and is picked up on screening. They may present clinically with a lump and calcification on radiology. They are characterised by hyperplastic distorted lobules of acinar tissue. They exhibit increased collagenous stroma. They have little or no malignant risk.

. B Neoadjuvant chemotherapy

Neoadjuvant chemotherapy is the treatment of choice for this patient who has locally advanced breast cancer. It makes inoperable tumours operable. Breast conservation therapy can also be performed in some cases after neoadjuvant therapy. It takes care of systemic micrometastasis.

Breast conservation therapy is indicated in a tumour size less than 4 cm. Absolute contraindications of breast conservation are multifocal and multicentric tumours, size of more than 4 cm, pregnancy and repeated positive margins on excision. Relative contraindications are collagen vascular disease, previous radiotherapy, abnormal tumour breast ratio and large volume breast. In locally advanced breast cancer, breast conservation therapy can be done after downsizing by neoadjuvant chemotherapy.

Radiotherapy is not commonly used as a neoadjuvant therapy. Presence of fungation and ulceration are relative contraindications for radiotherapy. Modified radical mastectomy in large lesions is often associated with positive resection margins and is not the best initial treatment. Palliative mastectomy is performed in systemically advanced breast cancer.

4. B Duct ectasia

Duct ectasia leads to dilatation of ducts of the breast with periductal mastitis. It often gives rise to a retroareolar mass. The secretions extravasate and give rise to an abscess and later a periareolar sinus.

Carcinoma of the breast usually presents with a lump in the breast with or without bloody discharge from the nipple. Any ulcer usually is fungating in type. Paget's disease is a superficial skin manifestation of an underlying breast cancer. It presents as an eczematous lesion involving primarily the nipple which is gradually eroded. The involvement of areola occurs subsequently. All patients must be screened for underlying cancers and the nipple should be biopsied if there is any doubt.

Benign cysts of breast are non-progressive lesions. They rarely rupture and lead to sinus formation. Tuberculosis is relatively uncommon in developed countries. The condition is usually secondary to pulmonary tuberculosis. Patients usually present with a lump, shallow ulcers and axillary lymphadenopathy. There may be associated systemic features like evening fever, chronic cough and weight loss.

5. C *BRCA2* gene

BRCA2 is the most likely gene to be mutated in the family. It is located in chromosome 13. Typically this gene mutation is associated with male breast cancer. The majority of breast cancers are sporadic and only 5% are inherited. The *APC* gene is specific for colorectal cancer and has no relationship with breast cancer. *BRCA1* is located at the long arm of chromosome 17. It occurs with greater frequency in Ashkenazi Jews. In these women breast cancer usually occurs at a younger age. In these women there is a lifetime risk of around 50% of developing ovarian cancer.

CHEK2 is a cell cycle check point kinase gene. It is also a variant of tumor suppressor gene. These mutations can cause breast cancer usually before the age of 60 years. Male association has not been found with *CHEK2* gene mutation. *p53* is a tumour suppressor gene. Mutation in *p53* gene leads to Li–Fraumeni syndrome. This is characterised by an inherited predisposition to develop multi organ cancers. There is a familial predisposition of early breast carcinoma associated with sarcomas and multiple cancers throughout their life.

Chapter 36

Musculoskeletal system

A 35-year-old woman presents with a history of symmetrical polyarthropathy affecting the small joints of both hands and both feet. Examination reveals swan neck and boutonniere deformities in the fingers of both hands. Radiographs of the affected joints demonstrate varying degrees of joint space narrowing and bony erosions.

Which finding would suggest Felty's syndrome?

A   Anaemia
B   Dry eyes and mouth
C   Neutropenia
D   Raised inflammatory markers (erythrocyte sedimentation rate, C-reactive protein)
E   Rheumatoid factor positive

A 63-year-old man presents with a painful left arm with no history of preceding trauma. Examination reveals pain over the proximal aspect of the left humerus and subsequent radiographs are consistent with a pathological fracture. A subsequent bone scan reveals further pathological lesions of the femur and spine.

Which primary malignancy is the most probable cause of the secondary bony metastases?

A   Colonic carcinoma
B   Gastric carcinoma
C   Hepatoma
D   Pancreatic carcinoma
E   Renal cell carcinoma

A 42-year-old man presents with a one week history of sudden onset of increasing pain, swelling and redness to his left great toe. On examination there is tenderness, swelling and erythema over the metatarsophalangeal joint of the left hallux with an associated cellulitis. Tophi are also present. Subsequent blood tests demonstrate an elevated uric acid level and a diagnosis of gout was made.

Which one of the following is a recognised risk factor for gout?

A   Liver disease
B   Raynaud's syndrome
C   Renal impairment
D   Smoking
E   Steroids

4. A 69-year-old woman presents with history of increasing pain in both hips. Examination reveals an antalgic gait and a restriction of movement in both hips. Pelvic radiographs are suggestive of osteoarthritis.

    Which one of the following is a recognised characteristic of osteoarthritis on plain radiographs?

    A   Brodie's abscess
    B   Joint space widening
    C   Osteophytes
    D   Sequestrum
    E   Subchondral collapse

5. A 25-year-old old man presents with significant pain and swelling to the left forearm that has developed after the past 2 hours after being kicked by an opponent during a football match. On examination, there is significant swelling throughout the volar compartment with significant pain on passive stretch of the left wrist but with no sensory or motor abnormalities noted. Radiographs of the forearm reveal no bony injury. Despite adequate analgesia, 2 hours later the patient has persisting pain and continuous intracompartmental pressure monitoring of the forearm is compatible with compartment syndrome.

    What is the most appropriate treatment for this patient?

    A   Administer intravenous fluids to increase diastolic pressure
    B   Elevate arm and continue close observation
    C   Fasciotomy of the left forearm on the next available trauma list
    D   Increase analgesia
    E   Urgent fasciotomy of the left forearm

6. A 38-year-old man presents with a painful left wrist following a fall from his bicycle. On examination, he has a tender anatomical snuff box. Radiographs reveal a minimally displaced fracture through the waist of the left scaphoid. Following 6 months of treatment with immobilisation and subsequent mobilisation, the patient still has pain at the fracture site and check radiographs reveal no bone growth at the fracture site with no cortex bridging.

    What is the most likely diagnosis?

    A   Atrophic non-union
    B   Delayed union
    C   Hypertrophic non-union
    D   Infected non-union
    E   Union

7. A 3-year-old boy presents with a limp but no history of preceding trauma. Examination reveals a decreased range of movement with severe pain in the left hip. The patient is pyrexial with raised inflammatory markers and subsequent imaging reveals a significant effusion that was aspirated. On microbiological analysis using chocolate agar Gram-negative, rod-shaped organisms were identified.

What is the most likely causative organism?

A   *Haemophilus influenzae*
B   *Neisseria gonorrhoea*
C   *Staphylococcus aureus*
D   *Staphylococcus epidermidis*
E   Streptococci

A 14-year-old boy presents with pain, tenderness and localised swelling to the mid-shaft region of his right femur. Radiographs reveal a lytic lesion with a classic 'onion skin' periosteal reaction.

What is the most likely diagnosis?

A   Chondrosarcoma
B   Ewing's sarcoma
C   Fibrosarcoma
D   Osteochondroma
E   Osteosarcoma

Answers

1. C Neutropenia

Felty's syndrome is characterised by rheumatoid arthritis, splenomegaly, and neutropenia, with lymphadenopathy, vasculitis, anaemia, and thrombocytopaenia also found.

The most frequent form of inflammatory arthropathy is rheumatoid arthritis. The peak incidence is between the ages of 30–50 years and the female to male ratio is quoted as approximately 3:1. The pathogenesis is not conclusively known, however, it is thought to be associated with an unidentified trigger in genetically susceptible individuals (link with HLA-DR4 and DR1). This leads to activation of an immune and inflammatory process with lymphocytes, plasma cells and macrophages leading to chronic joint and tissue inflammation. Clinical features include an exacerbating remitting symmetrical polyarthropathy, with stiffness (early morning) and swelling predominantly affecting the small joints of the hands and feet, although any joint can be involved. Classic deformities to the hands include:

- Swan neck deformity (proximal interphalangeal joint hyperextension, metacarpophalangeal joint and distal interphalangeal joint flexion)
- Ulnar and volar deviation of the fingers (synovial inflammation of the wrist and metacarpophalangeal joints)
- Boutonnière deformity (distal interphalangeal joint hyperextension and proximal interphalangeal joint flexion)
- Prominent ulnar styloid (wrist subluxation)

Known extra-articular and systemic features include vasculitis, rheumatoid nodules, dry eyes and dry mouth (Sjögren's syndrome), pericarditis, pulmonary fibrosis, lung nodules, normochromic normocytic anaemia, thrombocytosis and amyloidosis. Routine blood tests in rheumatoid arthritis patients demonstrate raised inflammatory markers including erythrocyte sedimentation rate and C-reactive protein, with immunological tests including Rheumatoid factor positive (75% cases positive), anti-cyclic citrullinated protein antibody positive (70% cases positive), and antinuclear antigen positive (50% cases positive). Classical findings on X-ray include bony erosion, periarticular osteoporosis, and joint space narrowing. Treatment is with disease-modifying anti-rheumatic drugs (e.g. methotrexate or sulfasalazine first-line), steroids, non-steroidal anti-inflammatory drugs, biologicals (e.g. antitumour necrosis factor therapy), joint injections and arthroplasty.

2. E Renal cell carcinoma

Secondary bone tumours often metastasise from:

- Prostate (sclerotic lesions)
- Breast (lytic lesions)
- Kidney (lytic lesions)
- Lung (lytic lesions)
- Thyroid (lytic lesions)

Patients with bony metastasis may present with symptoms from their primary lesion and/or with symptoms and signs of their secondary lesion(s) including bone pain, pathological fracture or spinal cord compression. Pathological fractures are characterised by fracture following a low energy injury, through a region of bone with a pre-existing abnormality due to destruction of the bone architecture. Investigation includes radiographs, blood tests (calcium and alkaline phosphatase), bone scan and bone biopsy. The Mirels scoring system is used to guide treatment of pathological lesions (prophylactic fixation ≥ 8) and is based on four categories each scored 1–3:

- Pain (mild, moderate, mechanical)
- Tumor location (upper limb, lower limb, peritrochanteric/proximal femur)
- Lesion type (blastic, mixed, lytic)
- Lesion size (< 1/3, 1/3–2/3, > 2/3 of cortex involved)

Treatment includes analgesia, bisphosphonates, radiotherapy, chemotherapy along with surgery to stabilise actual or impending pathological fractures are all possible management avenues.

3. C Renal impairment

Gout is characterised by hyperuricaemia (increased production or decreased excretion of uric acid) leading to the deposit of crystals within the joints and soft tissues, resulting in an inflammatory arthropathy. It predominantly affects men (8:1) and the peak age incidence is 20–40 years. Factors associated with increased production of uric acid include genetics (Lesch–Nyhan syndrome) and concomitant diseases (myeloproliferative and lymphoproliferative disorders). Factors associated with decreased excretion include renal impairment, thiazide diuretics and excess alcohol intake.

Investigations include blood tests (leucocytosis, raised C-reactive protein and erythrocyte sedimentation rate, abnormal urea and electrolytes, raised urate), imaging (bony erosions, loss of joint space, osteosclerosis) and joint aspiration (polymorphs, urate crystals, no organisms). Management for an acute attack requires rest, analgesia (e.g. non-steroidal anti-inflammatory drugs), colchicine and/or joint injection with steroid. Risk reduction strategies include lifestyle changes (alcohol reduction, avoid purine rich foods, weight loss) and medications (e.g. allopurinol, probenecid).

Pseudogout is a predominantly large joint inflammatory arthropathy characterised by calcium pyrophosphate crystals deposition within joints and is associated with osteoarthritis. Less commonly associated diseases include endocrine disorders (e.g. diabetes mellitus, hyperparathyroidism, hypothyroidism, and acromegaly) and liver disorders (e.g. haemochromatosis, Wilson's disease). It predominantly affects women and the peak age incidence is 60–80 years.

Investigations include blood tests (leucocytosis, raised C-reactive protein and erythrocyte sedimentation rate, raised calcium), imaging (chondrocalcinosis) and joint aspiration (polymorphs, rhomboid shaped CPP (calcium pyrophosphate) crystals, no organisms).

4. C Osteophytes

Osteoarthritis is characterised by joint cartilage damage with joint space narrowing, osteophytes, subchondral sclerosis and subchondral cysts found on radiographs of the affected joint(s). Subchondral collapse is characteristic of avascular necrosis, whereas sequestrem and a Brodie's abscess are associated with osteomyelitis.

Risk factors for osteoarthritis include obesity, manual occupation, previous trauma or septic arthritis, developmental dysplasia of the hip (DDH), hypermobility syndrome, Perthes disease and Paget's disease. The hips, knees, spine and hands are most commonly involved and presentation with pain, swelling (osteophytes, e.g. Bouchard's and Heberden's nodes in the hands) and stiffness of the affected joint(s) that is exacerbated by weight bearing and movement. Blood tests and joint aspirations are usually unremarkable.

Management includes lifestyle modification (weight loss, physiotherapy), analgesia (e.g. non-steroidal anti-inflammatory drugs), intra-articular steroid injection or surgery (arthroplasty).

5. E Urgent fasciotomy of the left forearm

Acute compartment syndrome is a surgical emergency. It occurs when the contents of a inelastic walled compartment of the body swell and so raise the pressure within that compartment. In this case the muscle has swollen within the fascia. Once the pressure reaches a critical level the capillaries then the veins draining the compartment (which are thin walled) collapse under the external pressure. Arterial blood continues to enter but venous drainage is blocked. Pressure will then rapidly rise to mean arterial pressure when circulation in the compartment ceases and ischaemia starts. The muscles most commonly affected are those in the lower leg, and forearm, less commonly the intrinsic muscles of the hand and foot.

There does not need to be a fracture for a compartment syndrome to develop. Crushing injuries and severe bruising are potent causes. Indeed open fractures are unlikely to cause this problem because the fascia is also likely to be breached. The diagnosis is a clinical one (intercompartmental pressure measurements are unreliable), but an intercompartmental pressure within 30 mmHg of diastolic pressure is claimed to be diagnostic. If there is severe pain especially on passively extending the affected muscles then a compartment syndrome is present and a fasciotomy must be performed whatever the intercompartmental pressures are found to be. The warm ischaemic time for limbs is not normally more than 3–6 hours so fasciotomy must be performed urgently if it is to succeed. Fasciotomy after 24–48 hours is likely to do more harm than good as a reperfusion syndrome will result and lead to myoglobinuria and renal failure.

When a fasciotomy is performed all the compartements which might be involved (four in the lower leg) must be fully decompressed along their whole length. The wounds should be left open and no attempt made to close them until the swelling has gone down. Regular inspections are needed to identify and remove dead tissue.

. A Atrophic non-union

Fractures of the proximal pole or waist of the scaphoid are a known risk factor for delayed or non-union of the scaphoid. Radiological union is frequently defined as the bridging of three out of the four cortices at the fracture site. Delayed union is defined as a persistent absence of clinical and radiological signs of fracture union, with the fracture taking longer than expected to unite. The time before a delayed union is defined as a non-union is fracture dependent. In a scaphoid fracture, this is often defined as the absence of trabeculae bridging the fracture site at 16 weeks. Non-union may be atrophic with no callus formed and thinning of the fractures ends. The cause is likely to be loss of blood supply. Excessive movement at the fracture site leads to hypertrophic non-union which is seen on radiographs as expansion of the bone ends and excessive callus formation but no bridging of the fracture site. Risk factors for delayed or non-union are shown in **Table 36.1**.

Table 36.1

Patient factors	Injury factors	Treatment factors
Age	Open fracture	Prolonged immobilisation
Smoking	Extensive soft tissue trauma	Poor fracture reduction
Diabetes mellitus	Infection	Poor fracture fixation
Medications, e.g. non-steroidal anti-inflammatory drugs	Neurovascular injury	
	Site of fracture (diaphysis/metaphysis)	
	Degree of bone loss	
	Polytrauma, e.g. head injury	
	Pathological fracture	

Table 36.1 Risk factors for delayed or union categorised according to patient, injury and treatment characteristics

. A *Haemophilus influenzae*

Bacterial infection of a native or prosthetic joint is an orthopaedic emergency. In the native joint it can lead to joint destruction and in all patients can lead to severe sepsis. Risk factors include co-existing joint diseases, e.g. rheumatoid arthritis, previous joint arthroplasty, extremes of age, immunosuppression, diabetes and social deprivation. Common infecting organisms include *Staphylococcus aureus*, *Streptococcus*, *Neisseria gonorrhoeae*, *Haemophilus influenzae* and *Staphylococcus epidermidis*. *Staphylococcus* and *Streptococcus* are gram-positive organisms. *Neisseria gonorrhoeae* infection is commonly seen in sexually active young adults and is associated with polyarthralgia, tenosynovitis, urogenital symptoms and a pustular rash. *Staphylococcus epidermidis* is the common causative organism following joint arthroplasty. The common affecting organisms in children are shown in **Table 36.2**.

Table 36.2

Age	Common organisms
<12 months	Staphylococcus
	Group B streptococcus
6 months – 5 years	Staphylococcus
	Haemophilus influenzae
5–12 years	Staphylococcus aureus
12–18 years	Staphylococcus
	Neisseria gonorrhoea

Table 36.2 Risk factors for delayed or union categorised according to patient, injury and treatment characteristics (adapted from Miller MD, Thompson SR and Hart J. Review of Orthopaedics (6th ed). Philadelphia: Elsevier; 2012).

8. B Ewing's sarcoma

Ewing's sarcoma is a particularly malignant very rare small round cell tumour of the bone that frequently affects male teenagers. A genetic translocation is associated with the tumour (t 11;22). Localisation is often in the diaphysis of long and tubular bones, e.g. femur, pelvis ribs, humerus or spine. Radiographs demonstrate bone destruction and soft tissue swelling with a characteristic 'onion-skin' periosteal reaction.

Osteochondroma is a common cartilage tumour of cartilage that predominantly affects the metaphyses of long-bones in children and adolescents. The majority of tumours are asymptomatic. They have a 'mushroom type' appearance on imaging. Chondrosarcoma is a rare malignant bone tumour that is predominantly seen in older people (peak incidence is around 45 years) rather than children. The majority are found within the medulla of the proximal femur, pelvis, proximal humerus, ribs and spine. Endosteal scalloping is seen on imaging. Osteosarcoma is the most common malignant bone tumour of both children and adults (excluding myeloma) Risk factors include male gender, Paget's disease, retinoblastoma and radiation exposure. The tumours are destruction in nature and are often localised to the metaphyseal ends of the long bones, e.g. distal femur. Skip lesions are common. Metastases to the lung can occur. Radiographs demonstrate sclerosis, bony destruction, Codman's triangle and sunray spicules.

Chapter 37

Lymphoreticular system and liver

. A 30-year-old woman, a recent immigrant from Africa, complains of an ulcer on the right side of her neck, which appeared 4 weeks ago. It was preceded by a matted lump, which first appeared 6 months ago. She has regular episodes of fever in the evenings.

What is the most likely diagnosis?

A   Branchial fistula
B   Hodgkin's lymphoma
C   Infected sebaceous cyst
D   Secondary cervical metastasis
E   Tuberculous sinus from tuberculous cervical lymphadenitis

. A 38-year-old man presents with a painless, solid, firm, mass on the right side of his neck, which has been slowly growing in size over the last 8 months. He has hepatosplenomegaly; he complains of malaise, evening pyrexia with night sweats, pruritus and has recently lost some weight.

What is the most likely diagnosis?

A   Branchial cyst
B   Carotid body tumour
C   Hodgkin's lymphoma
D   Secondary cervical metastasis
E   Tuberculous lymphadenitis

. A 40-year-old woman complains of malaise, tiredness and itching all over her body for almost 1 year. Her daughter noticed that for the last few months, she has a yellowish tinge to her conjunctiva. She has smooth hepatomegaly. Her serum bilirubin is 37 µmol/L and alkaline phosphatase is 720 units/L.

What is the most likely diagnosis?

A   Common bile duct stones
B   Portal hypertension
C   Primary biliary cirrhosis
D   Primary sclerosing cholangitis
E   Secondary metastases in liver

4. A 25-year-old man complains of recurrent intermittent jaundice for 2 years. He has episodes when he feels lethargic and unduly tired. He looks slightly jaundiced and has an enlarged spleen. On one occasion he had fever, abdominal pain, nausea and vomiting when he looked very anaemic. He has developed a 3 cm superficial ulcer on his leg.

What is the most likely diagnosis?

A   Chronic leukaemia
B   Hereditary spherocytosis
C   Idiopathic thrombocytopenic purpura
D   Myelofibrosis
E   Splenic infarction

5. A 65-year-old man complains of generalised aches and pains all over his body. Spinal X-rays showed some collapse of mid-thoracic vertebrae. Routine blood test showed:

Haemoglobin 9 g/dL
Neutropenia
Thrombocytopenia
Serum calcium 2.9 mmol/L
Serum potassium 5.9 mmol/L
Serum creatinine 210 μmol/L
Urea 16 mmol/L
HCO_3 16 mmol/L
C-reactive protein 212 mg/L
Erythrocyte sedimentation rate 70 mm in the first hour
Urine is positive for Bence-Jones protein

What is the most likely diagnosis?

A   Multiple myeloma
B   Myelofibrosis
C   Osteoporosis
D   Paget's disease
E   Skeletal metastases

Answers

E Tuberculous sinus from tuberculous cervical lymphadenitis

This woman from Africa has the typical features of tuberculous cervical lymphadenitis (it's old name was scrofula or the King's touch, as it was thought that this could heal it). This has resulted in cervical lymph node swelling preceding the formation of a sinus. The nodes are matted. She also has the classical feature of evening pyrexia. The bacillus enters through the tonsil. Humans can be infected by both the bovine and the human form. A primary pulmonary focus should be excluded.

The node caseates, breaks down and forms a cold abscess (**Figure 37.1**), so called because it is not warm or tender. The pus, initially confined by the deep cervical fascia, tracks through the fascia superficially to form a biloculated abscess called a 'collar-stud' abscess resembling a dumb-bell. Left untreated, it bursts forming a sinus (**Figure 37.2**) which typically has an overhanging edge. The diagnosis is confirmed by biopsy. This shows caseating necrosis in which the dead tissue lacks any structure; there is a granuloma containing multinucleated giant cells arranged in a horseshoe shape called Langhans cell. Tuberculosis elsewhere in the body, particularly in the lungs, should be excluded and appropriate treatment instituted.

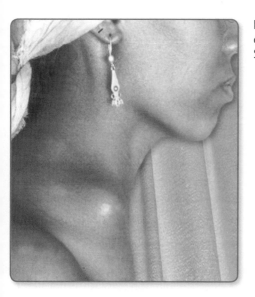

Figure 37.1 Cold abscess. Courtesy of Professor Ahmad Fahal, Khartoum Sudan.

C Hodgkin's lymphoma

This man has a neck lump typical of Hodgkin's disease – he has a mass of firm lymph nodes (**Figure 37.3**), slowly growing in size of several months duration and enlarged liver and spleen. He has constitutional symptoms, referred to as 'B' symptoms, such

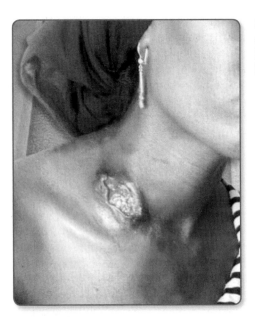

Figure 37.2 Tuberculous sinus with overhanging edge. Courtesy of Professor Ahmad Fahal, Khartoum, Sudan.

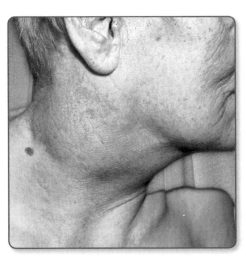

Figure 37.3 Lump on right side of neck: Hodgkin's lymphoma.

as fatigue, pruritus, and cyclical temperature (Pel–Ebstein fever). Sometimes there may be pain at the sites of involvement brought on by alcohol intake. The diagnosis is confirmed by lymph node biopsy; fine-needle aspiration cytology is not suitable as it will not give the full architecture. The extent of the disease is evaluated by haematological and biochemical investigations, imaging by chest X-ray, CT scan of the neck, chest and abdomen and bone marrow biopsy. This is a generalised disease of the reticuloendothelial system. Prior to definitive treatment the condition should be staged according to the Ann Arbor system devised in 1971. Pathologically four different types of Hodgkin's lymphoma are recognised: nodular sclerosis, mixed-cellularity, lymphocyte-rich and lymphocyte-depleted.

Macroscopically there is a homogenous white cut surface showing broad bands of fibrosis dividing the parenchyma into distinct nodules with foci of necrosis. Microscopically lymphocytes, eosinophils, macrophages, neutrophils, plasma cells, fibroblasts are present. Typically multi-nucleated (sometimes binucleate as mirror-image) cells with large nucleoli within a rich inflammatory background are seen. These cells are called Reed–Sternberg cells. The ideal management is by a multidisciplinary team consisting of radiotherapist, oncologist, pathologist and the surgeon.

. C Primary biliary cirrhosis

This patient has primary biliary cirrhosis. By far the vast majority of sufferers are women who present with gradual onset of fatigue and pruritus over a long period, jaundice being apparent later on. Hepatomegaly with scratch marks from pruritus is clinically apparent. Raised serum bilirubin and alkaline phosphatase should alert one to the diagnosis. This is confirmed by the presence of antimitochondrial antibodies, raised serum immunoglobulin (IgM). Eighty five per cent of patients with primary biliary cirrhosis have at least one other autoimmune disease such as chronic thyroiditis, rheumatoid arthritis, scleroderma, Sjögren's syndrome or systemic lupus erythematosus. Liver ultrasound shows altered architecture.

Ultimate confirmation is by liver biopsy. The condition is a chronic progressive cholestatic liver disease causing destruction of intrahepatic bile ducts. Three stages are recognised: ductal lesion, scarring and cirrhosis. In stage 1, there is chronic destructive cholangitis where the bile ducts are infiltrated by lymphocytes, plasma cells and macrophages with the formation of epithelioid granulomas. In stage 2, small bile ducts are destroyed with scarring of medium-sized bile ducts. There is florid proliferation of bile ductules within the portal tracts; severe cholestasis results. In stage 3, the end-stage, cirrhosis results with the liver becoming dark green in colour due to bile stasis, with scarcely any bile ducts left. The liver ultimately becomes a nodular green structure. Liver transplantation is the treatment of choice.

. B Hereditary spherocytosis

This young man with splenomegaly and intermittent jaundice, splenomegaly and a leg ulcer suffers from hereditary spherocytosis. It is also called acholuric jaundice as there is no bile pigment in the urine in the presence of jaundice. This is because, the jaundice is from unconjugated bilirubin that is not water soluble and hence is not excreted by the kidney. Absence of pruritus is also a feature of unconjugated hyperbilirubinaemia. The acute clinical episode in the patient of fever, abdominal pain, nausea and vomiting and extreme anaemia is caused by a haemolytic crisis. These patients have a high chance of developing pigment gallstones which might be silent.

In this condition, there is a premature destruction of red cells (extravascular haemolysis) caused by the monocyte/macrophage system in the spleen. The fundamental defect is an autosomal dominant hereditary disorder typified by a spherical red blood cell as opposed to the normal biconcave shape. The normal biconcave shape allows the red blood cell to be flexible helping it to circulate freely through the microcirculation and splenic vasculature. However, a deficiency in the cytoskeletal protein in the red blood cell causes it to be round (spherocyte) and rigid, and therefore unable to negotiate the splenic vasculature, predisposing it to a shortened life-span and haemolysis. The peripheral blood smear shows many spherocytes and reticulocytes and the osmotic fragility test is positive. Radioactive chromium labelled with technetium will demonstrate the extent of severity of red blood cell destruction by the spleen, and thus can predict the efficacy of splenectomy.

5. A Multiple myeloma

This patient suffers from multiple myeloma showing all the classical features: generalised bone pain, particularly in the axial skeleton, with vertebral collapse and clinical effects of bone marrow infiltration causing pancytopenia. Hypercalcaemia occurs from bone destruction and osteoclastic activity; the most frequently affected bones are the skull, spine, ribs and pelvis. Occasionally chronic renal failure results from the hypercalcaemia causing nephrocalcinosis. Presence of paraproteins in the blood and monoclonal light chains (Bence Jones protein) in the urine make the diagnosis obvious. There is humoral immune deficiency with reduction in serum immunoglobulin G (IgG) from suppression of normal B lymphocytes. This predisposes the patient to recurrent pneumonia and pyelonephritis. Confirmation of diagnosis is by bone marrow aspirate showing clusters of neoplastic and atypical plasma cells.

This condition is primarily a plasma cell neoplasia. Macroscopically the osseous lesions are well demarcated, greyish red with a fleshy or gelatinous consistency. The cortical bone is destroyed with extension of the tumour into the surrounding soft tissues. Sometimes, there is enlargement of the lymph nodes, spleen and liver. Microscopically the bone marrow is infiltrated by sheets of immature malignant plasma cells which are normally found in the bone marrow and produce immunoglobulin. The kidneys show nephropathy with deposits of amyloid, calcium uric acid crystals and light-chain casts resulting in renal failure. When the condition is localised as a discrete tumour it is called a plasmacytoma. The management is supportive with appropriate medical treatment to alleviate symptoms.

Section B

Principles of Surgery in General

Chapter 38

Perioperative care

Theme: American Society of Anaesthesiologists (ASA) classification

Options for Questions 1–4:

A   I-E
B   II-E
C   III-E
D   IV-E
E   V-E
F   VI-E

For each of the following cases, select the single most appropriate ASA class. Each option may be used once, more than once or not at all.

1. A 28-year-old man who is normally fit and well, has been declared brain dead following a head injury sustained during an alleged assault. He has no other injuries and is awaiting organ harvesting.

2. A 78-year-old man with a history of hypertension presents to the emergency department with abdominal pain and signs of hypovolaemic shock. He is not responding to fluid resuscitation. He has just arrived in theatre for emergency abdominal aortic aneurysm repair.

3. A 36-year-old woman requires laparoscopic cholecystectomy for acute cholecystitis. She has a goitre but is euthyroid on treatment with levothyroxine.

4. A 58-year-old woman is admitted as an emergency with a perforated sigmoid diverticulum for a Hartmann's procedure. She has a history of chronic obstructive pulmonary disease (COPD), presents dyspnoea on minimal exertion and requires treatment for exacerbations of COPD several times a year.

Theme: Nerve injury during anaesthesia

Options for Questions 5–8:

A	Common peroneal nerve	E	Radial nerve
B	Facial nerve	F	Supraorbital nerve
C	Femoral nerve	G	Tibial nerve
D	Median nerve	H	Ulnar nerve

For each of the following cases, select the single most likely nerve injury. Each option may be used once, more than once or not at all.

5. A 62-year-old man in the prone position for lumbar discectomy complains of loss of sensation to the anterior half of his scalp.

6. A 38-year-old woman has undergone low anterior resection. She complains of foot drop and sensory loss over the dorsal and lateral surface of her foot.

7. A 64-year-old man complains of sensory loss in the medial one-and-a-half digits of her hand following laparoscopic cholecystectomy.

8. A 52-year-old man complains of sensory loss over the lateral dorsal aspect of the hand and a wrist drop following open fasciectomy for an ipsilateral Dupuytren's contracture.

Theme: Monitoring of the anaesthetised patient

Options for Questions 9–11:

A	Airway pressure monitor	H	Intra-arterial blood pressure monitor
B	Bispectral analysis		
C	Electrocardiograph – lead II	I	Nasopharyngeal temperature probe
D	Electrocardiograph – lead V5		
E	End-tidal carbon dioxide analyser	J	Noninvasive blood pressure monitor
F	End-tidal anaesthetic agent analyser		
		K	Peripheral nerve stimulator
G	Inspired oxygen analyser	L	Pulse oximeter

For each of the following cases, select the single most useful monitor. Each option may be used once, more than once or not at all.

9. A 49-year-old man undergoing lumbar discectomy, to assess adequacy of ventilation.

10. A 27-year-old woman at the end of a laparoscopic cholecystectomy, to assess whether reversal of muscle relaxation is required.

11. A 74-year-old man undergoing femoral endarterectomy under spinal anaesthesia. He has had a recent MI to monitor myocardial ischaemia.

nswers

F VI-E

This patient has been declared brain dead and is waiting for organ harvest for the purpose of organ donation. He is therefore ASA VI. The E denotes the fact that it is an emergency not a planned procedure. The patient was normally fit and well prior to the assault but he is now no longer regarded, as ASA I. ASA classification is not a very sensitive predictor of anaesthetic mortality but it does offer a reasonable estimate of overall outcome. It does not require calculation of a complex scoring system. The predicted mortality following surgery by ASA class is shown in **Table 38.1**.

Table 38.1 Predicted mortality following surgery by ASA class.

ASA Class	Predicted mortality (%)
I	0.05
II	0.4
III	4.5
IV	25
V	50
VI	100

E V-E

This patient has haemorrhagic shock secondary to a ruptured abdominal aortic aneurysm. His haemodynamic status is not improving with fluid resuscitation and he is moribund so the only chance of survival is with operative management hence his ASA V status. The patient has a history of hypertension so before his aneurysm rupture, he would have been considered ASA II but this is no longer the case.

B II-E

This patient would be categorised as having mild systemic thyroid disease, i.e. an ASA II patient. This patient has a goitre so the anaesthetist will undertake careful preoperative assessment of the airway as the goitre may make management of the airway more challenging, e.g. by tracheal compression if it extends retrosternally. Ideally, hypothyroid patients should be rendered euthyroid before surgery to avoid the potential effects of hypothyroidism including myocardial depression, decreased ventilatory drive, abnormal baroreceptor function, reduced plasma volume, anaemia and altered hepatic drug metabolism. The perioperative risk is probably greater in hyperthyroidism especially in view of the cardiovascular effects, which include atrial fibrillation, congestive cardiac failure and ischaemic heart disease. Thyroid storm is a serious complication of hyperthyroidism where a life-threatening hypermetabolic crisis develops.

4. C III-E

This patient would be considered to have systemic disease which is severe but which is not a constant threat to life, i.e. ASA III. Her dyspnoea does not occur at res which would put her into an ASA IV category. It can be difficult to decide which cla patients are assigned to because the American Society of Anaesthesiologists does not provide any specific guidance but various groups of experts have suggested some consensus guidelines to help with this, for example, in the NICE preoperative investigation guidelines which can be read at http://www.nice.org.uk/nicemedia/live/10920/29094/29094.pdf.

5. F Supraorbital nerve

The supraorbital nerve is a terminal branch of the frontal nerve. It exits the skull via the supraorbital foramen after which it can be compressed by suboptimal head position during prone positioning. The areas to which it provides sensory supply include the conjunctiva of the eye and the skin from the forehead as far back as the vertex. Adequate padding of the bony prominences can prevent compression inju

6. A Common peroneal nerve

The common peroneal nerve is formed from the sciatic nerve. Its descent is obliqu along the lateral portion of the popliteal fossa to the head of the fibula, where it is palpable in slim subjects. It supplies sensation to the dorsum of the foot and moto innervation to the lateral compartment of the leg.

Positioning for low anterior resection requires access to the perineum to use an end-to-end anastomosis stapler. This is commonly achieved by using the lithotomy position. In this position, the common peroneal nerve can be compressed betwee the lateral head of the fibula and the bar holding of the legs. Great care must be taken to avoid this especially in patients with low body mass index and if surgery i likely to be prolonged.

7. H Ulnar nerve

The ulnar nerve originates from the medial cord of the brachial plexus (C8–T1) and descends on the posteromedial aspect of the humerus. At the elbow it passes posteriorly to the medial epicondyle of the distal humerus and is vulnerable to inju at this point.

During laparoscopic cholecystectomy, the arms are often placed by the patient's side to provide optimal surgical access to the abdomen. Devices used to secure the arms in this position can compress the ulnar nerve against the medial epicondyle of the humerus if they are not positioned appropriately. Damage to the ulnar nerv can produce a clawed hand and sensory loss in the little finger and medial half of t ring finger.

Whilst the ulnar nerve is derived from the brachial plexus, the signs and symptoms suggest damage at a specific point distal to the brachial plexus.

. E Radial nerve

The radial nerve originates from the posterior cord of the brachial plexus (C5–T1). During open fasciectomy for Dupuytren's contracture, a tourniquet is applied to the upper arm to minimise blood loss and provide optimal surgical conditions. If this tourniquet is not adequately padded or if the tourniquet pressure is excessively high (leading to damage from mechanical compression and ischaemia) or too low (resulting in passive congestion of the arm). Nerve tissue is more vulnerable to compression injury whereas muscle is more susceptible to ischaemia. Care should be taken to ensure that the minimum tourniquet pressure required to obtain bloodless field is used at all times and that the recommended time for tourniquet inflation is never exceeded. The highest risk of nerve damage is seen in patients who are cachectic, have flaccid skin or conical shaped arms.

E End-tidal carbon dioxide analyser

The end-tidal carbon dioxide analyser or capnography is one of the basic requirements for monitoring during anaesthesia according to the Association of Anaesthetists of Great Britain and Ireland. It is used to assess adequacy of ventilation, i.e. the clearance of CO_2 from the body. It does not provide any information about oxygenation. End-tidal CO_2 is a good proxy for alveolar CO_2 in normal anaesthetised patients with a difference of only 0.4–0.7 kPa. If end-tidal CO_2 is above the normal range, consideration should be given to increasing minute ventilation in patients who are receiving positive pressure ventilation. The capnograph trace rapidly drops or falls to zero with a decrease in cardiac output or after cardiac arrest. It is also useful in the detection of oesophageal rather than tracheal intubation and blockage or disconnection of the breathing system.

0. K Peripheral nerve stimulator

The degree of neuromuscular blockade can be assessed by applying a supramaximal stimulus to a peripheral nerve with a peripheral nerve stimulator, and then assessing the associated muscular response. It is important to assess neuromuscular function prior to waking the patient up and attempting tracheal extubation because complications such as residual airway obstruction, regurgitation and aspiration, weakness and respiratory failure may result from residual paralysis. Clinical assessment is also important and may include assessment of the tidal volume or ability to cough or achieve a sustained head lift. If required, non-depolarising muscle relaxants such as atracurium can be reversed by administering the anticholinesterase neostigmine. There is a relatively new drug called sugammadex which can be used to reverse a particular class of non-depolarising muscle relaxant which includes rocuronium by encapsulating rocuronium molecules and preventing their action at the neuromuscular junction.

1. D Electrocardiograph – lead V5

For real time perioperative monitoring, a continuous electrocardiograph trace is displayed on the monitoring screen. Most patients require only a 3-lead ECG with the electrodes being placed on the right arm, left leg and left arm. This allows recording of leads I, II and III with lead II being most commonly displayed on the monitor because it allows the best identification and interpretation of arrhythmias.

In patients who are at increased risk of myocardial ischaemia, a 5-lead ECG can be used to generate a V5-lead which will demonstrate 90% of detectable myocardial ischaemic changes and also provide arrhythmia monitoring. This 5-lead ECG set up is commonly used routinely in patients undergoing vascular and cardiac surgery an would be considered in high cardiac risk patients under going noncardiac surgery.

Electrocardiograph monitoring during surgery can be difficult as lead placement may be suboptimal to allow better surgical access and interference from diathermy is common despite an electromagnetic filter being used to try and reduce this. The presence of an ECG trace does not mean that there is a cardiac output, e.g. in cardiac arrest due to pulseless electrical activity.

Chapter 39

Postoperative management and critical care

heme: Hypoxaemia in surgical patients

ptions for Questions 1–4:

A	Acute lung injury	E	Opioid induced respiratory depression
B	Acute respiratory distress syndrome	F	Pulmonary embolism
C	Atelectasis	G	Pneumonia
D	Fat embolism		

or each of the following cases, select the single most likely diagnosis. Each option may e used once, more than once or not at all.

. A 25-year-old man attends the emergency department following a road traffic accident. A femoral shaft fracture is seen on X-ray and femoral nailing is carried out the following morning. Six hours postoperatively, he develops pyrexia, confusion and petechial rash on the anterior chest wall.

. A 42-year-old woman is admitted to the surgical ward with acute pancreatitis, and is receiving 10 litres per minute of oxygen via a non-rebreathe mask (estimated FiO_2 0.80). PaO_2 is 8 kPa. Bilateral infiltrates are visible on a chest X-ray taken that morning.

. A 34-year-old woman is in the recovery room following an elective laparoscopic cholecystectomy for biliary colic. She complains of being in severe abdominal pain. She is obese (BMI = 33) and smokes 20 cigarettes a day but is otherwise well. Respiratory rate is 16 breaths per minute, heart rate is 103 beats per minute and blood pressure is 142/84 mmHg. She requires 6 L/min of oxygen to maintain $SpO_2 > 94\%$.

. A 67-year-old man is in the surgical high dependency unit 72 hours following anterior resection for bowel cancer. He complains of breathlessness at rest and some right-sided pleuritic chest pain but denies other cardiorespiratory symptoms. He does not appear to be sedated or in pain and is receiving analgesia via a patient controlled morphine pump (PCA). He is haemodynamically stable but is hypoxic and tachypnoeic. His chest sounds clear. An arterial blood gas has shown PaO_2 of 6.8 kPa and $PaCO_2$ of 3.6 kPa on 5 L/min of oxygen.

Theme: Electrolyte disturbances

Options for Questions 5–8:

A	Hypercalcaemia	F	Hypocalcaemia
B	Hyperchloraemia	G	Hypochloraemia
C	Hyperkalaemia	H	Hypokalaemia
D	Hypermagnesaemia	I	Hypomagnesaemia
E	Hypernatraemia	J	Hyponatraemia

For each of the following cases, select the single most likely electrolyte disturbance. Each option may be used once, more than once or not at all.

5. An 87-year-old man is in the recovery room following transurethral resection of the prostate. He shows signs of restlessness, visual disturbance and hypertension.

6. A 64-year-old man is admitted to the emergency department following a road traffic accident. He has been fluid resuscitated using a large volume of 0.9% sodium chloride.

7. A 38-year-old woman is an inpatient in the surgical unit following total thyroidectomy 12 hours ago. She previously had difficulty breathing and circumoral paraesthesia.

8. A 45-year-old man is reviewed at the pre-assessment clinic prior to a inguinal hernia repair and noted to be in atrial fibrillation. He has a history of significant alcohol excess. Serum potassium is 4.5 mmol/L.

Theme: Cardiovascular complications following surgery

Options for Questions 9–12:

A	Broad QRS complexes, tented T waves	E	P waves unrelated to QRS complexes
B	Disorganised waveform, broad QRS complexes	F	Regularly irregular rhythm P waves present
C	Irregularly irregular rhythm, absent P waves	G	Sinus tachycardia, low-voltage QRS complexes
D	Lead I: prominent S wave, lead III: Q wave, inverted T wave	H	ST elevation in the anterior leads

For each of the following cases, select the single most likely ECG finding. Each option may be used once, more than once or not at all.

9. A 68-year-old man is in the high dependency unit 48 hours following an oesophagogastrectomy for cancer. There is concern regarding anastamotic breakdown.

0. A 55-year-old man in the high dependency unit 72 hours following an elective abdominal aortic aneurysm repair. He gets an episode of severe chest pain which is not relieved by glyceryl trinitrate spray.

1. A 32-year-old woman presents to the emergency department. She was trapped in a car for several hours following a road traffic accident with extensive soft tissue injuries to both legs. She is tachycardic and her creatine kinase is 6300 mmol/L.

2. A 65-year-old female is in the orthopaedic ward 48 hours after left total hip arthroplasty. She complains of shortness of breath and pleuritic chest pain. Her chest is clear. A recent blood gas shows hypoxaemia and a recent chest X-ray detected no abnormality.

Answers

1. D Fat embolism

Fat emboli can be a found in lung parenchyma and peripheral circulation after long bone or other trauma. In some patients this causes a syndrome with severe neurological and respiratory sequelae. It is not clear whether the emboli exert their effects by a mechanical obstruction or whether a reaction involving toxic intermediaries is to blame. Non-traumatic causes of fat embolism, e.g. pancreatitis, diabetes mellitus and steroid treatment are less common.

This case describes the classic triad of symptoms seen in fat embolism in the context of a high risk injury. This triad generally presents 24–72 hours postinjury:

- Respiratory compromise: this is generally the first sign to present; 50% of patients develop severe hypoxaemia and may require intubation.
- Neurological dysfunction: this caused by cerebral emboli, which can cause an acute confusional state or focal neurological deficit, which are generally transient and fully reversible.
- Petechial rash: this occurs last and only in 60% cases. Not only does it appear on the anterior chest wall, but may also be seen on the conjunctiva and oral mucous membranes.

The only management of fat embolism is supportive so efforts should be made to prevent it occurring by limiting intraosseous pressure and avoiding cement and reaming when possible. Overall mortality remains between 5 and 15%.

Despite the pyrexia, it is too early for an infective cause for hypoxaemia in this case and the petechial rash is almost pathognomonic for fat embolism.

2. B Acute respiratory distress syndrome

Acute pancreatitis can be complicated by multiple organ dysfunction. The respiratory complications can be severe and often herald a poor outcome.

There are a number of causes of hypoxaemia in acute pancreatitis:

- Acute respiratory distress syndrome (ARDS)
- Pneumonia
- Pleural effusion
- Atelectasis
- V/Q mismatch with no radiological abnormality

The diagnostic criteria for ARDS were determined by the 1994 American European Consensus Conference Committee. They are:

- Acute onset
- Bilateral infiltrates on chest X-ray
- No evidence of left atrial hypertension, with pulmonary artery occlusion pressure of ≤18 mmHg if measured
- PaO_2/FiO_2 ratio ≤27 kPa

ARDS and acute lung injury (ALI) are both on a spectrum of refractory hypoxaemia so have identical criteria aside from a different threshold for diagnosis. For ALI it is a PaO_2/FiO_2 ratio ≤ 40 kPa as it is associated with less severe hypoxaemia. In this case, the PaO_2/FiO_2 ratio $= 8$ kPa/0.8 $= 10$ making the diagnosis most likely to be ARDS.

The treatment of ARDS is supportive with attention paid to treating the underlying cause where possible. Patients generally require intubation and ventilation in the intensive care unit to optimise oxygenation and to manage other failing organ systems.

ARDS is associated with diffuse damage to the alveoli and endothelial leakage and injury. The early phase lasting from days 1–5 is characterised as being 'exudative' with leakage of protein rich fluid into the interstitium and air spaces. The later phase is typically 'fibroproliferative' in nature with architectural changes including emphysema and pulmonary fibrosis developing.

3. C Atelectasis

Hypoxaemia in the recovery room can be multifactorial. The hypoxaemia is not severe enough and the clinical setting not indicative of acute lung injury or acute respiratory distress syndrome. It is an elective procedure so pneumonia or pulmonary embolism are unlikely. The patient remains in pain so opioid induced respiratory depression is also unlikely.

The hypoxic respiratory drive is blunted by residual anaesthetic agents and analgesia; they can also cause hypoventilation. The airway can become obstructed due to a reduced conscious level. Ventilation perfusion mismatching can be caused by a reduction in functional residual capacity caused by general anaesthesia and the supine position combined with poor secretion clearance due to a reduced cough reflex and impaired ciliary function.

Atelectasis describes the absence of gas from part of, or the entire, lung. It is caused by obstruction of aeration of the alveoli. The gas trapped within the alveoli is eventually absorbed leaving nothing to splint open the alveoli so they collapse. Gas exchange and oxygenation are then markedly decreased. This occurs in the dependent region of normal lungs during anaesthesia. Other causes include endobronchial intubation. In this patient, smoking will make the sputum thick and sticky putting her at risk of sputum retention. Her uncontrolled pain will reduce chest movement and subsequently aeration of that area of lung postoperatively the failure to reinflate the lung produces atelectasis.

There is already supplemental oxygen therapy in situ. The priorities should now be: a) getting the patient to sit up to improve respiratory mechanics and increase functional residual capacity, b) optimising analgesia so the patient can freely cough and take a deep breath and c) arranging chest physiotherapy to ensure that the collapsed areas of lung are reinflated to avoid chest sepsis postoperatively.

4. F Pulmonary embolism

Pulmonary embolism is mechanical obstruction of a pulmonary artery or arteriole with thrombus which is often derived from a deep vein thrombosis in the legs or pelvis. It may present with pleuritic chest pain, tachynpnoea, tachycardia and cyanosis unless the PE is massive in which case hypotension or cardiac arrest may occur.

This patient has a number of risk factors for pulmonary embolism including malignancy, major abdominal/pelvic surgery and immobility. He should have been given venous thromboembolism prophylaxis including an anticoagulant, e.g. low molecular weight heparin and mechanical prophylaxis, i.e. graduated compression stockings.

The patient has been receiving opioid analgesia, but the history is not compatible with opioid related respiratory depression as there is no sedation and the patient is tachypnoeic. The arterial blood gas also does not support opioid related respiratory depression as in that scenario; one would expect the $PaCO_2$ to be increased. Pneumonia would also be part of the differential diagnosis, but there are no changes on auscultation of the chest and there is no cough or sputum production.

Arterial blood gas abnormalities in patients with pulmonary embolism can vary dependent on the size and duration of the embolism. The patient's underlying cardiorespiratory fitness status will also have an effect. Hypoxia and hypocarbia are seen due to a number of factors including ventilation perfusion mismatching.

Confirmation of the diagnosis using either CT pulmonary angiography or ventilation-perfusion scanning should occur followed by treatment with low molecular weight heparin or unfractionated heparin if concerns about postoperative bleeding persist.

5. J Hyponatraemia

This patient has hyponatraemia secondary to transurethral resection of the prostate (TURP) syndrome. This occurs when irrigation fluid is absorbed through open prostatic vessels. The ideal irrigation fluid must not conduct electricity to prevent dispersion of diathermy current and be transparent to allow good surgical visibility. It therefore must be electrolyte free so often contains glycine.

TURP syndrome is characterised by cardiorespiratory and neurological dysfunction due to changes in plasma osmolality and circulating volume, together with the effects of glycine, caused by the absorption of the irrigation fluid. Whilst hyponatraemia is common and an easily measured laboratory finding, it is thought that hypo-osmolality is more important than hyponatraemia in contributing to the neurological dysfunction. Risk factors include:

- Long procedure (inexperienced surgeon, technically difficult case, large prostate)
- Large volume of fluid absorbed (more open venous sinuses, higher pressure infusion of irrigation fluid, low venous pressure)
- Co-morbidity (pre-existing heart failure)

Principles of treatment are:
- ABC approach
- Stop infusion of intravenous fluids and administer furosemide
- Further prostatic resection should cease and surgery should end once haemostasis is secured

- Haemoglobin and sodium should be checked
- Manage complications, e.g. arrhythmias, seizures

If sodium is less than 120 mmol/L, then 3% sodium chloride can be given under expert direction with the aim of correcting the sodium to between 125–130 mmol/L. The sodium concentration should not increase by more than 12 mmol/L in the first 24 hours.

5. B Hyperchloraemia

When chloride rich solutions are administered in large quantities, hyperchloraemia and acidosis may develop. Stewart's theory of acid–base balance can be used to explain the mechanism behind this.

Hyperchloraemia is usually asymptomatic, but there may be symptoms of an associated acidosis if this is severe. It is unclear what impact this has but in recent years, there has been increased recognition that hyperchloraemic acidosis can develop after chloride rich solutions are administered in large quantities and efforts have been made to consider alternatives.

The current British consensus guidelines on intravenous fluid therapy for adult surgical patients support using a more physiological 'balanced' solution for resuscitation. These are now commonly available in both crystalloid (e.g. Hartmann's solution) and colloid (e.g. Geloplasma) formations.

Other causes of hyperchloraemia include endocrine causes, e.g. hyperparathyroidism, renal causes, e.g. renal tubular acidosis and gastrointestinal causes, e.g. diarrhoea, loss of pancreatic secretion and drugs, e.g. acetazolamide.

7. F Hypocalcaemia

Hypocalcaemia following thyroid surgery is caused by damage to the parathyroid glands which produce parathyroid hormone (PTH), which is integral to the regulation of serum calcium.

Deficiency in PTH leads to hypocalcaemia which in the post-thyroidectomy setting may be permanent (0.4–13.8% of patients) due to direct trauma, (inadvertent) surgical removal or compromise of blood supply; or it may be transient (2–53% of patients) due to reversible ischemia or hypothermia.

Risk factors for hypocalcaemia following thyroidectomy

- Indication for thyroidectomy (Graves' disease and malignancy)
- Extent of procedure performed
- Amount of parathyroid tissue removed

Most patients are asymptomatic. Classic symptoms include: circumoral paresthesiae, tetany, carpopedal spasm, laryngospasm, seizures, prolonged QT interval on ECG, and cardiac arrest.

Routine postoperative check of PTH and calcium will identify patients at risk of hypocalcaemia following thyroidectomy. Asymptomatic patients do not necessarily require treatment as this may interfere with the stimulation of the stunned parathyroid glands to produce PTH.

In early symptomatic postoperative hypocalcaemia, replacement should be by the intravenous route titrated to symptoms and blood levels. Oral calcium supplementation should then be commenced alongside replacement of vitamin D.

8. J Hypomagnesaemia

Patients with a history of alcohol excess have a number of reasons for developing atrial fibrillation one of which is electrolyte imbalance. Other causes of hypomagnesaemia are listed below:

- Reduced intake: prolonged parenteral nutrition, alcohol excess, anorexia
- Increased gastrointestinal loss: malabsorption, prolonged vomiting or diarrhoea
- Increased renal loss: either drug induced or due to intrinsic renal disease

The clinical features can be divided into:
- Neuromuscular: tetany, muscle weakness, seizures, nystagmus
- Cardiovascular: ST depression, T wave inversion, prolonged QT interval, arrhythmias, e.g. atrial fibrillation, ventricular fibrillation

Atrial fibrillation needs to be controlled prior to surgery so this should prompt further assessment of the patient.

Magnesium replacement can be either intravenous or oral. Severe symptomatic hypomagnesaemia should be treated intravenously with up to 50 mmol magnesium given over 8–24 hours. The efficacy of this treatment is limited by the magnesium reabsorption in the loop of Henle and up to 50% of this dose may be excreted. Oral magnesium supplementation should be used in asymptomatic patients, but this may cause diarrhoea. With both intravenous and oral replacement, it is important to monitor patients for signs and symptoms of hypermagnesaemia.

Hypomagnesaemia is often seen in combination with hypokalaemia and hypocalcaemia so these electrolytes should also be corrected.

9. C Irregularly irregular ventricular rhythm, absent P waves

The description 'irregularly irregular ventricular rhythm with absent P waves' is suggestive of atrial fibrillation. Atrial fibrillation is a supraventricular tachycardia where there is uncoordinated atrial contraction. If atrioventricular conduction remains intact, the ventricular response is rapid and irregular. Causes of atrial fibrillation can be divided into cardiac causes which include: postmyocardial infarction, hypertension, valvular heart disease, congenital heart disease.

Other causes which include: alcohol excess, pulmonary embolism, lower respiratory tract infection and hyperthyroidism

In postoperative patients, atrial fibrillation can be a sign of surgical sepsis. In a patient who has recently undergone oesophagectomy, priorities are management of the arrhythmia and looking for an underlying cause which may be anastamotic breakdown or pneumonia.

Management of the arrhythmia should focus on controlling the ventricular rate and if possible, restoration of sinus rhythm. The method of choice is dependent on haemodynamic status; the main options are either chemical or electrical cardioversion. Once haemodynamic stability has been achieved, consideration should be given to preventing recurrence of atrial fibrillation and preventing thrombotic complications.

0. H ST elevation in the anterior leads

The description 'ST elevation in the anterior leads' is suggestive of anterior myocardial infarction. The perioperative period can be associated with large and unpredictable changes in atherosclerotic plaque biology with an increased risk of plaque rupture. It also can lead to a mismatch of myocardial oxygen supply and demand with significant variation in heart rate, blood pressure, anaemia and hypoxaemia.

Perioperative ischaemia is a significant predictor of mortality and morbidity from non-cardiac surgery. Perioperative ischaemia can be silent and very difficult to treat due to the increased risk of bleeding with anticoagulants, antiplatelet agents and thrombolysis.

A more effective strategy may be to identify high risk patient preoperatively and investigate them according to either the European Society of Cardiology or the American Hearth Association guidelines. Optimisation of pharmacological treatment and revascularisation options can then be considered. This will not avoid all risk as unpredictable plaque rupture may still occur.

1. A Broad QRS complexes, tented T waves

The description 'broad QRS complexes, tented T waves' is suggestive of hyperkalaemia. This is a clinical emergency and treatment should be instituted immediately with 10 mL calcium gluconate 10% as a slow bolus to stabilise the myocardium with continuous ECG monitoring, then treatments such as insulin/ dextrose infusion to drive potassium intracellularly.

In this scenario, it is related to the development of rhabdomyolysis. Rhabdomyloysis may be:

- Traumatic: following crush injury, excessive muscle activity, electrocution
- Nontraumatic: infective causes, electrolyte disturbances, metabolic and immune mediated disorders

Irrespective of the aetiology, the final common pathway is release of myocyte components into the systemic circulation which causes hyperkalaemia, acidosis and acute renal failure.

Creatine kinase should be checked and if this is greater than 5000 mmol/L, acute renal failure should be expected in approximately 50% of cases. The urine may be dark and test positively for blood on urinalysis. Urinalysis can not differentiate between myoglobin and haemoglobin.

Prompt crystalloid fluid resuscitation should be commenced and consideration given to alkalinisation of the urine with sodium bicarbonate to increase the solubili† of myoglobin and reduce the severity of renal dysfunction. Renal replacement therapy may be required.

12. D Lead I: prominent S wave, lead III: Q wave, inverted T wave

The description 'Lead I: Prominent S wave, lead III: Q wave, inverted T wave' is consistent with suspected pulmonary embolism (PE). The most common ECG findin‡ in PE is a sinus tachycardia. The classical 'S1Q3T3' ECG changes shown in **Figure 39.1** are not as commonly seen in clinical practice. Right heart strain patterns, e.g. right axis deviation, right bundle branch block and T wave inversion in leads V1–V4 may also occur. ECG is of limited diagnostic value in PE but can be helpful in ruling out obvious myocardial ischaemia from the differential diagnosis.

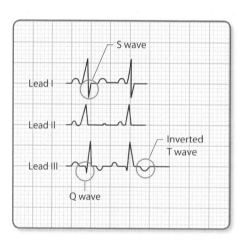

Figure 39.1 S1Q3T3 ECG pattern.

Hip arthroplasty is major surgery and the incidence of postoperative deep vein thrombosis diagnosed on venography is 70% with <1% fatal PE, if no prophylaxis is given. This rate significantly decreases with prophylaxis.

Clinical features depend on the severity of PE with pleuritic chest pain, dyspnoea and haemoptysis in milder cases and hypotension, cyanosis and raised jugular venous pressure in more significant PEs. Smaller PEs have less haemodynamic effect‡ but infarction of an area of lung tissue may occur. Multiple PEs can cause pulmonary‡ hypertension.

Chapter 40

Surgical technique and technology

heme: Types of suture material used with needles

ptions for Questions 1–3:

A	Chromic catgut 4/0	**E**	Polydioxanone 5/0
B	Metal clips	**F**	Polygalactin 2/0
C	Plain catgut 3/0	**G**	Polypropylene 5/0
D	Polyamide 4/0	**H**	Silk 1/0

or each of the following scenarios, select the single most appropriate suture material.
ach option may be used once, more than once or not at all.

. A 35-year-old man undergoes an open suprapubic cystolithotomy for removal of a
large bladder calculus. The bladder is repaired in two layers.

. A 19-year-old man falls from height and is brought to the emergency department
with a scalp laceration. The laceration is closed.

. A 56-year-old man undergoes a reversed saphenous vein femoropopliteal bypass
for occlusive disease of the superficial femoral artery. An arterial anastomosis is
carried out.

heme: Surgical wound closure and anastomotic technique

ptions for Questions 4–6:

A	Continuous suture	**E**	Single layer interrupted serosub-mucosal (extramucosal) suture
B	Horizontal mattress	**F**	Subcuticular suture
C	Interrupted suture	**G**	Tension suture
D	Laparostomy and use of Bogota bag	**H**	Vertical mattress suture

or each of the following scenarios, select the single most appropriate suturing
echnique. Each option may be used once, more than once or not at all.

. A 65-year-old man is undergoing colorectal anastomosis after anterior resection. A
hand-sewn anastomosis is performed.

5. A 70-year-old woman on the 6th postoperative day following a mid-line laparotomy for a perforated duodenal ulcer has developed a wound dehiscence. The patient is on steroids and is taken to theatre for resuture of the abdomen.

6. A 56-year-old man is known to suffer from chronic obstructive airways disease and presents with perforated appendicitis. After laparotomy, appendicectomy and peritoneal lavage, it is difficult to approximate the abdominal wall with conventional suturing technique due to gross abdominal distension.

Theme: Sterilisation techniques

Options for Questions 7–9:

A	Autoclaving	D	Ethylene oxide gas
B	Cetrimide and chlorhexidine solution	E	Formaldehyde
		F	Povidone iodine solution
C	Chlorine dioxide solution	G	Ultraviolet rays

For each of the following implements used at surgery, select the single most appropriate method of sterilisation. Each option may be used once, more than once or not at all.

7. Abdominal drain.

8. Deaver's retractor.

9. Gastroscope.

Theme: Energy sources

Options for Questions 10–12:

A	Argon beam coagulator	E	Monopolar coagulation current
B	Bipolar current	F	Monopolar cutting current
C	Chemical cautery	G	Thermal cautery
D	Cryotherapy	H	Ultrasonic shears

For each of the following scenarios, select the single most likely energy source. Each option may be used once, more than once or not at all.

10. A 25-year-old man presents to the emergency department with a crush injury to his hand. His wound is being explored under tourniquet and Bier's block. Haemostasis needs to be achieved.

11. A 40-year-old woman is due to have a right hemicolectomy for carcinoma of the caecum. The operation is due to be carried out by the usual open procedure.

12. A 70-year-old woman with a pacemaker and left-sided hemiarthroplasty of her hip has to undergo laparotomy for suspected colonic perforation from carcinoma. Haemostasis needs to be achieved by special technique in view of the presence of a prosthesis and a pacemaker.

Answers

1. F Polygalactin 2/0

Polygalactin is a synthetic multifilament absorbable suture material. Absorbable sutures are preferred for bladder closure so that no foreign material stays in the bladder wall avoiding a nidus for any subsequent stone formation. Bladder closure is usually done in two layers and is water tight with 2/0 or 1/0 suture.

2. H Silk 1/0

Scalp is a tough layer of the skin and is closed with a nonabsorbable suture like silk. Silk is easier to knot and does not slip. This quality is a great help in the presence of profuse bleeding. Due to the strength of the skin of the scalp and to avoid suture breakage during knotting a thicker suture like 1/0 or 2/0 is to be used.

3. G Polypropylene 5/0

Fine monofilament polypropylene suture is used for vascular anastomosis. Size of the suture varies from a finer 4/0 or 5/0 in femoral or popliteal arteries to heavier sutures like 2/0 or 3/0 for the abdominal aorta.

4. E Single layer interrupted serosubmucosal (extramucosal) anastomosis suture

In colorectal surgery this method of anastomosis is now regarded as the method of choice. Interrupted nonabsorbable sutures taking bites of the serosa and submucosa but excluding the mucosa are taken. This will preserve the blood supply and not narrow the lumen after the anastomosis. This technique would ensure a water-tight anastomosis that heals well in spite of the inherent tenuous blood supply of the colon.

5. G Tension suture

For resuture of a wound dehiscence tension sutures are used. The term 'tension suture' is a misnomer because they are never tied under tension. They are so called because they are tied in such a way that they should relieve abdominal tension. Strictly speaking they should be called 'through-and-throughs' as they go through all the layers of the abdominal wall including skin. The suture is taken at least 2 cm from the wound edge and the knot tied over a fine rubber tube so that the nylon suture does not dig into the abdominal skin. The sutures are left in place for 2 weeks. Sometimes such sutures are used prophylactically in patients such as the immunocompromised, the jaundiced, those with chronic renal failure and patients on steroids, who are vulnerable to developing burst abdomen.

6. D Laparostomy and use of Bogota bag

Any attempt to close the abdomen forcibly under tension causes increased pressure in the abdominal cavity risking the possibility of abdominal compartment syndrome. This condition leads to reduced venous return (from pressure on inferior vena cava) and severely affects respiration (from diaphragmatic splinting) resulting in Type 2 respiratory failure. In such cases, the abdominal wall is left open (laparostomy) and the exposed bowel can be covered with a soft plastic bag (Bogota bag) cut into a size to fit the defect and sutured to the rectus sheath all around. This was devised from a sterilised urology fluid bag in 1984 by Dr Oswaldo Borraez, a trauma surgeon while he was a resident in Bogota. Once the acute stage of oedema and infection has settled, it is usually possible to approximate the abdominal wall or leave it for closure by secondary intention.

7. D Ethylene oxide gas

Ethylene oxide gas is used for disposable material such as plastic tube drains and catheters made of polyvinylchloride, latex or rubber. This highly penetrative gas requires 12 hours to be effective which includes the time for aeration to rid the article of the residual toxic gas. It is also used for instruments that cannot withstand temperatures above 60°C.

8. A Autoclaving

Autoclaving is steam under pressure used for metallic instruments except for sharp objects such as scissors which would become blunt by this method. Used at 134°C at 30 per square inch (psi) for 3 minutes or 121°C at 15 psi for 15 minutes, this technique is one of the most reliable and efficient methods of sterilisation.

9. C Chlorine dioxide solution

Chlorine dioxide solution is used to disinfect gastroscopes. This is an oxidising and germicidal agent, ClO_2, a clear colourless and odourless solution (called Tristel) used to disinfect fibreoptic endoscopes. In the past 2% glutaraldehyde was used for this purpose. A 20 minute immersion would get rid of most micro-organisms but not spores. It was extremely irritant and toxic to the skin; hence it has been replaced with chlorine dioxide.

10.   B Bipolar current

Bipolar current is a safe current as the path of the current is limited between the two poles and no stray current passes to the patient's tissues. It is used where the blood vessel is an end artery particularly in fingers and toes. There is no patient electrode. The active and return electrodes are at the operation site – the two blades of the forceps perform both functions. It is ideally used in a patient with a pacemaker and for delicate surgical procedures.

1. E Monopolar coagulation current

Monopolar coagulation current is the one most commonly used in conventional open surgery. The active electrode is at the surgical site; the return electrode is usually on patient's thigh. The pad is $70\,cm^2$; before it is applied the hair at the site is shaved. Other precautions to be taken are: there should be no fluid in the vicinity; the patient should not touch any metal objects; and in a patient with prosthesis, the patient electrode should be as far away as possible from the prosthesis.

2. H Ultrasonic shears

Ultrasonic shears achieves haemostasis using vibration at ultrasonic frequency. There is no passage of electrical current through the patient's tissues. Hence, it is safe in patients who have implanted pacemakers or metallic prostheses.

Chapter 41

Management and legal issues in surgery

Theme: Breaking bad news

Options for Questions 1–3:

A The environment was not appropriate

B A check should have been made as to whether the patient wanted someone with them

C The interviewer should have found out how much patient wanted to know before starting

D Adequate time should have been left to complete the task

E Simpler language could have been used

F This was handled correctly

For each of the following scenarios, select the single most appropriate critique. Each option may be used once, more than once or not at all.

1. A 60-year-old retired man has smoked all his life. He developed a cough and an X-ray shows a suspicious shadow. Tracheal cytology confirms the presence of an adenocarcinoma. On scanning, there is evidence of metastases in the brain and in the vertebrae. An interview is arranged with the patient and his wife. It is explained that there is a cancer in his lungs and that it has spread throughout his body, such that only palliative treatment would be appropriate. He is shown both the scans and it is explained where metastases can be seen. The patient and his wife seem shocked, but have no questions. But the wife does mention that she had not wanted her husband told just at this moment since he was being treated for depression.

2. A 30-year-old married woman has had a breast lump removed. At clinic 1 week later she is told that the lump was an aggressive form of cancer and that she needs a mastectomy and radiotherapy. She is very upset by the news and needs a great deal of support and reassurance. The clinic nurse phones her husband to arrange for her children to be collected from school and to ask him to come and collect her from the clinic as she feels too upset to drive.

3. A 30-year-old man has a phaeochromocytoma. It is explained that surges in hormones released by the tumour are leading to instability in the blood pressure homeostasis mechanisms and that these fluctuations are responsible for his symptoms. The doctor then goes on to explain how difficult the tumour can be to find and that there may be rebound side-effects after it has been successfully removed. The patient seems a little dissociated from the interview but has no questions.

Theme: Communication skills

Options for Questions 4–5:

A　Acknowledge good work
B　Acknowledge that there is a problem as soon as possible
C　Get the facts first
D　Give the people involved a severe ticking off
E　Make sure that everyone who needs to know is informed
F　Make sure that you have a quiet room where you will not be disturbed
G　Make sure that you know everyone's names and their responsibilities
H　Remain calm, delegate duties
I　Set some ground rules for discussion
J　Take copious notes

For each of the following situations, select the single most appropriate initial action, which is most likely to achieve a successful outcome. Each option may be used once, more than once, or not at all.

4.　There is a dispute between two members of staff over duties on the ward. Both have given their side of the story. A meeting is called to try to resolve the issue.

5.　Four ambulances arrive simultaneously at the emergency department with four seriously injured patients from a car crash. They have not given any notice of their arrival.

Theme: Evidence-based surgical practice

Options for Questions 6–8:

A　Enter keywords into an internet search engine
B　Perform a literature review for the Cochrane collaboration
C　Perform an audit
D　Perform a randomised controlled trial (RCT)
E　Give a presentation based on the patients seen
F　Search for NICE or SIGN guideline

For each of the following situations, select the single most appropriate action, which is most likely to give a clinically useful answer. Each option may be used once, more than once, or not at all.

6.　A consultant has designed a new method for ligating perforating varicose veins, using a small metal coil which he has had designed and had made for him by a local company. He is now going to start implanting these.

7.　There are two different knee replacements used in the hospital, and it has been agreed that the unit should only use one. But it cannot be decided which is the one which should be used.

8.　There appear to be too many cases of wound infection on the ward. This may be a result of there being no hand-gel available at the end of each patient's bed.

Theme: Ethics and medical negligence

Options for Questions 9–11:

A   There was a breach of duty of care

B   On the balance of probabilities there is negligence

C   The patient has come to harm, but so far no more than this can be said

D   There is no legal issue here

E   There is no negligence as there is no breach of care

For each of the following situations, select the single most likely conclusion that will be drawn when legal advice is sought. Each option may be used once, more than once, or not at all.

9. A 30-year old woman has a swab left in her abdomen following a laparotomy, but she is otherwise well.

10. A 10-year old boy is given penicillin. It was not thought that the patient was allergic to penicillin. He comes out in a rash, which settles within hours.

11. A 70-year old man has a total hip replacement. On rounds the following morning it is noticed that he has a foot drop. This subsequently turns out to be permanent.

Theme: Handling a complaint

Options for Questions 12–14:

A   Acknowledge as soon as possible before you know the facts

B   Arrange a meeting and explain what has happened

C   Apologise first even before you have the facts

D   Bring the case up first at a clinical governance meeting on a 'no-name' basis

E   Gather the facts together before calling a meeting

F   Keep the complaint on a 'need to know' basis so that morale in the unit is maintained

G   Promise to learn from what has happened

H   Write immediately that 'You are sorry that you feel this way'

For each of the following situations, select the single most appropriate action. Each option may be used once, more than once, or not at all.

12. A 70-year-old man had a total hip replacement 2 weeks ago. He has now been told that the joint is infected and that it will need to be changed. His wife complains about this and says that lots of the patients treated by this service have become infected. This is checked with the consultant and the infection control officer. A recent audit of the unit shows that the unit has had three infections in the 150 hip replacement operations performed in the last year. The national infection rate is reported as being between 1 and 3%. All measures which should be taken to prevent infection have been taken.

13. A 90-year-old woman falls out of bed when slightly confused. This occurred because the cot sides were down at the time of the accident. There are instructions

in the nursing notes that the sides should be kept up at all times. The sides were apparently down because the nurses were all busy with another patient who had collapsed.

14. A 60-year-old man complains because he has to return to theatre after a ligature has slipped on a large vessel. The ligature had not been double tied. The doctor proposes to see the patient and apologise personally for what has happened.

Answers

C The interviewer should have found out how much patient wanted to know before starting

Breaking bad news is not a simple business. It is important to find out how much the patient wants to know at that time before proceeding. It may be that they want to take the information in smaller pieces separated by time so that they have a period to digest the change in their life. The wife's wishes that her husband should not be told at that time do not take priority over his wishes, but they need to be taken into account.

B A check should have been made as to whether the patient wanted someone with them

Most people would like to have someone that they trust and respect with them when they are coping with bad news. In this case, it might have been better for this patient to have her husband with her while she was given the news.

E Simpler language could have been used

Language which may be simple to you, and which is used in everyday work conversation, may be completely incomprehensible to the patient. Conversely, highly educated patients, especially doctors, may find layman's language patronising. It is therefore important to check regularly that you are using language appropriate to the patient's needs.

I Set some ground rules for discussion

When setting up a meeting for 'conflict resolution' there need to be clear ground rules. These must be agreed before negotiation starts as otherwise the situation can be made worse not better. Examples might be:

- There is to be no abusive language
- Either side can call 'time-out' if they feel that the meeting is going out of control

H Remain calm, delegate duties

This is another form of crisis where the ability of the department to respond is at risk of being overwhelmed by the medical need. You may well need to triage the casualties (decide the order of priority in which they are treated), and you will certainly need to calmly allocate your staff to where they can do the most good for the maximum number.

6. E Give a presentation based on the patients seen

There will be nothing in the literature. So, the first thing to do is to review the result which this technique has achieved. Presentation of these results and comparison with those achieved by other units using other techniques has no scientific validity but is useful because it will show what questions need to answered by a properly set-up prospective trial.

7. D Perform a randomised controlled trial (RCT)

This issue could be resolved simply by choosing the cheapest implant, but it would be much better if a check was made first on whether there was any difference in outcome attributable to the implant, not the surgeon or any other confounding factor. Large numbers will be needed if this study is to give a valid result so the trial may need to be organised as a multi-centre one.

8. C Perform an audit

This is a clear example of where an audit is needed. First you need to find out what exactly is your infection rate, and how this compares with other units. Then, if your rate is high, you need to try an intervention (such as putting hand gel at the end of each bed) and review to see if your rate has now fallen. This process of identifying a problem, implementing a solution and then checking the results is sometimes calle closing the audit loop.

9. A There was a breach of duty of care

It falls below an acceptable standard of care for a swab to have been left in the abdomen after surgery, so there is a 'breach of care'. This is the first 'hurdle' that has to be crossed by the plaintiff if medical negligence is to be proven. We do no yet know from this scenario whether the other preconditions of negligence have been met.

10. C The patient has come to harm, but so far no more than this can be said

The patient has come to harm as a result of the penicillin being given. It is not yet proven that there is a breach of care (perhaps the patient did not admit to being allergic to penicillin despite being asked). Nor is it clear that the patient has 'consequences' as a result of this harm, e.g. he has had to take time off school. 'Coming to harm' is a second condition for medical negligence which needs to be proven in British law for a case to suceed.

11. D There is no legal issue here

Here, there are consequences of the surgery performed: the patient is going to be left with a permanent foot drop. 'Consequences' is the third condition which is required if medical negligence is to be proved, but the scenario does not yet tell us whether the other conditions ('breach of care' and 'harm') have occurred, as we do not yet know why the patient has a foot drop. It is likely that the sciatic nerve was damaged (harmed) at surgery, but other possibilities have not yet been excluded.

2. B Arrange a meeting and explain what has happened

You know the facts. This appears to have been an 'act of God'. All reasonable precautions have been taken, and there is no need for an apology. Your figures for infection appear to be in the middle of the national average. However a meeting is now needed to explain the situation carefully to the patient and his wife. This should help everyone come to terms with what has happened. If the patient's wife continues to blame the service for what has happened, you should not say 'I am sorry that you feel this way' (option H). That is not an apology (nor should it be), it is a rather irritating way of saying that you disagree with their view.

3. C Apologise first even before you have the facts

This patient should not have fallen out of bed. It is important to apologise for this mistake. Contrary to popular belief an apology does not lay you open to litigation. The evidence is that frequently a full and heart-felt apology satisfies the patient and prevents litigation. Additionally, it would be good to explain that measures are to be taken to ensure that this does not happen again, and to bring the subject up at the next clinical governance meeting to remind everyone to check cot sides all the time.

4 G Promise to learn from what has happened

It appears that you know the facts. You will meet with the patient. You are going to apologise because an error has been made. Now you need to apply the most important measure to ensure that the patient feels happier about things and, if possible, litigation is avoided. This is to explain that every possible measure is to be taken to ensure that this 'never happens again'. One way in which this can be done is to hold a clinical governance meeting to explore what has happened in a 'no blame' environment and explore what extra measures (training, double checks, check-sheets, etc.) could be introduced to prevent a recurrence.

Chapter 42

Clinical microbiology

Theme: Pathogen likely to be isolated

Options for Questions 1–3:

A β-lytic *Streptococcus*
B *Candida albicans*
C *Clostridium welchii*
D *Escherichia coli*

E *Staphylococcus aureus*
F *Staphylococcus epidermidis*
G *Streptococcus pyogenes*

For each of the following cases, select the single most likely organism to be cultured. Each option may be used once, more than once or not at all.

A 70-year-old woman has a routine hip replacement. All goes well initially but over the next few months, she complains of increasing pain in the hip. Her C-reactive protein is raised at 50 mg/L and she is apyrexial. A needle aspiration of the hip joint is performed.

A 70-year-old man has a repair of a recurrent inguinal hernia. Within 48 hours the wound is red and swollen and the patient is pyrexial. Blood cultures are sent for.

A 70-year-old woman has been receiving chemotherapy for carcinoma of the breast. She is put on a broad spectrum antibiotics for a chest infection which takes 10 days to clear. On day 8, while she is still on antibiotics, she complains of a red and sore mouth with white plaques on the tongue and cheeks. A swab is taken from one of these plaques.

Theme: Appropriate treatment of infections

Options for Questions 4–6:

A Amoxicillin
B Cefuroxime
C Clotrimoxazole (Canesten)
D Flucloxacillin
E Gentamycin

F Nitrofurantoin
G Oral penicillin
H Penicillin V
I Vancomycin

For each of the following cases, select the single most appropriate therapy. Each option may be used once, more than once or not at all.

A 65-year-old man is scheduled for a total hip replacement which needs to be covered by a prophylactic antibiotic.

5. A 70-year-old woman has had a mastectomy develops a purulent discharge from the wound. Two other patients on the ward have also developed wound infections

6. An 18-year-old man has cut his hand on a tin that he was opening. The wound has been closed, but cellulitis is spreading in pink streaks up the arm from the wound.

Theme: Preventing cross-infection

Options for Questions 7–9:

A   Autoclaving
B   Disposable instruments
C   Peritoneal washout
D   Skin cleaning with povidone iodine

E   Universal precautions or standard precautions (health care)
F   Washing instruments before autoclaving

For each of the following cases, select the single most appropriate technique for the prevention of cross-infection. Each option may be used once, more than once or not at all.

7. A 70-year-old man undergoes an emergency Hartmann's resection for perforated diverticulitis with faecal peritonitis.

8. A 25-year-old healthy man sustains a needle stick injury while clearing up a trolley following a lumbar puncture. The patient on whom the lumbar puncture was performed is known to be hepatitis B-positive.

9. A 20-year-old man attends the emergency department with a laceration to his forehead involving the eyebrow. This needs to be sutured.

Theme: Side effects of antibiotics

Options for Questions 10–11:

A   Aplastic anaemia
B   Hearing loss
C   Pseudo-membranous colitis
D   Staining of teeth
E   Skin rash

For each of the following cases, select the single most likely side-effect. Each option may be used once, more than once or not at all.

10. An 80-year-old woman is being treated with gentamycin for a pseudomonas infection of a leg ulcer. Routine blood results show a raised blood level of the antibiotic.

11. A 5-year-old girl with tonsillitis is given tetracycline in case there is a bacterial component to the infection.

Theme: Management in accidental contamination

Options for Questions 12–14:

A Conference of all ward staff immediately

B Incise the wound at point of injury to make it bleed freely

C Post exposure prophylaxis treatment started immediately

D Suck the wound followed by post exposure prophylaxis

E Post exposure prophylaxis and cessation of treatment, if subsequently risk is found to be low

F Wash the area and report the incident

For each of the following cases, select the single most appropriate management option. Each option may be used once, more than once or not at all.

12. A 30-year-old woman, a ward auxilliary receives a needle stick injury from a discarded needle while emptying a rubbish bag in the main treatment room. There are no known 'high risk' patients on the ward.

13. A 22-year-old female student nurse is clearing away a trolley just used to take a bone marrow sample from a patient who is known to be HIV-positive. She receives a needle stick injury but is worried that it was her fault and does not report it for 4 hours.

14. A 25-year-old female nurse is taking down an intravenous infusion from a patient, who is not known to be carrying HIV, or any form of hepatitis, but is a patient with a potentially high-risk lifestyle. She receives a deep needle stick injury from the intravanous cannula, which is covered in the patient's blood. There is no information in the notes to suggest that the patient has an HIV infection, and there is nothing to suggest that they are high-risk.

Answers

1. F *Staphylococcus epidermidis*

Total joint replacements are performed under super-sterile conditions, but it is never possible to remove all the skin commensals from the operating field. The one most likely to contaminate the wound and then infect the implant is *Staphylococcus epidermidis*, which under normal circumstances is not a pathogen.

2. E *Staphylococcus aureus*

Staphylococcus aureus is the organism most likely to infect a wound in hospital. In some cases, this will be methicillin-resistant *Staphylococcus aureus* (MRSA) an organism of low virulence but high infectivity which spreads from patient-to-patient in hospitals and nursing homes where there are patients with low resistance to infection.

3. B *Candida albicans*

Antibiotic treatment may destroy the body's natural bacterial flora and leave the patient open to attack by fungi such a thrush (oral candidiasis). The mucous membranes will be red and sore with plaques of white material on them.

4. B Cefuroxime

When giving prophylactic antibiotics it is important to cover the most likely infecting organism as well as other less likely culprits. It is therefore usually wise to give a broad spectrum antibiotic such as cefuroxime rather than a narrow spectrum one such as flucloxacillin which will cover *Staphylococcus* (the most likely infective organism) but may not be of any value against gram-negative organisms.

5. I Vancomycin

A hospital acquired infection is likely to be resistant to first line antibiotics and so a special antibiotic such as vancomycin needs to be considered as it is much more likely to be effective. The sensitivity of the organism will need to be checked by taking cultures, preferably when the patient is not on any antibiotic (so that there is no masking).

6. G Oral penicillin

The organism here is likely to be *Streptococcus pyogenes* which is very sensitive to penicillin. Rather than sticking any more needles into the patient, it would be quite reasonable to give the penicillin orally.

C Peritoneal washout

In this procedure for perforated large bowel, the surgeon would be working in a field contaminated with *Escherichia coli*. Washing out the peritoneal cavity with several litres of warm normal saline will reduce the contamination load, and give the body a better chance of combating the effects of faecal peritonitis and further effects of sepsis.

E Universal precautions or standard precautions (health care)

Universal precautions or standard precautions (health care) consist of a whole system of behaviour geared towards preventing staff and patients from being cross infected. They are especially valuable for avoiding needle stick injuries, which are a potent cause of hepatitis infection.

B Disposable instruments

Prions are not reliably destroyed by any conventional sterilisation technique such as autoclaving or ionising radiation. The only way to be certain of not transmitting prions between surgical cases is to have disposable instruments.

. B Hearing loss

Gentamycin has a very narrow therapeutic range: too low a concentration and it is ineffective, too high and it causes deafness. It is excreted by the kidneys and so the dose needs to be very carefully titrated in patients with any renal insufficiency.

. D Staining of teeth

Tetracycline is taken up by growing bone and teeth, and can be used in histological studies of both. However in children, it also has the side-effect of staining teeth yellow and so should be avoided in children.

. F Wash the area and report the incident

Any contamination from a patient should be treated with copious washing with soap and water. There is no place for sucking the wound or for vigorous scrubbing (B). The guidelines for post exposure prophylaxis (PEP) should then help to decide the chances of contamination containing HIV and the chance of this being transmitted. If there is no broken skin and mucous membranes are not involved then the risk is so low that the complication risk of PEP outweigh the benefits. Again if the source of contamination is a low risk patient, then again PEP should not be given as the risks outweigh the benefits. It will be valuable to have a clinical governance meeting on this case and to use the problems raised to heighten everyone's awareness that they need to be careful. The staff member will need support and counselling.

13. E Post exposure prophylaxis and cessation of treatment if subsequently risk is found to be low

This is a high risk injury (penetrating injury from a positive patient). Therefore, PEP should be given, starting as soon as possible. PEP is thought to be effective if given within 72 hours of the exposure, so this patient is well within the time limits, but will require counselling and reassurance.

14. E Post exposure prophylaxis and cessation of treatment if subsequently risk is found to be low

The risk here is uncertain but might be 'high' risk as the patient comes from a high risk group (intravenous drug user, homosexual contact, those living in parts of the world where HIV is known to be common). Therefore, consent should be obtained from the patient to test for HIV. However, post exposure prophylaxis should be started right away. If the HIV test result on the patient comes back negative then PEP can be stopped.

Chapter 43

Emergency medicine and trauma management

Theme: Pathophysiology of trauma

Options for Questions 1–3:

A	Acute respiratory distress syndrome	F	Class III hypovolaemic shock
		G	Class IV hypovolaemic shock
B	Anaphylactic shock	H	Fat embolism syndrome
C	Cardiogenic shock	I	Neurogenic shock
D	Class I hypovolaemic shock	J	Septic shock
E	Class II hypovolaemic shock	K	Tension pneumothorax

For each of the following cases, select the single most appropriate diagnosis. Each option may be used once, more than once or not at all.

A 22-year-old man presents with multiple injuries following a fall from his motorcycle at high speed. Injuries identified include a significant head injury, splenic rupture and an open right tibial diaphyseal fracture. He undergoes urgent splenectomy, with wound debridement and intramedullary nailing of his tibial fracture. He returns to the intensive therapy unit intubated and ventilated on inotropic support. On day 2 postoperatively his oxygen and ventilator requirements increase and chest radiographs reveal diffuse fluffy pulmonary infiltrates with a $PaO_2/FiO_2 < 200$ mmHg.

A 74-year-old man presents with a sudden onset of abdominal pain radiating to the flanks. In the emergency department, he has a palpable abdominal mass, a tachycardia of 125 beats per minute, a blood pressure of 80/40 mmHg, a urine output of less than 5 mL/h, a respiratory rate of 35 breaths per minute, and is confused.

An 18-year-old man presents with an isolated femoral shaft fracture following a road traffic accident (passenger) and is placed in traction while waiting for definitive intramedullary nailing. On day 2 post-admission, he is reviewed on the pre-theatre ward and found to be confused, hypoxic, pyrexial and has developed a petechial rash over his anterior chest wall.

Theme: Trunk and neurological trauma

Options for Questions 4–7:

A Anterior cord syndrome	**F** Intracerebral haemorrhage
B Brown-Séquard syndrome	**G** Pneumothorax
C Central cord syndrome	**H** Subarachnoid haemorrhage
D Cardiac tamponade	**I** Subdural haemorrhage
E Extradural haemorrhage	**J** Tension pneumothorax

For each of the following cases, select the single most appropriate diagnosis. Each option may be used once, more than once or not at all.

4. A 48-year-old man with a background of alcohol excess presents following a fall whilst intoxicated. On examination, he is found to have substantial abrasions around the right side of his head, but with no other injuries found and is lucid wit a Glasgow coma score 14/15 (eye opening 4, verbal response 4, motor response 6) Following 2 hours in the emergency department, his score falls with an associated bradycardia and hypertension, and is found to have a fixed and dilated pupil on the right hand side.

5. A 32-year-old woman presents complaining of thoracic pain following a fall from horse whilst out riding. On examination, she is tender in the region of T6–T8 with evidence of swelling and bruising in this region. Imaging reveals compression fractures of T6 and T7 with impingement of the fragments on the vertebral canal. On detailed neurological assessment, she is found to have loss of power below the level of the fracture, with an associated loss of power and temperature sensation. Proprioception and touch remain intact.

6. A 24-year-old man presents following a penetrating wound to his anterior chest wall following an altercation. On examination, he is found to have 2 cm penetrating wound on the anterior chest wall in the region of the 5th intercostal space mid-clavicular line. He is a tachycardia with a pulse of 132 beats per minute, a blood pressure of 76/42 mmHg, with a raised jugular venous pressure and muffled heart sounds.

7. A 28-year-old woman presenting following a fall from a height of approximately 30 ft. On primary surgery she is found to have high oxygen requirements and cardiovascular instability with a raised jugular venous pressure, tracheal deviation to the right and diminished breath sounds on the left hand side of the chest. Radiological findings include multiple left sided rib fractures, a pelvic fracture, an open long bone fracture and a significant head injury.

heme: Orthopaedic trauma

ptions for Questions 8–10:

A	Cannulated screw fixation	H	Total hip replacement
B	Dynamic hip screw fixation	I	Traction
C	External fixation	J	Wound debridement and washout
D	Hip hemi-arthroplasty	K	Wound debridement and washout
E	Intramedullary fixation		with fracture fixation
F	Nonoperative treatment	L	Wound debridement, washout
G	Open reduction internal fixation		and closure with fracture fixation

or each of the following cases, select the single most appropriate management. Each ption may be used once, more than once or not at all.

A 31-year-old man presents with an open fracture of his right tibia following a direct blow from a horse to his right leg. On examination, there is 5 cm wound over the anteromedial aspect of his right leg with evidence of contamination. No distal neurovascular deficit is found.

A 48-year-old woman presents following a simple twisting injury to her left ankle. She has no past medical history of note and it is an isolated injury. On examination, it is a closed injury and she is neurovascularly intact. Anteroposterior and lateral radiographs of the left ankle reveal an undisplaced lateral malleolus fracture at the level of the syndesmosis, with no disruption of the ankle mortice.

0. A 78-year-old woman presents following a simple mechanical fall whilst out doing her shopping and is complaining of right sided hip pain and an inability to weight bear. She has a past medical history of osteoarthritis, hypertension, hypothyroidism and hyperlipidaemia. It is an isolated injury. On examination, her right lower limb is shortened and externally rotated. Radiographs demonstrate evidence of a right intertrochanteric neck of femur fracture with moderate to severe arthritic changes in the ipsilateral hip.

heme: Burns

ptions for Questions 11–12:

A	18% body surface area affected, 0.9 litres in first 24 hours	E	28% body surface area affected, 5 litres in first 24 hours
B	18% body surface area affected, 1.8 litres in first 24 hours	F	28% body surface area affected, 10 litres in first 24 hours
C	28% body surface area affected, 1.8 litres in first 24 hours	G	36% body surface area affected, 5 litres in first 24 hours
D	28% body surface area affected, 3.6 litres in first 24 hours	H	36% body surface area affected, 10 litres in first 24 hours

or each of the following cases, select the single most appropriate diagnosis and fluid esuscitation management (using the Parkland formula, excluding maintenance fluids). ach option may be used once, more than once or not at all.

11. A 28-year-old fit and well man presents after being trapped in a house fire. He is found to have burns to both arms (circumferential) and anterior torso. His weight is 70 kg and his height is 1.75 m. Current urine output is 15 mL/h.

12. A 4-year-old fit and well girl presents after jumping into a bath full of hot water. She is found to have circumferential burns to both legs. Her weight is 16 kg and her height is 1 m. Current urine output is 8 mL/h.

Answers

. A Acute respiratory distress syndrome

Acute respiratory distress syndrome is defined as the acute onset of severe refractory hypoxaemia following either direct or indirect injury to the lungs in the absence of evidence of cardiac failure. Two phases of injury are described with an acute inflammatory exudative phase (complement activation), followed by abnormalities in lung mechanics leading to decreased lung compliance. Potential causes include:

- Direct lung contusion, fat embolus, aspiration, inhalation injury, near drowning
- Indirect trauma, sepsis, burns, massive blood transfusion, pancreatitis, cardiac bypass

efined criteria for diagnosis include:

- Identified precipitating factor
- Acute onset of symptoms
- Refractory hypoxaemia
  - $PaO_2/FiO_2 < 200$ mmHg
  - $PaO_2/FiO_2 < 300$ mmHg = acute lung injury
- Absence of cardiac failure
  - Pulmonary artery wedge pressure <18 mmHg
- Bilateral diffuse 'fluffy' pulmonary infiltrates on chest radiograph

Management is supportive including ventilation with high positive end-expiratory pressure and steroids, along with treatment of the underlying cause. The mortality rate is 50–60%.

. F Class III hypovolaemic shock

Shock is defined as acute circulatory failure leading to inadequate tissue perfusion pressure, thus resulting in the inability to meet the metabolic requirements for aerobic cellular respiration. Types of shock include:

- Hypovolaemic (tachycardia, hypotensive)
- Cardiogenic (tachycardia, hypotensive)
- Neurogenic (bradycardia, hypotensive)
- Septic (tachycardia, hypotensive)
- Anaphylactic (tachycardia, hypotensive)

For trauma patients, hypovolaemic shock is most commonly seen. Hypovolaemic shock is classified as laid out in **Table 43.1**.

Table 43.1

	I	II	III	IV
Blood loss (mL)	< 750	750–1500	1500–2000	2000+
% blood volume (70 kg adult)	15	15–30	30–40	40+
Pulse rate (beats per minute)	< 100	>100	>120	140+
Blood pressure	↔	↔	↓	↓
Pulse pressure	↔	↓	↓	↓
Respiratory rate (breaths per minute)	14–20	20–30	30–40	> 40
Urine output (mL/h)	> 30	20–30	5–15	Anuric
CNS	Restless	Anxious	Anxious and confused	Confused and lethargic
Fluid required	Crystalloid	Crystalloid and colloid	Colloid and blood	Colloid and blood

Table 43.1 Classification of hypovolaemic shock.

## 3.	H Fat embolism syndrome

Fat embolism is a rare complication that can occur following a fracture of a long bones, e.g. femoral shaft fracture, soft tissue injury or burns. Early stabilisation of long bones fractures is preventative.

The pathogenesis is thought to be:

- Mechanical, with direct obstruction by microemboli (e.g. lipid globules from bone marrow adipocytes) of end organ capillaries, e.g. brain and lungs
- Metabolic, with the release of fatty acids and subsequent activation of the clotting cascade (e.g. platelets) and granulocyte activation, leading to endothelial vascular damage

The onset of symptoms and signs is commonly within the first week after injury, with a peak at 24–72 hours post injury. These are related to the organs affected but commonly include shortness of breath, hypoxia, tachycardia, pyrexia, agitation/delirium/coma, subconjunctival or retinal bleeds and a petechial haemorrhagic rash (axilla or chest wall). Blood tests reveal anaemia and thrombocytopenia, with urine and sputum analysis showing evidence of fatty infiltrates. Chest radiographs finding include pulmonary oedema and peripheral patchy consolidation. Management is supportive including ventilation (high positive end-expiratory pressure), fluids (albumin) and steroids. Complications include acute respiratory distress syndrome, with a mortality rate of 10–15%.

4. E Extradural haemorrhage

Patients who sustain significant head injuries may suffer from intracranial bleeding. This can be categorised into:

- Extracerebral (extradural, subdural, subarachnoid; **Table 43.2**)
- Intracerebral

Table 43.2

Type	Cause	Clinical presentation
Extradural	Bleed between skull and dura matter. Low energy trauma possible. Associated with fracture and subsequent injury to artery or dural venous sinus, e.g. middle meningeal artery injury secondary to temporal fracture.	Boggy swelling, e.g. in temporal region Concussion followed by lucid interval Rapid decline (↓Glasgow coma score, bradycardia, ↑blood pressure) Dilated ipsilateral pupil Contralateral hemiparesis CT appearance is a biconvex lens
Subdural	Bleed between dura matter and arachnoid. Associated with shearing injury to bridging veins. Chronic presentation in elderly patients after minor trauma, with better prognosis.	Initial injury Rapidly worsening headache and ↓ Glasgow coma score CT appearance is a crescent shape

Table 43.2 The contrasting presentations of extracerebral haemorrhages. Subarachnoid bleeds occur between the pia and arachnoid, presenting with headache, meningeal irritation and with blood (xanthochromia) present in the cerebrospinal fluid on lumbar puncture.

5. A Anterior cord syndrome

Injuries to the spinal cord can be classified as shown in **Table 43.3**.

6. D Cardiac tamponade

Cardiac tamponade (pericardial tamponade) is a trauma emergency and occurs when there is a rapid accumulation of fluid within the fibrous pericardial sac, leading ultimately to obstructive shock. The most common cause is a penetrating injury to the chest, with the left and right ventricle frequently injured. Clinical findings include:

- Tachycardia, tachypnoea, declining Glasgow coma score
- Beck's triad

Table 43.3

Category	Cause	Clinical presentation
Complete cord	Complete transection of spinal cord	Total irreversible paralysis and loss of sensory distal to level
Anterior cord	Involvement of the corticospinal and spinothalamic tracts with preservation of the dorsal columns	Loss of motor function below level (corticospinal tract)
		Loss of pain and temperature below level (spinothalamic tract)
	Associated with anterior spinal artery occlusion, anterior dislocations, disc herniation, vertebral compression fractures	Touch and proprioception remain intact (dorsal columns)
Posterior cord	Involvement of the dorsal columns only	Loss of touch and proprioception with ataxia
	Hyperextension injuries, posterior vertebral fractures, posterior spinal artery occlusion	Pain, power and temperature intact below level
Central cord	Spinothalamic and corticospinal involvement	Loss of pain and temperature below level. Loss of upper limb power
	Associated with trauma in young patients, elderly patients with cervical spondylosis, syringomyelia, spinal tumours	Some preservation lower limb sensation and power
		Touch and proprioception remain intact (late involvement only)
Brown–Séquard	Lateral cord hemisection or mass with ipsilateral pyramidal tract and dorsal column involvement	Loss of power and proprioception below lesion on ipsilateral side
	Associated with penetrating injuries, tumours affecting one side, infection, multiple sclerosis	Loss of pain and temperature below level on contralateral side

Table 43.3 Classification of spinal cord injuries.

- Hypotension (↓ stroke volume), raised jugular venous pressure (impaired venous return), muffled heart sounds (blood in pericardial sac)
- Pulsus paradoxus
  - ↓ ≥10 mmHg in blood pressure on inspiration
- Kussmaul's sign
  - Raised jugular venous pressure on inspiration

- ECG
  - Small amplitude QRS complexes, ST segment change
- ECHO
  - Small or collapsed ventricle, distended pericardium

Without urgent treatment with pericardiocentesis, pulseless electrical activity arrest will result.

J Tension pneumothorax

A pneumothorax occurs when there is air within the pleural cavity. A tension pneumothorax occurs when there is a 'one way valve' at the site of air entry into the pleural cavity, where air is entering the pleural cavity on inspiration (valve open), but with no expulsion of air on expiration (valve closed).

Clinical findings include:

- Tachycardia, raised jugular venous pressure, hypotension, tachypnoea, hypoxia,
- Ipsilateral signs
  - Diminished breath sounds, hyper-resonance, expanded, decreased movement
- Chest X-ray
  - Lung collapse, trachea deviated away from side of injury

Without urgent needle decompression, pulseless electrical activity arrest will result. Decompression involves insertion of a large bore cannula in the second intercostal space (mid-clavicular line) on the affected side, followed by chest drain insertion.

K Wound debridement and washout with fracture fixation

The Gustilo–Anderson classification of open fractures is:

- I: wound less than 1 cm, clean, minimal soft tissue damage, no periosteal stripping
- II: wound greater than 1 cm, moderate soft tissue damage, no periosteal stripping
- IIIA: extensive soft tissue damage, periosteal stripping, but adequate coverage no flap needed
- IIIB: extensive soft tissue damage, periosteal stripping, inadequate coverage and flap needed, massive contamination
- IIIC: open fracture associated with arterial injury requiring repair

Irrespective of the size of the wound or soft tissue damage, some injuries are classified as a grade III, e.g. high-energy, segmental fracture, traumatic amputation, heavy contamination (e.g. farm injuries, gunshot wounds).

Assessment of and management of open fractures includes:

- Initial assessment following advanced trauma life support guidelines
- Immediate management
  - Photograph, wound lavage, iodine-soaked gauze and sterile dressing
  - Reduction of fracture if required, e.g. for skin compromise or neurovascular compromise
  - Immobilisation
  - Antibiotics +/– tetanus

- Theatre
  - For open fractures, urgent exploration, washout and debridement is considered best practice, although the timing is open to controversy
  - Adequate debridement involves extending the wound, debridement of all contaminated or devitalised tissues, delivering of the fracture ends and copious lavage (e.g. 9–10 L of saline)
  - Stabilisation of the fracture, either temporary (e.g. external fixation) or definitive (e.g. intramedullary nail) is normally carried out at the primary surgery
  - The wound is routinely left open, with a return to theatre for further assessment (e.g. delayed closure, further debridement, consideration of flap coverage) 48 hours later

9. F Nonoperative treatment

The ankle joint is a hinge type mortice joint with an articulation between the body of the talus and the distal aspects of the tibia (tibial plafond and medial malleolus) and fibula (lateral malleolus). Injuries commonly occur following a twisting mechanism. On examination there is tenderness, swelling and ecchymosis over the lateral and/or medial sides of the ankle joint. Integrity of the skin may be compromised and urgent reduction should be carried out if found. Assessment of neurovascular status is essential.

Classification of ankle fractures is with the AO–Weber classification using anteroposterior and lateral radiographs of the ankle joint. The classification is:

- Weber A: Horizontal avulsion fracture of lateral malleolus below the level of the syndesmosis
- Weber B: Fracture of the lateral malleolus at the level of the syndesmosis
- Weber C: Fracture of the lateral malleolus above the level of the syndesmosis

This classification can help guide treatment. Isolated Weber A fractures are stable injuries and can be treated nonoperatively. Isolated stable Weber B fractures, with no evidence of medial ligament disruption (undisplaced ankle mortice on radiographs) can be treated nonoperatively. Unstable Weber B and Weber C fractures or best treated with open reduction and internal fixation.

10. B Dynamic hip screw fixation

Proximal femoral fractures frequently occur following a low energy fall in elderly osteoporotic women. The mean age at the time of injury is approximately 80 years of age and almost a third of patients die within the first year following fracture. Fractures of the hip can be classified according to disruption of the capsular blood supply to the femoral head:

- Intracapsular or subcapital
- Extracapsular
  - Intertrochanteric
  - Subtrochanteric

Intracapsular neck of femur fractures is commonly classified according to the Garden classification:

- Garden I: incomplete or valgus impacted fracture

- Garden II: complete undisplaced fracture
- Garden III: complete fracture with partial displacement but contact between fracture fragments
- Garden IV: complete fracture with total displacement

Treatment of proximal femoral fractures is described in **Figure 43.1**. Undisplaced intracapsular hip fractures are routinely managed with fixation. Consideration of co-morbidities including osteoporosis and alcohol excess in patients less than 60 years of age with displaced intracapsular hip fractures is needed as some may be better managed with a hip arthroplasty.

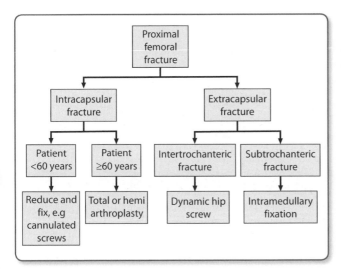

Figure 43.1 A management algorithm for proximal femoral fractures.

1. H 36% body surface area affected, 10 litres in first 24 hours

Two arms = 18%, anterior torso = 18%, total 36% body surface. Fluids = 4 mL x 36 x 70 = 10.08 L. (See details under answer 12, below.)

2. C 28% body surface area affected, 1.8 litres in first 24 hours

Burns can be classified according to type, depth, severity and surface area. Types of burns include:

- **Thermal burns**, which are most frequently seen and are commonly due to hot liquids or gases.
- **Chemical burns** are caused by strong acids or alkalis, e.g. sodium hydroxide, sulphuric acid, hydrofluoric acid. Alkali burns are known to be more severe.
- **Radiation burns** are caused by exposure to radiofrequency energy, e.g. sunlight, or ionising radiation, e.g. radiotherapy.
- **Electrical burns**, e.g. following an electric shock.

How the depth of burns is determined is shown in **Table 43.4**.

The assessment of surface area is according the rule of nines:

- Adults
  - 9% for head (4.5% anterior, 4.5% posterior)
  - 9% for each arm (4.5% anterior, 4.5% posterior)
  - 18% for each leg (9% anterior, 9% posterior)
  - 36% for torso (18% anterior, 18% posterior)
- Children
  - 18% for head (9% anterior, 9% posterior)
  - 9% for each arm (4.5% anterior, 4.5% posterior)
  - 14% for each leg (7% anterior, 7% posterior)
  - 36% for torso (18% anterior, 18% posterior)

The size of a patient's hand is defined as 1% of their total body surface area (TBSA). Burns of ≥10% TBSA in children or ≥15% in adults are consider major and potentially life-threatening. The American Burn Association defines burns to mild, moderate or severe depending on age, types, depth, body surface area and associated features.

The management of burns follow the ABCDE assessment with consideration for airway burns and compromise, hypovolaemic shock, burns care, analgesia and if

Table 43.4

Category	Clinical presentation	Time to repair and complications
Superficial	Involves only the epidermis and is painful, dry with associated erythema.	Repair is within 7 days Complications are very rare
Superficial partial thickness	Involves the epidermis and superficial dermis and is painful, moist, erythematous (blanching) and often associated with blisters.	Repair is within 14–21 days Local infection or cellulitis
Deep partial thickness	Involves the epidermis, superficial dermis and deep dermis. The burns are painful and moist with a pink-white appearance that has minimal blanching. Associated with blisters that may be blood filled.	Repair is within 1 month Local infection or cellulitis Contractures Scarring/skin grafting
Full thickness	Involves the epidermis and all of the dermis. The burns are painless and dry with a stiff black-white. Minimal/no sensation over affected area.	Require debridement/excision Local infection or cellulitis Contractures Scarring/skin grafting Amputation

Table 43.4 Assessment of the severity of burns according to depth.

necessary surgery. Intravenous fluid resuscitation in the first 24 hours is often guided by the Parkland formula (or equivalent):

= 4 mL x (percentage of TBSA) x weight in kilograms.

NB: 50% of the volume calculated should be given over the first 8 hours, with the remainder given over the subsequent 16 hours.

Chapter 44

Principles of surgical oncology

Theme: Aetiology of malignant tumours

Options for Questions 1–3:

A   Chemical carcinogens
B   Fungal and plant toxins
C   Genetic inheritance
D   Infections
E   Physical carcinogens

For each of the following situations, select the single most likely aetiology. Each option may be used once, more than once or not at all.

1. An 8-year-old boy, a recent arrival from Uganda, has been brought by his parents with a swelling arising from his cheek of 3 weeks duration. This is painful. When the child was much younger, he had suffered from malaria. On examination, he has a diffuse, tender, inflamed looking lump over his right maxilla.

2. A 55-year-old man has been referred to the one-stop haematuria clinic with periodic, profuse and painless haematuria for the past 2 months. On examination, there are no physical findings except for slight anaemia.

3. A 50-year-old man complains of anorexia, weight loss, upper abdominal pain and occasional vomiting. On oesophagogastroduodenoscopy he has a fungating mass in the pylorus from which biopsies have been taken.

Theme: Pathological types of malignant tumours

Options for Questions 4–6:

A   Adenocarcinoma
B   Basal cell carcinoma
C   Malignant melanoma
D   Osteosarcoma
E   Soft tissue sarcoma
F   Squamous cell carcinoma
G   Teratoma
H   Transitional cell carcinoma

For each of the following situations, select the single most likely pathological diagnosis. Each option may be used once, more than once or not at all.

4. A 35-year-old woman complains of a mole over her left shoulder region. She noticed that recently it has become itchy and has started bleeding. She would like it removed because of blood-staining of her clothes.

5. A 60-year-old man complains of haematuria in the form of passing clots and pain in his right loin for the past 4 months. On examination, he looks anaemic and has a mass in his right loin which moves with respiration, is bimanually palpable and ballotable.

6. A 65-year-old man underwent removal of a lump from the front of his left thigh. After 6 months a similar lump at the same site has returned. On examination, he has a firm, fairly fixed lump arising from the muscles of his thigh.

Theme: Tumour markers

Options for Questions 7–9:

A	α-fetoprotein	D	Cancer antigen 125
B	β-human chorionic gonadotrophin	E	Carcinoembryonic antigen
		F	Erythropoietin
C	Calcitonin	G	Prostate specific antigen

For each of the following situations, select the single most suitable tumour marker. Each option may be used once, more than once or not at all.

7. A 25-year-old man complains of a hard lump in his right testicle, which he found as he felt a sense of heaviness in his scrotum. Ultrasound of the testis showed a solid lump and in the abdomen a solid firm mass was felt in the umbilical region.

8. A 62-year-old man complains of increasing constipation. A barium enema showed a shouldered deformity in his upper descending colon. Colonoscopic biopsy showed a well-differentiated adenocarcinoma and the liver was free of secondaries. He is due to undergo a radical left hemicolectomy.

9. A 55-year-old woman complains of gradual painless abdominal distension, malaise and weakness. On examination, she has shifting dullness and fluid thrill. On abdominal ultrasound ascites are confirmed and she has bilateral solid ovarian masses about 6 cm in diameter.

Theme: Systemic effects of cancer

Options for Questions 10–12:

A	Anaemia	E	Endocrine syndromes
B	Amyloidosis	F	Polycythaemia
C	Cachexia	G	Pyrexia
D	Cutaneous manifestations	H	Venous thrombosis

For each of the following situations, select the single most suitable type of systemic effect. Each option may be used once, more than once or not at all.

10. A 70-year-old man complains of anorexia, weakness and intermittent vomiting. An urgent oesophagogastroduodenoscopy and biopsy was carried out which showed a mucin-producing carcinoma of the pyloric antrum.

. A 58-year-old man complains of gradual weight loss over 4 months. He has anorexia with epigastric dull ache radiating to the back. He gets some relief from his pain by leaning forwards whilst sitting up in bed. On examination, there is nothing to find except evidence of weight loss in the form of ill-fitting loose clothes.

. A 50-year-old man, a heavy smoker of many years, complains of cough with streaks of blood in his sputum for 4 months. He also complains of pain in the right side of his chest. A chest X-ray shows a large shadow in the mid-zone of his right lung. His family has noticed that he has become obese, particularly swollen facial features. His doctor found that recently he has become a type 2 diabetic.

heme: Palliation in malignant disease

ptions for Questions 13–15:

A	Adjuvant therapy	E	Radiotherapy
B	Chemotherapy	F	Stenting
C	Drugs and medical treatment	G	Surgery
D	Interventional radiology		

r each of the following situations, select the single most suitable palliative ocedure. Each option may be used once, more than once or not at all.

3. A 75-year-old man has channel transurethral resection of prostate for cancer prostate with bladder outflow obstruction. At the time of diagnosis he was found to have sclerotic bone secondaries in his lumbar vertebrae and pelvis. His prostate-specific antigen is raised.

4. A 60-year-old woman presents with quite severe features of carcinoid syndrome in the form of flushing, explosive watery diarrhoea, colicky abdominal pain and episodic sudden attacks of shortness of breath. She has a much raised urinary 5-hydroxyindoleacetic acid and liver ultrasound shows multiple solid tumours. Almost 6 years ago she underwent a right hemicolectomy for an ileal carcinoid tumour.

5. An 80-year-old man complains of intense pruritus. His family noticed that he is extremely icteric and his urine very dark yellow. On abdominal examination, he has a smooth, globular mass in the right hypochondrium and an enlarged liver.

heme: Cancer screening

ptions for Questions 16–18:

A	Barium enema	E	Oesophagogastroduodenoscpy
B	Colonoscopy	F	Smear test
C	Faecal occult blood testing	G	Tumour markers
D	Genetic screening		

r each of the following situations, select the single most suitable cancer screening odality. Each option may be used once, more than once or not at all.

16. A 30-year-old woman, who is completely asymptomatic has an elder brother who underwent an extended right hemicolectomy for Dukes stage B transverse colon carcinoma. Their father died from liver secondaries at the age of 68 years after an anterior resection at the age of 65 years.

17. A 35-year-old woman is concerned about her family history of breast cancer. Her mother died of secondaries from breast cancer at the age of 62 years. She has a sister who had breast cancer diagnosed and treated at the age of 42 years.

18. A 50-year-old woman has suffered from ulcerative colitis for 10 years during which time she has been on medical treatment with mesalazine, intermittent steroids and azathioprine. At present she has two to three bowel actions a day with some blood and mucus, a clinical situation which is no different over the last year or so.

Answers

D Infections

This young boy, a recent immigrant from Uganda, has Burkitt's lymphoma caused by infection with Epstein–Barr virus (EBV). This is a human herpesvirus that is widely found in humans all over the world. Adults develop antibodies to it. EBV infects B lymphocytes converting them into lymphoblasts. This conversion initially manifests as infectious mononucleosis. The B-lymphocyte proliferation stimulated by EBV is controlled by suppressor T cells. Chronic malaria prevents an adequate T-cell response causing uncontrolled B-cell proliferation leading to the development of lymphoma. The sequence of events forming the tumour could be summarised as: EBV infection → B lymphocytes into lymphoblasts → infectious mononucleosis → superimposed malarial infection → inadequate suppressor T-cell response → proliferation of a malignant clone of B cells → Burkitt's lymphoma.

Nasopharyngeal carcinoma is also ascribed to EBV.

A Chemical carcinogens

This patient has urinary bladder cancer unless otherwise proven. The aetiology is a chemical carcinogen, aromatic amines and azo dyes. Workers in the aniline dye, leather, rubber, paint and organic chemical industries are highly susceptible to urinary bladder cancer. Polycyclic hydrocarbons from cigarette smoke are an important risk factor of urinary bladder carcinoma as is β-naphthylamine to which dye industry workers are exposed. The aromatic amines and azo dyes are metabolised in the liver to form hydroxylamino derivative; these are then detoxified by conjugation with glucuronic acid. In the bladder, hydrolysis of glucuronide releases hydroxylamine causing DNA damage to the urothelial cell and cancer.

D Infections

This patient has a carcinoma of the stomach, the cause of which in the vast majority is *H. pylori* infection. In gastric cancer patients there is a high incidence of *H. pylori* infection found serologically many years before the onset of the disease. Patients who are seropositive for *H. pylori* are 3 times more likely to develop the condition. The organism affects almost 70% of the world's population. In some parts of the world almost 9 out of 10 in the population are infected. It is thought to cause atrophic gastritis, peptic ulceration, mucosa-associated lymphoid tissue tumours (MALTomas) and cancer. The stomach is the most common site of extra-nodal lymphoma. Most gastric lymphomas are B-cell tumours and have been known to regress after eradication of *H. pylori* infection.

C Malignant melanoma

This patient's history and description of the lesion is typical of a malignant melanoma which is a neoplasm arising from the melanocytes. Exposure to sun and persistent sunburn is associated with this condition; therefore, ultra-violet radiation is the responsible physical carcinogen. Malignant melanoma occurs mostly in white-skinned people. The skin of darker races is protected from the harmful effects of ultraviolet radiation by the greater amount of melanin.

The changes in the skin lesion that makes one suspect transformation into malignant melanoma can be summarised as **ABCDE:** geometrical **A**symmetry in two axes, irregular **B**order, lesion showing at least 2 different **C**olours, maximum **D**iameter >6 mm and **E**levation of lesion. The types of malignant melanoma are:

- Superficial spreading (70%)
- Nodular melanoma (15%)
- Lentigo maligna melanoma (5–10%)
- Acral lentiginous melanoma (2–8% in white-skinned, more common in the dark-skinned)

5. A Adenocarcinoma

This patient has the classical triad of an adenocarcinoma of the kidney – pain in the loin, haematuria and a loin mass. The mass has the features of an enlarged kidney – moving with respiration, bimanually palpable and ballotable. Sometimes, the patient may present from a secondary: an epileptic seizure from a cerebral secondary, haemoptysis from pulmonary secondary, or bone pain and/or pathological fracture from a skeletal metastasis in a long bone. The tumour is an adenocarcinoma arising from the tubular epithelial cells. The macroscopic appearance is that of a solid, yellow mass with cystic and haemorrhagic areas with necrosis (**Figure 44.1**); microscopically it is a clear cell carcinoma because of the presence of abundant glycogen.

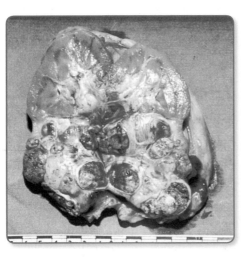

Figure 44.1 Adenocarcinoma of the kidney.

6. E Soft tissue sarcoma

This man has a soft tissue sarcoma because he has a recurrent firm, fairly fixed lump arising from the muscles of the thigh (**Figure 44.2**). The tumour may originate from

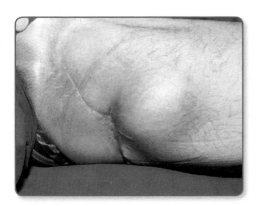

Figure 44.2 Soft tissue sarcoma.

connective tissue, muscle, fascia, periosteum or tendons. The tumour is well-demarcated with areas of necrosis and haemorrhage. Microscopically there are haphazardly arranged fibroblasts with dark, irregular, elongated nuclei of variable size. A magnetic resonance imaging is done followed by an incision biopsy to confirm the diagnosis. Excision of the tumour and reconstruction is carried out aided by frozen section to make sure that all tumour tissue has been removed. These tumours must be managed in a tertiary cancer centre.

A α-Fetoprotein

This young man has a solid mass in his testicle which is a testicular tumour. In view of his age, this is most likely a teratoma (non-seminomatous germ cell tumour). The tumour marker is α-fetoprotein (AFP). Blood should be sent to estimate this as soon as the diagnosis is suspected. The abdominal mass is a pre- and para-aortic group of lymph node secondaries. With such a clinical picture elevation of AFP is almost certain. The tumor marker level also helps in the staging of the tumour. T1M staging indicates that there are no secondaries but elevated marker level. Having done the tumour marker level preoperatively, it should be repeated shortly after orchidectomy. There is a protocol for follow-up at which this is repeated. If levels are elevated, secondaries should be sought on chest X-ray and CT of the abdomen and liver.

E Carcinoembryonic antigen

Carcinoembryonic antigen is the tumour marker that should be routinely carried out in colorectal carcinoma. It should be done as a baseline prior to surgery, in this radical left hemicolectomy. Thereafter, it is repeated at every follow-up. Elevated levels should alert one to the possibility of secondaries particularly in the liver or a recurrence or a metachronous carcinoma. Investigations should be carried out to look for recurrence and appropriate management instituted.

Carcinoembryonic antigen is also a tumour marker in medullary carcinoma of thyroid and mucinous adenocarcinoma of pancreas.

9. D Cancer antigen 125

This woman has bilateral ovarian carcinoma. The tumour marker in this condition is cancer antigen (CA) 125. This is an ovarian cancer related protein used routinely to help recognise early recurrence. CA 125 is detectable in about 50% of epithelial tumours confined to the ovary and about 90% of those that have disseminated.

A tumour marker is a circulating biochemical substance that can be detected in the cells or in the body fluids indicative of a malignant neoplasm. A marker is most useful when it is specific, sensitive and proportional to the tumour load. They are useful to screen, diagnose, assess prognosis, follow response to treatment and monitor for recurrence. Various types are known (**Table 44.1**).

Table 44.1

Type of tumour	Use(s) of tumour marker
Gastrointestinal	· Carcinoembryonic antigen in colorectal cancer
Hepatobiliary	· α-fetoprotein in hepatoma
Genitourinary	· Erythropoietin in Wilms' tumour
	· Prostate-specific antigen in prostate cancer
	In testicular tumours:
	· β-human chorionic gonadotropin
	· α-fetoprotein
Endocrine	· Calcitonin in medullary thyroid carcinoma
	· Other endocrine tumours
Gynaecology	· CA 125 in ovarian cancer

Table 44.1 Use of tumour markers.

10. H Venous thrombosis

Armand Trousseau, a French Physician, described venous thromboembolism and thrombophlebitis in him as he died from pancreatic cancer, although he thought he had gastric cancer. Venous thrombosis in the leg in gastric cancer is therefore referred to as Trousseau's sign. In pancreatic cancer and in gastric mucinous adenocarcinoma a hypercoagulable state exists which commonly leads to venous thromboembolism in the deep veins of the leg, often a cause of death from pulmonary embolism.

11. C Cachexia

This patient has weight loss, anorexia and backache relieved by bending forward. This is very suggestive of a carcinoma of the body of the pancreas; by bending forward the patient tries to relieve pressure on the coeliac plexus by the growth. Cachexia is a classical presentation of pancreatic cancer probably brought on by their decreased caloric intake from anorexia and abnormalities of taste. The diminished food intake does not always explain the significant wasting. This is thought to be due to tumour necrosis factor-α) and cytokines (interferons, interleukin-6) producing a wasting syndrome.

2. E Endocrine syndromes

This patient has all the features of a carcinoma of the right lung. The clinical features noticed by his family are suggestive of Cushing's syndrome, a diagnosis strengthened by the recent onset of diabetes. Small cell lung carcinoma, also known as 'oat cell' carcinoma, accounts for about one-fifth of all bronchogenic cancers. This is a highly malignant epithelial tumour often demonstrating paraneoplastic syndromes due to the ectopic secretion of adrenocorticotropic hormone, resulting in the cushingoid appearance with hypokalaemia, hyperglycaemia, hypertension and weakness.

3. E Radiotherapy

This patient has pain from bony secondaries from his cancer prostate which is being palliated locally by channel transurethral resection of prostate. This is also corroborated by his raised prostate-specific antigen. He should be palliated by radiotherapy to his lumbar vertebrae and pelvis. He should that not relieve his pain or there is recurrent pain in future, bilateral subcapsular orchidectomy is an option.

4. D Interventional radiology

This woman has classical carcinoid syndrome from multiple hepatic secondaries. The diagnosis is strongly supported by a raised urinary 5-hydroxyindoleacetic acid which confirms secondaries. The enzyme serotonin elaborated from the secondaries cause very distressing symptoms. The ideal palliative treatment is interventional radiology and hepatic artery embolisation. This renders the secondaries ischaemic, thereby making them non-functional.

5. F Stenting

This elderly man is extremely bothered by pruritus as a result of obstructive jaundice from a carcinoma of the head of the pancreas. Normally, the icterus does not bother the patient as much as his family members. He is not suitable for resection. The ideal palliation is endoscopic retrograde insertion of a stent into his common bile duct. Rarely, if this is not possible for technical reasons, the second option would be to do a cholecystojejunostomy and a gastrojejunostomy to prevent gastric outlet obstruction in future.

16. B Colonoscopy

This 30-year-old woman should be offered regular colonoscopic surveillance (at least annually). She belongs to a family with hereditary non-polyposis colorectal cancer. This is an autosomal dominant inherited disease accounting for 3–5% of all large bowel cancers. The clinical features of these patients are: onset at a young age, colon proximal to splenic flexure mostly affected, may have synchronous cancers and may develop extracolonic cancers – of the endometrium, ovary, stomach, and hepatobiliary tract and transitional carcinoma of the upper urinary tract.

17. D Genetic screening

This woman has a strong family history of breast cancer with two first degree relatives suffering from the condition. This risk is enhanced if the relatives had the disease at a young age or had bilateral disease. *BRCA1* (breast cancer-1) and *BRCA2* are the two high-risk genes that account for 20–50% of these cancers. *BRCA1* and *BRCA2* are tumour suppressor genes that are important in repair of DNA and regulation of mitotic phases. Mutations in these genes create the instability in cells of the breast and ovary encouraging the formation of cancer. Hence this woman should be offered genetic screening. If the patient proves to be 'gene positive' she could be given the choice of bilateral prophylactic mastectomy.

18. B Colonoscopy

As this woman has suffered from ulcerative colitis for 10 years, she has an enhanced chance of developing colorectal cancer. She should be subjected to annual colonoscopic surveillance and biopsy. Those that have high grade dysplasia should have the colon removed to prevent cancer. This risk is higher when the disease starts at a young age, when there is a very severe first attack and if the entire colon is involved. Often there may be a synchronous colon cancer when it occurs in ulcerative colitis.

Chapter 45

The abdomen

Theme: Abdominal pain

Options for Questions 1–2:

A   Carcinoma of stomach
B   Chronic cholecystitis
C   Chronic pancreatitis

D   Duodenal ulcer
E   Gastro-oesophageal reflux disease

For each of the following situations, select the single most likely diagnosis. Each option may be used once, more than once or not at all.

1   A 50-year-old woman complains of epigastric pain radiating to the back associated with heartburn of 4 months' duration. The pain does not have any regular pattern and not specifically related to food. She feels occasionally nauseous and is rarely sick. She has water brash and suffers from cough although she is not a smoker. On examination, she is overweight and has signs of basal crepitus in her lungs.

2   A 40-year-old man complains of epigastric pain radiating to the right upper quadrant for the last 6 months. He has noticed that the pain comes on a couple of hours or so after having had a meal. He has found that he gets relief by drinking milk and eating biscuits. Occasionally, he is woken up at night by his abdominal pain and again gets relief by either eating biscuits or drinking milk. He has put on some weight during this time. There are no physical findings.

Theme: Abdominal masses

Options for Questions 3–4:

A   Abdominal aortic aneurysm
B   Carcinoma of ascending colon
C   Carcinoma of stomach

D   Hydronephrosis
E   Mucocele of the gallbladder

For each of the following situations, select the single most likely diagnosis. Each option may be used once, more than once or not at all.

3   A 55-year-old woman suffered from an acute abdominal pain 6 weeks ago which was associated with nausea and vomiting. The pain lasted for 3 days during which time she was treated at home by her general practitioner with analgesics and anti-emetics. The pain subsided and subsequently she was referred to the surgical outpatient clinic. She was found to be pain free but abdominal examination showed a globular, non-tender mass in the right upper quadrant moving with respiration.

4. A 65-year-old man complains of recent shortness of breath whilst going about his daily routine activities for the last 2 months. On examination, he looks pale and abdominal examination reveals a mass in the right lumbar region which is mobile and non-tender.

Theme: The acute abdomen

Options for Questions 5–6:

A   Acute appendicitis
B   Acute biliary colic
C   Acute pancreatitis

D   Leaking abdominal aortic aneurysm
E   Perforated peptic ulcer

For each of the following situations, select the single most likely diagnosis. Each option may be used once, more than once or not at all.

5. A 70-year-old man complains of sudden onset of very severe abdominal pain radiating to the back and left side of the abdomen of 4 hours duration. He has a distended abdomen with a blood pressure of 90/60 mmHg, pulse rate of 120 beats per minute is cold and clammy and looks pale. Abdominal examination shows a grossly distended abdomen more on the left side with tenderness and guarding.

6. A 45-year-old man complains of sudden onset of severe epigastric pain radiating to the back of 6 hours duration. The pain has gradually spread to the rest of the abdomen and now has pain in his right shoulder tip. On examination, he has thoracic respiration, and the abdomen shows board-like rigidity.

Theme: Intestinal obstruction

Options for Questions 7–8:

A   Gallstone ileus
B   Incarcerated femoral hernia
C   Large intestinal obstruction from left colonic carcinoma

D   Upper small intestinal obstruction from adhesions
E   Volvulus of the sigmoid colon

For each of the following situations, select the single most likely diagnosis. Each option may be used once, more than once or not at all.

7. A 78-year-old man from the geriatric medical ward has been referred with gradual abdominal distension, particularly on the left side of almost a week's duration. His last bowel movement was 5 days ago. He complains of generalised abdominal pain. On examination, he is short of breath from his distended abdomen. His blood pressure is 110/80 mmHg and pulse is 100 beats per minute. The abdomen tympanitic; rectal examination reveals an empty ballooned rectum.

8. A 65-year-old woman complains of colicky abdominal pain, distension and vomiting of 36 hours duration. The vomitus is bile-stained to start with, but over the last 6

hours has become faeculent. On examination, she is dehydrated with a distended abdomen and a tender lump in her right groin below the inguinal ligament.

Theme: Peritonitis and abdominal and pelvic abscess

Options for Questions 9–10:

Acute perforated appendicitis   D Perforated diverticulitis
Pelvic abscess   E Subphrenic abscess
Pelvic inflammatory disease

For each of the following situations, select the single most likely diagnosis. Each option may be used once, more than once or not at all.

A 70-year-old woman complains of sudden onset of severe lower abdominal pain spreading to the entire lower half of abdomen of 6 hours duration. She has been suffering from constipation for several months prior to this acute episode. On examination she has septic shock with tenderness, rigidity and rebound tenderness all over her lower abdomen.

A 50-year-old woman underwent a laparoscopic closure of a perforated duodenal ulcer one week ago. Immediately following the operation she progressed satisfactorily for 4–5 days. After that she developed swinging pyrexia, complaining of pain in her right shoulder tip. She is breathless and tender in the right upper quadrant. A chest X-ray shows right pleural effusion.

Theme: Gastrointestinal haemorrhage

Options for Questions 11–12:

Aortoenteric fistula   D Mallory–Weiss syndrome
Bleeding peptic ulcer   E Oesophageal varices
Leiomyoma of stomach

For each of the following situations, select the single most likely diagnosis. Each option may be used once, more than once or not at all.

A 60-year-old man, a smoker, has been admitted as an emergency with sudden-onset severe acute haematemesis preceded by a few days of loose black stools. He has suffered on and off for years with indigestion for which he self-medicated. Recently, he took some nonsteroidal anti-inflammatory drugs for his arthritic knee. On examination he has features of hypovolaemic shock.

A 70-year-old man has been brought to the emergency department with sudden-onset severe acute haematemesis in the form of clots. He has hypovolaemic shock. On abdominal examination he has a well-healed mid-line scar extending from the xiphisternum to the pubic symphysis for an elective abdominal aortic aneurysm operation 6 years ago.

Theme: Hernia

Options for Questions 13–14:

A   Epigastric hernia

B   Femoral hernia

C   Incisional hernia

D   Inguinal hernia

E   Obturator hernia

For each of the following situations, select the single most likely diagnosis. Each option may be used once, more than once or not at all.

13.   A 68-year-old man complains of discomfort in his lower abdomen of 8 months duration. His discomfort dates back to the finding of a lump in his right groin which is slightly tender. On examination, he has a 3–4 cm lump at the medial end of his inguinal ligament. This lump is mobile, slightly tender, not reducible, situated below the inguinal ligament and lateral to the pubic tubercle.

14.   A 65-year-old woman complains of pain in her left knee of about 6 months duration. The pain starts in the groin and radiates down the inner side of the thigh and is made worse on coughing or any form of straining. On examination, she looks in some discomfort in her left groin and finds relief from the pain when she keeps her hip flexed, abducted and externally rotated. There is fullness under the pectineus muscle where a cough impulse can be felt.

Answers

. E Gastro-oesophageal reflux disease

This 50 year old woman has abdominal pain with heartburn, water brash and features of chest infection – tell tale features of gastro-oesophageal reflux disease. Her chest infection is due to aspiration of stomach contents from reflux. She needs an oesophagogastroduodenoscopy to see the degree of reflux and oesophagitis, look for any shortening of the oesophagus, and biopsies taken to look for dysplasia. There are various grades of oesophagitis, the commonest being streaks of mucosal inflammation (**Figure 45.1**). Initially she should be on medical treatment. This should be followed by regular endoscopies and a biopsy to make sure that the condition is healing and there is no metaplasia and dysplasia.

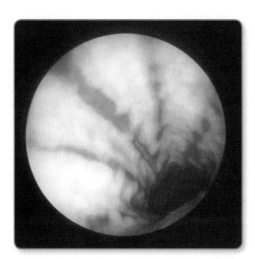

Figure 45.1
Oesophagogastrodudenoscopy showing streaks of mucosal inflammation from gastro-oesophageal reflux disease.

. D Duodenal ulcer

This man has the typical symptoms of a patient with duodenal ulcer – upper abdominal and right upper quadrant pain which comes on when he has an empty stomach. He eats in between meals to get relief from his pain. This has resulted in his gaining weight. The only physical finding is some tenderness over the region of the duodenum. He needs an oesophagogastroduodenoscopy and a urease test to confirm *Helicobacter pylori*, as well as a biopsy. While awaiting the results he should be started on the full course of anti-*Helicobacter pylori* treatment. After the course of treatment he should be re-endoscoped to make sure that the ulcer has healed.

. E Mucocele of the gallbladder

This woman had an attack of biliary colic 6 weeks ago. The pain subsided after 3 days of conservative treatment at home. On referral to the surgical outpatient she is found to have a globular mass in the right upper quadrant which moves with respiration – a typical finding of a distended gallbladder which is painless. This is pathognomonic of a mucocele of the gallbladder. This is produced by a gallstone impacted at the mouth of the cystic duct thereby obstructing it. The gallbladder cannot empty the bile; it distends due to the secretion of mucus – hence the name mucocele. The gallbladder wall is thinned and the bile is replaced by white mucus (**Figure 45.2**). The patient requires an ultrasound to confirm the diagnosis followed by a laparoscopic cholecystectomy.

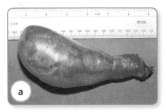
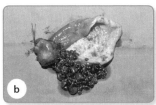

Figure 45.2 Mucocele of gallbladder.
(a) Unopened mucocele and (b) the same gallbladder, opened specimen, showing clear mucus and no green bile

4. B Carcinoma of ascending colon

This man has a carcinoma of the ascending colon. He has typical symptoms of anaemia – undue shortness of breath from daily normal activities. On examination, he has a mass in the region of the ascending colon. Anaemia is a classical elective clinical presentation of right-sided colonic carcinoma. This is because of chronic bleeding resulting in iron deficiency anmia. The patient would have low haemoglobin, his stools would be positive for faecal occult blood and a barium enema would show a typical apple-core deformity or an irregular filling defect (**Figure 45.3**). After confirmation, staging and bowel preparation he should undergo a radical right hemicolectomy.

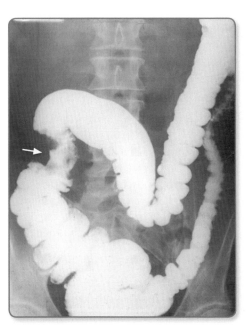

Figure 45.3 Barium enema showing irregular filling defect in ascending colon (arrow), typical of polypoid carcinoma.

D Leaking abdominal aortic aneurysm

This 70-year-old man has had an acute abdominal catastrophic pain with features of hypovolaemic shock – pallor, hypotension, tachycardia, and cold clammy skin. He has a distended abdomen, more marked on the left side with tenderness and rigidity. This man has a leaking abdominal aortic aneurysm. He needs immediate resuscitation with crystalloids using 2 wide-bore intravenous cannulae, an indwelling catheter and transfer to theatre for immediate operation. Rarely, some vascular surgeons may have a CT done on the way to the theatre. However, time should not be wasted over this if the diagnosis is obvious.

E Perforated peptic ulcer

This man has all the features of a perforated peptic ulcer which in most instances is a duodenal ulcer. His abdominal wall does not move with respiration, a typical sign of peritonitis. He has board-like rigidity and thoracic respiration. His right shoulder tip pain is due to diaphragmatic irritation. On percussion the liver dullness will be obliterated due to air in the subphrenic space. Note that these patients in the early stages are not shocked. He needs analgesia, intravenous line, nasogastric suction and a chest X-ray (erect) which may show gas under the right dome of the diaphragm (**Figure 45.4**). He should be operated upon as an emergency and the perforation closed with an omental patch and thorough peritoneal lavage. Postoperatively he should have the full course of anti-*Helicobacter pylori* regime.

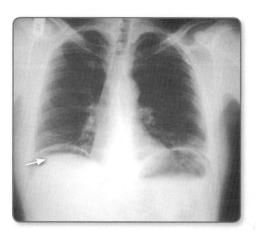

Figure 45.4 Chest X-ray erect showing free gas under right dome of diaphragm (arrow).

E Volvulus of the sigmoid colon

This elderly man has features of acute-on-chronic large bowel intestinal obstruction. His symptoms have been going on for almost a week. He has constipation and abdominal distension and some pain. He does not have features of strangulation such as hypotension, temperature or marked tachycardia. His abdominal distension is mainly on the left side. Pain is not a prominent feature as would happen in a patient who has a closed-loop large bowel obstruction from a left colonic carcinom. This patient needs an intravenous line, indwelling urinary catheter, confirmation of the diagnosis by a plain abdominal X-ray which would show a massively dilated and twisted sigmoid colon (**Figure 45.5a**); a Gastrografin enema can also be done. Initial management is by colonoscopic deflation. If conservative management is unsuccessful, operation will be necessary at which sigmoid colectomy (**Figure 45.** is done as a Hartmann's type procedure.

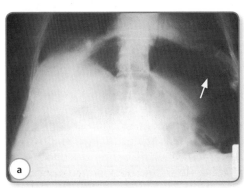
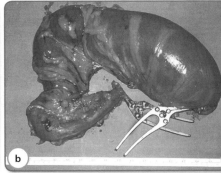

Figure 45.5 (a) Plain abdominal X-ray showing massively distended sigmoid colon (arrow). (b) A sigmoid colectomy specimen of sigmoid volvulus from the same patient.

8   B Incarcerated femoral hernia

This woman has the typical features of distal acute small bowel obstruction with abdominal pain, distension and faeculent vomiting which is a sign of distal ileal obstruction. The lump in the groin denotes an irreducible hernia which is a femora hernia as it is below the inguinal ligament. She has advanced signs of dehydration. She needs immediate resuscitation with intravenous fluids, indwelling catheter, nasogastric suction, central venous pressure (CVP) line. Once optimised, she needs an urgent operation.

9   D Perforated diverticulitis

This 70-year-old obese woman has lower abdominal peritonitis with features of septic shock. Her previous history of constipation and her obesity should alert one the possibility of diverticular disease. Features of peritonitis in the presence of sep shock should suggest faecal peritonitis from perforated diverticulitis, a very seriou condition. She should be resuscitated with analgesia, intravenous fluids, indwellir catheter, central venous pressure line and intravenous antibiotics. An erect chest X-ray may show gas under the right dome of the diaphragm. Once she is optimise she should be taken to the theatre for laparotomy.

At laparotomy she should undergo a Hartmann's operation – resection of the sigmoid colon with a terminal left iliac colostomy, closure of the rectum and thorough peritoneal lavage. She would require postoperative care in the intensive treatment unit and high-dependency unit.

0. E Subphrenic abscess

After laparoscopic closure of a perforated duodenal ulcer, this patient made a good recovery initially. However, a week later she has pyrexia with signs of intra-abdominal sepsis. She has pain in the right shoulder tip from diaphragmatic irritation and signs in the right upper quadrant with pleural effusion. She has a right subphrenic abscess. On chest X-ray she would have an elevated right dome of the diaphragm under which there would be a fluid level (**Figure 45.6**). She next needs an ultrasound and/or CT scan of the subphrenic spaces to localise the abscess. This would most probably be in the right anterior subdiaphragmatic space or in the hepatorenal pouch (Morrison's pouch). She would require a CT-guided drainage of the abscess. This may need to be done more than once as the abscess may be multi-loculated. Rarely, it may require the open operation of extraperitoneal drainage.

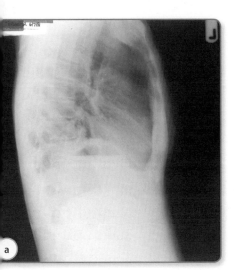
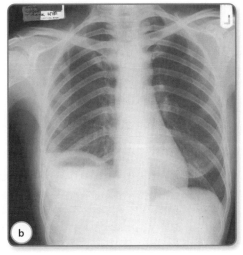

Figure 45.6 Two chest X-rays. Lateral (a) and anteroposterior (b) views showing raised right dome of diaphragm, under which there is a large air-fluid level.

1. B Bleeding peptic ulcer

This 60-year-old man has features of long-standing peptic ulceration as evidenced by his long-term indigestion for which he takes proprietary medicines. He is a smoker as the most sufferers of peptic ulceration are. He now has hypovolaemic shock with upper abdominal tenderness. He is bleeding from a peptic ulcer, the most probable site being a duodenal ulcer.

He needs immediate resuscitation: two wide bore intravenous cannulae through which crystalloids are infused followed by blood transfusion, indwelling catheter to monitor urinary output, central venous pressure line and urgent oesophagogastroduodenoscopy. In the case of a bleeding duodenal ulcer, this would show an ulcer crater on the posterior wall of the first of the duodenum. Attempts may be made to stop the bleeding with minimal access surgical methods such as lasers, argon diathermy and injection methods. As a rough guide, if a patient has had six units of blood, he needs an operation. If bleeding is from a spurting vessel from the ulcer base (from the gastroduodenal artery), this will require an open operation – pyloromyotomy, under-running the vessel and closure as a pyloroplasty. In all cases, the patient will need a full course of medical treatment for *Helicobacter pylori*. The overall management of acute upper gastrointestinal haemorrhage is summarised in **Figure 45.7**.

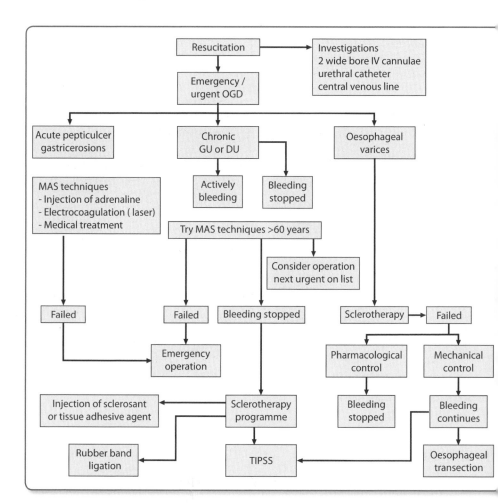

Figure 45.7 Management of acute upper gastrointestinal haemorrhage. OGD, oesophagogastroduodenoscopy; MAS, minimal access surgery; GU, gastric ulcer; DU, duodenal ulcer; TIPSS, transhepatic portosystemic stent shunt.

2. A Aortoenteric fistula

Any patient who has a vascular graft and a gastrointestinal bleed should be presumed to have an aortoenteric fistula unless otherwise proven. This man who had an operation for AAA in the past has now an acute haematemesis. This patient requires urgent resuscitation on the same lines as the preceding patient to be followed by oesophagogastroduodenoscopy. The latter may be difficult because of severe bleeding from the duodenum. If the bleeding has stopped, the experienced endoscopist may see the site of fistula between the duodenum and the aortic graft. This patient needs an immediate operation by an expert vascular surgeon. At operation the fistula has to be disconnected, the aortic graft removed, the duodenal hole closed, the ends of the aorta closed off followed by an axillobifemoral extra-anatomic bypass graft.

3. B Femoral hernia

This patient has an irreducible tender lump at the medial end of his right groin. This lump is below the inguinal ligament and lateral to the pubic tubercle, the site of the femoral canal. He therefore has a femoral hernia which probably contains irreducible omentum that is the cause of his lower abdominal discomfort. He needs an operation. Whilst there are several approaches, the simplest elective procedure is to do a low approach. An oblique incision is made along the medial half and 2 cm below the inguinal ligament, the hernial sac is isolated, opened, the contents reduced and the sac transfixed, ligated and removed. The femoral ring is obliterated by approximating the medial part of the inguinal ligament to the pectineal ligament. Femoral hernia is more common in the female, although inguinal hernia is more common than femoral in the female.

4. E Obturator hernia

Obturator hernia is six times more common in women. The pain of the hernia is referred along the geniculate branch of the obturator nerve to the knee. A swelling is not easily felt because the hernia is covered by the pectineus. A swelling is rarely obvious unless the limb is flexed, abducted and externally rotated; in this position, a hernia may be felt. On vaginal examination, a tender swelling may be felt in the region of the obturator foramen. A CT of the pelvis may be necessary, if the diagnosis is in doubt. Operation is the treatment of choice as strangulation in the form of a Richter's hernia is not uncommon.

Chapter 46

Upper gastrointestinal surgery

heme: Oesophageal conditions

ptions for Questions 1–5:

A Achalasia
B Barrett's oesophagus
C Carcinoma of oesophagus
D Hiatus hernia

E Oesophageal varices
F Pharyngeal diverticulum
G Schatzki's ring
H Scleroderma

or each of the following situations below, select the single most likely diagnosis. Each ption may be used once, more than once or not at all.

A 50-year-old man complains of intermittent difficulty in swallowing (dysphagia) with food sticking in the lower retrosternal region for the past 8 weeks; the dysphagia is usually for solid foods. This was preceded by heart-burn for several months for which he underwent an oesophagogastroduodenoscopy (OGD) with biopsy and was put on proton pump inhibitors. He is due for another OGD after 6 weeks.

A 60-year-old woman complains of repeated bouts of coughing when lying in bed and sensation of food material spilling over into her gullet. She suffers from recurrent chest infections for which she is treated with antibiotics. She has occasional dysphagia and is embarrassed by halitosis.

A 45-year-old man complains of dysphagia of almost 2 years duration. This is more marked with liquids. Sometimes there is regurgitation of undigested food and foul-smelling frothy sputum. He suffers from intermittent cough, chest infections and retrosternal discomfort. He has lost 10 kg in weight in 6 months.

A 65-year-old man, a heavy smoker and drinker, complains of progressive dysphagia of 8 weeks duration. He has difficulty swallowing solids, which tends to stick in the middle of his retrosternal region. He has lost so much weight that his belt has gone up two notches within the last 8 weeks and his clothes feel very loose.

A 55-year-old woman complains of heartburn, discomfort in the epigastrium after meals, and nausea with a feeling of pressure behind her breast bone after meals for several months. The feeling is relieved by belching; sometimes there is regurgitation of food and acid in the lower retrosternal region. She has occasional dysphagia and she has been treated for recurrent chest infections.

Theme: Gastric and duodenal conditions

Options for Questions 6–9:

A	Carcinoma of stomach	E	Gastric outlet obstruction
B	Duodenal adenocarcinoma	F	Gastric ulcer
C	Duodenal diverticulum	G	Gastritis
D	Gastric lymphoma	H	Leiomyoma of stomach

For each of the following situations, select the single most likely diagnosis. Each option may be used once, more than once or not at all.

6. A 60-year-old man underwent cardiac bypass surgery 2 months ago. The procedure was uneventful and he returned home after 10 days. Because of the pain of his sternotomy he took nonsteroidal anti-inflammatory drugs (NSAIDs) for relief. Recently, he has felt unwell, with a small haematemesis and epigastric discomfort. His doctor advised him to stop his NSAIDs and referred him for an oesophagogastroduodenoscopy.

7. A 60-year-old woman, a smoker, complains of bouts of epigastric pain for the past 8 months. The pain comes on 10–15 minutes after meals. Vomiting relieves her pain. Although her appetite is good, she is frightened to eat for fear of the pain. These bouts of pain are cyclical: there are periods when she is pain-free. From time to time she has taken over-the-counter medicines with some benefit. On examination, there is nothing to find except for some epigastric tenderness.

8. A 60-year-old man presents to his general practitioner with intermittent non-bilious vomiting for the past couple of months. The vomitus is foul-smelling and contains undigested food taken a few days before. He has suffered from indigestion for many years for which he takes over-the-counter drugs. He has lost 12 kg in weight during this period. He looks dehydrated, unwell with a succussion splash and a visible gastric peristalsis.

9. A 55-year-old man complains of recent loss of appetite, epigastric pain, intermittent vomiting and weight loss for the last 6 weeks. The vomitus at times is dark red. He recently noticed that his left leg is swollen with a tender cord-like structure along his calf diagnosed as thrombophlebitis.

Theme: Gastric and duodenal conditions

Options for Questions 10–12:

A Carcinoma of stomach	E Gastric outlet obstruction
B Duodenal adenocarcinoma	F Gastric ulcer
C Duodenal diverticulum	G Gastritis
D Gastric lymphoma	H Leiomyoma of stomach

For each of the following situations, select the single most likely diagnosis. Each option may be used once, more than once or not at all.

10. A 35-year-old woman complains of upper abdominal discomfort of 6 weeks duration. She is otherwise well and has not been off work as a medical secretary. Her general practitioner had a barium meal carried out and referred her for a surgical opinion.

11. A 65-year-old woman presented with undue shortness of breath of recent origin and intermittent vomiting of 3 months duration. On examination, her general practitioner found that she has iron deficiency anaemia with a haemoglobin of level of 8 g/dL. She is jaundiced and complains of recent itching. The serum biochemistry shows a picture of obstructive jaundice.

12. A 70-year-old man presents to his general practitioner, since he suddenly vomited blood clots and a couple of days later noticed that he had black tarry stools. The general practitioner felt a vague lump in the epigastrium. The patient was not keen on hospital admission. Therefore, he had haematological tests carried out which showed haemoglobin of 10 g/dL and a barium meal showed a space-occupying lesion. He was then persuaded to be admitted to the surgical ward.

Answers

1. B Barrett's oesophagus

This patient has had heartburn for several months for which he underwent oesophagogastroduodenoscopy, biopsy and is now being treated medically. This is a typical history in gastro-oesophageal reflux disease (GORD). The patient's dysphagia could well be due to stricture within Barrett's oesophagus. The condition, described by Norman Barrett of St Thomas's Hospital, London in 1950, is a metaplastic response to chronic GORD. Here the squamocolumnar junction moves proximally where strictures can occur. Such patients should be under regular endoscopic surveillance to exclude dysplasia or in situ cancer. In the presence of intestinal metaplasia, the increased risk of adenocarcinoma is 25–30 times that of the general population.

The relative risk of cancer increases with the increasing length of abnormal mucosa so that the following terms are used:

- Classic Barrett's – 3 cm or > columnar epithelium
- Short-segment Barrett's – < 3 cm of columnar epithelium
- Cardiac metaplasia

Management depends on the findings: balloon dilatation for strictures, antireflux surgery for severe symptoms of GORD, surveillance for dysplasia and resection for severe dysplasia (some authorities consider severe dysplasia as in situ carcinoma) or carcinoma.

2. F Pharyngeal diverticulum (Zenker's diverticulum)

This patient has the classical symptoms of a pharyngeal diverticulum – recurrent chest infections from aspiration of food contents into the tracheobronchial tree. This is more marked when the patient is in the recumbent position and food spills over from the diverticulum. Dysphagia is a late symptom due to external pressure on the cervical oesophagus. Very rarely when the diverticulum is large, it may be felt on the left side of the neck and the contents emptied with a gurgling sound.

The diverticulum occurs through a weakness between the oblique thyropharyngeus part and the circular cricopharyngeus part of the inferior constrictor muscle. The gap, triangular in shape, is called the Killian's dehiscence (Gustav Killian, 1860–1921, Professor of Laryngology, Freiburg and Berlin). It is thought to occur due to incoordination between the constrictor muscles of the pharynx and the cricopharyngeal sphincter.

Results from a barium swallow shows arrest of barium in a smooth pouch which may contain food residue shown as filling defects within the pouch (**Figure 46.1**). The picture may also show spillage of barium into the tracheobronchial tree.

While open excision used to be the mode of treatment, endoscopic stapling diverticulotomy with cricopharyngeal myotomy is the treatment of choice. Through

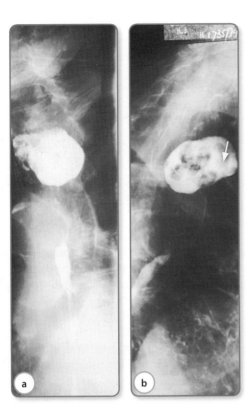

Figure 46.1 (a) and (b) Barium swallow showing arrest of barium in a smooth pouch with food residue (arrow) – typical of a pharyngeal diverticulum.

a bivalved pharyngoscope a linear cutting stapler is used to divide the septum between the diverticulum and upper oesophagus, so that the diverticulum becomes a part of the oesophageal lumen. This minimal access surgical treatment should only be carried out once a squamous carcinoma within the diverticulum, a rare occurrence, is excluded.

3. A Achalasia

Long-standing dysphagia, particularly for liquids, is the hallmark of achalasia. It may be associated with odynophagia (painful swallowing). Chest pain may occur, mimicking angina. Repeated chest infections from regurgitation of food, especially at night, are common. The condition is the result of the absence of ganglion cells in the myenteric plexus of Auerbach (Leopold Auerbach, 1828–1897, Professor of Neuropathology in Breslau), which is situated between the muscle layers and forms part of the enteric nervous system. This causes failure of relaxation of the gastro-oesophageal junction resulting in massive dilatation of the proximal oesophagus with large amount of food residue.

Barium swallow shows a classical 'bird's beak' appearance distal to a massively dilated oesophagus containing food residue (**Figure 46.2**) with absence of the gastric air bubble. Such an appearance is referred to as megaoesophagus. It is important to exclude malignancy, a complication that occurs in 3%, by

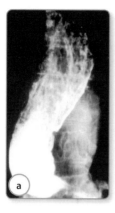
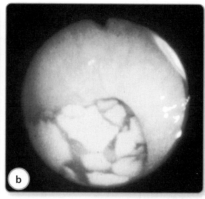

Figure 46.2 (a) Barium swallow shows a classical 'bird's beak' appearance distal to a massively dilated oesophagus containing food residue. (b) Oesophagogastro-dudenoscopy view showing food residue in oesophagus.

oesophagogastroduodenoscopy (OGD) and biopsy. On OGD, the endoscopist feels like they are entering a huge cave and finds that the gastro-oesophageal junction is eccentric in position. Depending upon the severity, balloon dilatation can be attempted initially. The definitive treatment is Heller's (Ernst Heller, 1877–1964, Surgeon in Leipzig) cardiomyotomy, carried out laparoscopically or thoracoscopically. Some surgeons add an anti-reflux procedure to the operation to prevent gastro-oesophageal reflux, which is a complication of the operation. The procedure can also be carried out through a laparotomy or left thoracotomy.

4. C Carcinoma of oesophagus

Progressive dysphagia of short duration in a heavy smoker and chronic alcoholic is due to carcinoma unless otherwise proven. Clinical examination would not show much other than evidence of weight loss. There will be features of malnutrition and, if the condition is advanced, a secondary liver or a left supraclavicular lymph node may be felt.

Besides all routine haematological and biochemical blood tests, a barium swallow will show an irregular stricture with shouldering (**Figure 46.3a**). An urgent oesophagogastroduodenoscopy carried out shows a polypoid growth (**Figure 46.3b**) at the same time an endoluminal ultrasound (EUS) is done to assess the local extent of the growth and the state of mediastinal lymph nodes. Biopsy should follow EUS. A CT of the chest should follow to look for local spread and assess the possibility of resection; CT of the liver is also done. If at this stage of the investigations, resection is regarded as possibility then laparoscopy and laparoscopic ultrasound is carried out as a final staging procedure to exclude peritoneal secondaries.

If the carcinoma is resectable, then a two-stage Ivor-Lewis operation is done. In suitable cases, a trans-hiatal oesophagectomy may be carried out. If the growth is inoperable, as most of them are, then a self-expanding metallic stent is inserted. This is followed by palliative radiotherapy which is effective in squamous cell carcinoma. Palliative chemotherapy may also be considered and other palliative methods, such as laser ablation, are also available. Rarely, adjuvant chemotherapy and radiotherapy may be given followed by further assessment for a possible resection.

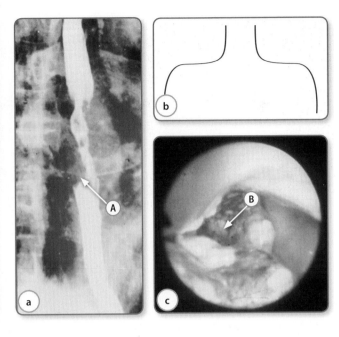

Figure 46.3 (a) Barium meal showing shouldering (A and schematic line in diagram b), typical of carcinoma. (c) Oesophagogastro-dudenoscopy showing polypoid growth in oesophagus (B).

. D Hiatus hernia

This middle-aged woman has clinical features of gastro-oesophageal reflux disease (GORD) from a hiatus hernia – heartburn, epigastric discomfort, feeling of pressure in the retrosternal region and belching. Chest infections suggest regurgitation whilst dysphagia might be the result of oesophagitis or early stricture. The commonest type of hiatus hernia is the sliding variety (85%) where the gastro-oesophageal junction is in the chest, as a result of which the oesophagus is shortened. The normal gastro-oesophageal junction is 40 cm from the incisors. In this situation the junction may be encountered at 36 cm or 37 cm. The other variety of hiatus hernia is the paraoesophageal (rolling) type where the cardia remains in its normal anatomical position. This is rare. The third variety is the mixed type where the cardia is displaced into the chest along with the greater curve of the stomach, which can be seen on barium meal (**Figure 46.4**).

She should undergo an oesophagogastroduodenoscopy during which the site of the gastro-oesophageal junction, the type and quantity of refluxing fluid, the degree of oesophagitis (see Figure 45.1) and the state of the hiatus are noted; biopsy is taken to exclude metaplasia. As she has dysphagia, balloon dilatation may need to be considered. 24-hour pH monitoring is an accurate method to diagnose GORD. Medical treatment in the form of life-style changes and a proton pump inhibitor to which sometimes a H_2-receptor antagonist may need to be added. Surgery is considered when there is failure of medical treatment.

. G Gastritis

This patient has erosive gastritis caused by nonsteroidal anti-inflammatory drugs that have disturbed the gastric mucosal barrier. An oesophagogastroduodenoscopy

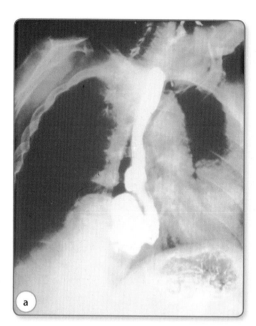 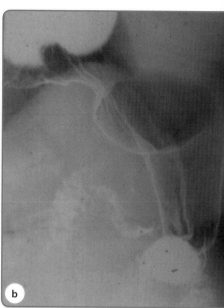

Figure 46.4 (a) and (b) Barium meal showing shortened oesophagus with gastro-oesophageal junction and part of greater curvature in the chest. These symptoms are typical of a mixed type of hiatus hernia.

to confirm the diagnosis is the next step. It is also possible that his gastritis could be from stress ulceration having recently had cardio-pulmonary bypass surgery. Following such surgery, reduced blood supply to the superficial gastric mucosa may induce ulceration which manifests itself as haematemesis. In intensive care units, prevention of stress ulceration is routinely carried out by the use of H2-receptor antagonists with barrier agents such as sucralfate.

Gastritis can be of two types – type A and type B. Type A gastritis is an autoimmune condition causing atrophy of the parietal cell mass resulting in hypochlorhydria and achlorhydria. The parietal cell also produces intrinsic factor; hence there is B_{12} malabsorption with resultant pernicious anaemia. This predisposes to gastric cancer.

Type B gastritis is associated with *Helicobacter pylori* infection. It affects the pyloric antrum causing peptic ulceration. This may go on to form pangastritis which is a precursor of cancer. Intestinal metaplasia is associated with chronic pangastritis. When associated with dysplasia, intestinal metaplasia has a high chance of turning malignant. Therefore, patients with type A and type B gastritis should be on regular endoscopic surveillance. There are other types of gastritis (**Figure 46.5**), e.g. Ménétrier's disease, where there is gross hypertrophy of gastric mucosal folds, hypochlorhydria, hypoproteinaemia and anaemia. It is pre-malignant and the treatment is gastrectomy.

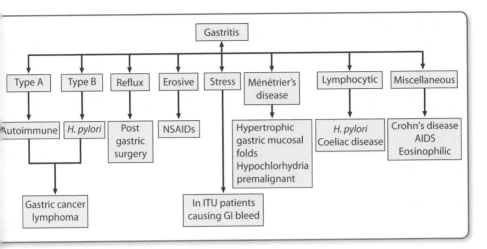

Figure 46.5 Types of gastritis.

. F Gastric ulcer

This patient has features of peptic ulceration in the stomach as the pain comes on shortly after food. Periodicity is a typical feature of the pain; the period when pain is absent, is regarded as due to spontaneous healing of the ulcer. She needs an oesophagogastroduodenoscopy (OGD) and multiple biopsies. A gastric ulcer should be regarded as malignant unless otherwise proven conclusively by an experienced endoscopist and histopathologist. In case of a benign gastric ulcer *H. pylori* infection should be sought for by doing the Campylobacter-like organism test, also called rapid urease test, or biopsy. Biopsy may be negative if the patient already has had empirical treatment from her general practitioner. *H. pylori* infection can be successfully eradicated in the vast majority by the regime consisting of a proton pump inhibitor with metronidazole, amoxycillin and clarithromycin. Advising on lifestyle changes, in particular stopping smoking, is essential but not often followed by the patient. After the course of medical treatment, even if symptoms have abated, an OGD should be done to confirm that the ulcer has healed. If the ulcer has not healed, a gastrectomy should be done. The macroscopic appearance is that of a punched out ulcer with a clear-cut edge which overhangs the base (**Figure 46.6**). Very rarely a benign gastric ulcer can turn malignant.

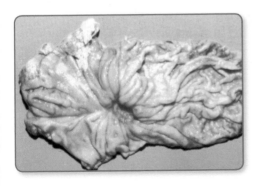

Figure 46.6 Stomach showing punched out ulcer with overhanging edge – a benign gastric ulcer.

8. E Gastric outlet obstruction

The history of indigestion for many years with vomiting, dehydration, weight loss, succussion splash and visible gastric peristalsis is typical of gastric outlet obstruction from a cicatrised, healed duodenal ulcer. The effects of dehydration are loss of skin turgor, dry tongue and sunken eyes. This patient will have serious metabolic effects of hypochloraemic, hypokalaemic, metabolic alkalosis. Long-standing alkalosis may cause reduction in the ionised serum calcium resulting in clinical tetany. There is also incipient renal dysfunction which is the outcome of prolonged dehydration. Because of the dehydration, the body tries to retain sodium in preference to potassium and hydrogen; this results in paradoxical aciduria exacerbating the hypokaleamia.

This patient will need resuscitation, confirmation of the diagnosis followed by definitive treatment. The patient should have vigorous intravenous rehydration using normal saline with added potassium; this is monitored by an indwelling urinary catheter and a central venous pressure line. The barium meal will show a huge stomach with a large amount of food residue (**Figure 46.7**). The stomach should be emptied by a large bore orogastric tube with repeated washouts followed by oesophagogastroduodenoscopy to confirm the diagnosis and exclude carcinoma of the pylorus.

As definitive treatment, during endoscopy, depending upon the tightness of the stricture, balloon dilatation may be attempted. This may have to be repeated and may not be successful in the long-term. The definitive surgical treatment of posterior, retrocolic, isoperistaltic gastrojejunostomy should be carried out.

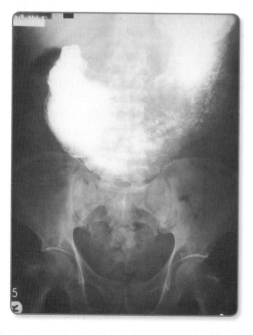

Figure 46.7 Barium meal showing a huge stomach with a large amount of food residue, typical of gastric outlet obstruction.

9. A Carcinoma of stomach

Anorexia, asthenia and anaemia (the 3 As) are the hallmarks of cancer stomach. This man complains of abdominal pain, intermittent vomiting of blood [from gastric outlet (outflow0 obstruction] and weight loss. He has Trousseau's sign, usually a sinister finding of visceral cancer. He has a gastric cancer unless otherwise proven.

In this particular patient, in view of Trousseau's sign, radical curative treatment may be unlikely. The patient should have a CT scan followed by oesophagogastroduodenoscopy (OGD) and biopsy. It is better to do the biopsy after the CT as biopsy may distort the CT findings. An endoluminal ultrasound done at the same time as OGD will assess accurately the local extent. If investigations thus far indicate the possibility of a radical curative resection, then a laparoscopy and laparoscopic ultrasound as a staging procedure is appropriate.

When feasible, radical curative total gastrectomy is carried out. In distal growths, confined to the pylorus (**Figure 46.8**) a subtotal gastrectomy can be carried out. When a curative resection is done with removal of the N1 and N2 group of lymph nodes, the resection is referred to as D2 gastrectomy. Neo-adjuvant chemotherapy

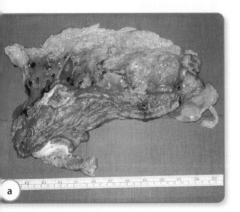
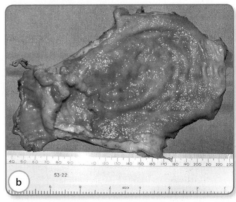

Figure 46.8 (a) and (b) Tissue removed during a subtotal gastrectomy for carcinoma of he pylorus.

improves prognosis in patients in whom the growth has been resected. In advanced cases palliation can be achieved by partial gastrectomy. Where that is not possible, in gastric outlet obstruction, a stent can be inserted or an anterior gastrojejunostomy performed. Histologically two types are identified: intestinal type where the prognosis is better and diffuse anaplastic type, also called linitis plastica (**Figure 46.9**) which has a dismal outcome.

10. C Duodenal diverticulum

The barium meal shows the C of the duodenum with an outpouching of the contrast seen inside a smooth-lined pouch on the mesenteric border (**Figure 46.10**).This is typical

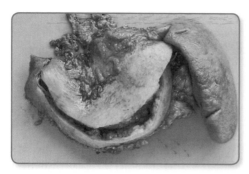

Figure 46.9 Linitis plastica. Courtesy of Dr James McPhie.

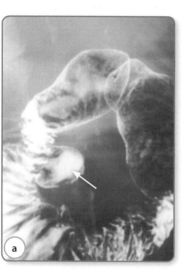
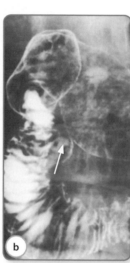

Figure 46.10 (a) and (b) Barium meal showing duodenal diverticulum (arrows).

of a congenital duodenal diverticulum. A congenital diverticulum is one where all the coats of the bowel- mucosa, muscularis and serosa – go to form the diverticulum. It is found at the entrance of the ampulla of Vater which is the junction of the foregut and hindgut and the site of maximum weakness. The position is described as 'paravateric'.

These do not produce any symptoms. A duodenal diverticulum can be regarded as 'the diagnostic scapegoat of the upper abdomen'. If a patient with upper abdominal symptoms has been found have a duodenal diverticulum on oesophagogastroduodenoscopy, the clinician should look for other causes as the diverticulum is an innocent bystander. However, the condition has a clinical significance. It may be difficult to do an endoscopic retrograde cholangiopancreatography and hazardous to attempt papillotomy. Rarely the diverticulum may be intra-pancreatic. The cause of an acquired duodenal diverticulum is a chronic duodenal ulcer.

11. B Duodenal adenocarcinoma

This woman's presenting symptom of shortness of breath is due to anaemic hypoxia. She has intermittent vomiting and has been found to have clinical itching and biochemical features of obstructive jaundice. These features point to an obstruction in the duodenum causing block of the ampulla of Vater – a periampullary carcinoma. This is the commonest site of adenocarcinoma of the small bowel. Patients are anaemic because they bleed from the ulcerated tumour. The jaundice may wax and wane. This is because when the tumour outgrows its blood supply, part of the tumour necroses opening up the ampulla allowing the bile to drain.

The management is confirmation of the diagnosis by oesophagogastroduodenoscopy and biopsy; a barium meal will show an 'apple-core' deformity with a hugely dilated stomach (**Figure 46.11**); staging is carried out by CT scan, chest X-ray, laparoscopy and laparoscopic ultrasound. If the growth is localised without any distant spread, curative resection (possible in 70%) is performed by Whipple's pancreaticoduodenectomy; the 5-year survival rate is about 20%. Palliation is carried out by stenting of the common bile duct to alleviate jaundice and an anterior gastrojejunostomy for gastric outlet obstruction. If stenting of the common bile duct is not feasible then the triple bypass procedure of cholecystojejunostomy, jejunojejunostomy and anterior gastrojejunostomy is done.

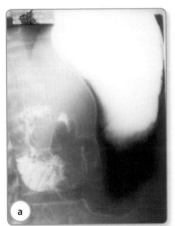
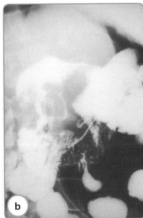

Figure 46.11 (a) and (b) Barium meal showing 'apple-core' deformity in the duodenum with a dilated proximal stomach – duodenal carcinoma.

2. H Leiomyoma of stomach

Acute upper gastrointestinal tract haemorrhage is the classical presentation of a leiomyoma of stomach. The possibility of the presence of an epigastric mass may denote a gastric cancer; this is unlikely in the absence of weight loss. Oesophagogastroduodenoscopy (OGD) is the investigation of choice, but as the patient refused hospital admission initially, a barium meal was carried out. This shows a smooth filling defect in the body of the stomach, typical of a submucosal tumour (**Figure 46.12**). In the centre of the filling defect there is a patch of barium due to ulceration of the tumour which causes the acute bleeding – the typical

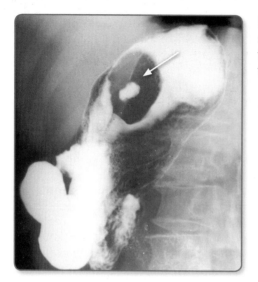

Figure 46.12 Barium meal showing smooth filling defect in the body of the stomach with mucosal ulceration, typical of a leiomyoma (arrow).

presenting feature. These tumours are referred to as gastrointestinal stromal tumours.

The patient needs an urgent OGD which would show a tumour in the posterior wall of the stomach; this is followed by a CT. The treatment is local excision.

Chapter 47

Hepatobiliary and pancreatic surgery

Theme: Acute hepatobiliary presentations

Options for Questions 1–4:

A   Acute cholecystitis
B   Acute pancreatitis
C   Crigler–Najjar syndrome
D   Gallstone ileus

E   Liver fluke
F   Mirizzi's syndrome
G   Viral hepatitis

For each of the following situations, select the single most likely diagnosis. Each option may be used once, more than once or not at all.

A 59-year-old man presents with acute severe central abdominal pain radiating to the back. This had been preceded by several weeks of intermittent right upper quadrant pain. He has no significant past medical history, although is mildly obese.

A 72-year-old woman presents with symptoms of obstructive jaundice. She is known to have a solitary large gallstone, but has been managed conservatively due to significant comorbidity.

A 45-year-old obese woman presents with severe constant right upper quadrant pain. Over the past 3 years she has been experiencing similar intermittent episodes which previously have always resolved sponatenously.

An 80-year-old woman presents with a 2-day history of increasing vomiting and abdominal distension. She has not passed any stool or flatus for 24 hours. This patient was diagnosed with a large solitary gallstone some years previously, but surgery was not performed due to severe comorbidity.

Theme: Classification of jaundice

Options for Questions 5–7:

A	Blood transfusion jaundice	**E**	Physiological jaundice
B	Hepatic (hepatocellular)	**F**	Posthepatic (cholestatic)
C	Infective jaundice	**G**	Prehepatic
D	Mixed hepatic and posthepatic		

For each of the following situations, select the single most likely diagnosis. Each option may be used once, more than once or not at all.

5. A 74-year-old woman fell 2 weeks previously which resulted in a large haematoma on her left thigh. The haematoma has gradually reduced in size, however she has noticed that her skin has a yellow tinge. Blood tests show an isolated raised bilirubin with normal coagulation screen.

6. A 60-year-old woman has been admitted as an emergency with a 4-day history of severe right upper quadrant pain, vomiting, jaundice and intense pruritus. She is found to have a high temperature with rigors and hyperdynamic circulation.

7. An 18-year-old woman presents with jaundice and pallor. She reports that she has always looked pale and on previous blood tests she has been anaemic. Her anaemia was previously thought due to menorrhagia, although her periods have never been particularly heavy. On examination, her abdomen is soft and non-tender with a palpable spleen.

Theme: Hepatobiliary investigations

Options for Questions 8–10:

A	Abdominal ultrasound scan	**E**	Magnetic resonance cholangiopancreatography
B	Computerised tomographic scan		
C	Endoscopic ultrasound scan	**F**	Operative cholangiogram
D	Endoscopic retrograde cholangiopancreatography	**G**	Percutaneous transhepatic cholangiogram

For each of the following situations, select the single most likely diagnosis. Each option may be used once, more than once or not at all.

8. A 46-year-old moderately obese woman presents with severe right upper quadrant pain which has gradually increased in severity. This episode was preceded 6 month of intermittent right upper quadrant pain and nausea. On examination, she is pyrexial and Murphy's sign is positive. Liver function tests are normal.

9. A 68-year-old man presents with right upper quadrant pain and mildly deranged obstructive liver function tests. Abdominal ultrasound scan demonstrated gallstones in the gallbladder, but the common bile duct could not be seen.

0. A 53-year-old woman presents for elective cholecystectomy following a long history of intermittent right upper quadrant pain. Ultrasound scan had demonstrated gallstones within the gallbladder but no other significant abnormalities. Preadmission blood tests had shown mildly raised bilirubin, alkaline phosphatase and gamma-glutamyl transpeptidase. She is currently well and pain free.

heme: Hepatobiliary tumours

Options for Questions 11–12:

A	Adenoma	D	Hepatocellular carcinoma
B	Angiosarcoma	E	Liver metastasis
C	Cholangiocarcinoma		

'or each of the following situations, select the single most likely diagnosis. Each option nay be used once, more than once or not at all.

1. A 43-year-old man with cirrhosis due to alcoholic liver disease presents with constant right upper quadrant pain which has increased over several months. On examination, the liver edge is palpable and found to be firm and irregular.

2. A 70-year-old man, who is a long-term smoker, presents with vague right upper quadrant pain. He has lost considerable weight over the past 6 months and for the past year has been experiencing worsening haemoptysis. On examination, an irregular liver edge is palpable.

Theme: Benign conditions

Options for Questions 13–14:

A	Liver trauma	D	Primary sclerosing cholangitis
B	Polycystic liver disease	E	Right heart failure
C	Primary biliary cirrhosis		

'or each of the following situations, select the single most likely diagnosis. Each option nay be used once, more than once or not at all.

3. A 42-year-old woman presents with fatigue, itch and constant mild right upper quadrant pain. These symptoms have been present for several months but have recently increased in severity.

4. A 56-year-old man is referred by his GP with an irregular palpable liver edge approximately 5 cm below the costal margin. He had presented for a routine check up and had not complained of any abdominal discomfort, was systemically well with no weight loss.

Answers

1. B Acute pancreatitis

Acute pancreatitis usually presents with upper/central abdominal pain radiating to the back. On examination, there may be Cullen's sign and Grey Turner's sign (**Figure 47.1**). It is more common in men. Aetiology varies across the world but gallstones and alcohol account for the majority of presentations. The key blood test is serum amylase which would typically be elevated greater than three times normal in an episode of pancreatitis. Amylase levels rise within 2–12 hours of onset of abdominal pain and peak after 1–3 days. It should be notes that in patients presenting late the amylase level may be falling. Serum lipase level may remain elevated for longer and can be a useful addition to the investigation profile. Levels of these enzymes do not provide prognostic information. The clinical course in acute pancreatitis may be protracted with risks of subsequent complications related to the systemic inflammatory response. Mild acute pancreatitis usually results in pancreatic oedema followed by complete resolution. At the more severe end of the scale pancreatic necrosis may occur with varying degrees of local tissue destruction. Scoring systems are used in an attempt to predict those patients who are likely to deteriorate. These include the Glasgow scoring system and Ranson's criteria. Pancreatic necrosis may become infected or an abscess may develop, risking generalised sepsis, multiorgan failure and death. A fluid collection may develop in the lesser omental sac known as a pseudocyst. This may resolve with time, or persist and become and infected.

The main differential here is acute cholecystitis, however the pain is central suggesting pancreatitis as a more likely diagnosis. Gallstone ileus would likely present with signs of obstruction.

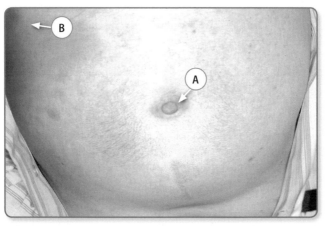

Figure 47.1 Patient with acute severe pancreatitis showing bruising around the umbilicus (Cullen's sign, A) and bruising of the flanks (Grey Turner's sign, B).

F Mirizzi's syndrome

A single large gallstone will be unlikely to pass through the cystic duct into the common bile duct. However, the stone within the gallbladder may cause pressure on the common hepatic duct leading to biliary obstruction and jaundice (**Figure 47.2**). In the chronic setting a fistula may develop between the gallbladder and common hepatic duct. Fistula can also develop between the gallbladder and small bowel. If a large stone passes into the small bowel then gallstone ileus may occur as the stone can lead to small bowel obstruction.

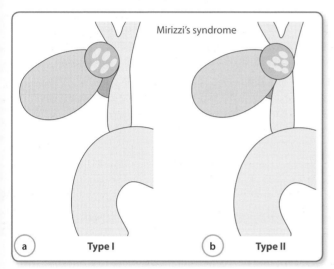

Figure 47.2 The two types of Mirizzi's syndrome. (a) Type I, Mirizzi's syndrome with a large gallstone pressing on the common hepatic duct. (b) Type II, progression of Mirizzi's syndrome with the gallstone fistulating into the common hepatic duct.

A Acute cholecystitis

This is inflammation of the gallbladder causing acute pain in the right upper quadrant and sometimes round to the epigastrium. The pain may have variable presentation, including sharp, dull, constant or cramp-like pain, radiate to the back or to the right scapula. In the overwhelming majority this is associated with gallstones; however acute cholecystitis can occur without gallstones, termed acalculous cholecystitis. This may occur as a manifestation of severe illness rather than a primary condition. On examination, Murphy's sign may be positive. This sign is elicited by the examiner placing their hand below right costal margin and asking the patient to breathe in. If the gallbladder is acutely inflamed, inspiration will lead to inferior displacement of the gallbladder which comes into contact with anterior abdominal wall, causing exacerbation of pain and the patient to 'catch their breath'. For a positive test the examiner should also test below the left costal margin for absence of pain. Ultrasound scan is generally the favoured imaging modality for diagnosis, enabling assessment of gallbladder wall thickness, presence of gallstones and calibre of the common bile duct. **Figure 47.3** shows an acutely inflamed gallbladder. Figure 45.2 shows a mucocele of the gallbladder caused by

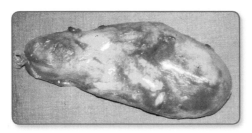

Figure 47.3 Acute cholecystitis. Ho~~w~~ gall bladder removed as an urgent open cholecystectomy.

obstruction of the gallbladder outlet via the cystic duct with stones. The gallbladder becomes distended with mucus and can present with similar symptoms as acute cholecystitis. Rarely carcinoma of the gallbladder may be found. Given the possibil~~ity~~ of carcinoma, it is important to avoid perforation during cholecystectomy. If the gallbladder is perforated there is a risk of disseminating the malignancy.

It is important to understand the difference between cholecystitis and cholangitis. The latter describes ascending infection within the biliary tree. Patients can deteriorate rapidly, requiring prompt diagnosis and intervention.

4. D Gallstone ileus

Gallstone ileus is an infrequent complication of gallstones. It develops in the chronic setting where a fistula develops between the gallbladder and duodenum. The gallstone then passes into the duodenum. If the stone is large it may obstruc~~t~~ the ileum. The stone passes down to the ileocaecal valve where it finally obstruct~~s~~ the small bowel. Although most gallstones are radio-opaque, occasionally this unusual cause for obstruction may be seen on an abdominal radiograph. The original fistula may enable gas to enter the biliary tree causing pneumobilia. This is seen as gas in the right upper quadrant (**Figure 47.4**). Larger gallstones are predominantly cholesterol based (around 80%); pigment stones are smaller

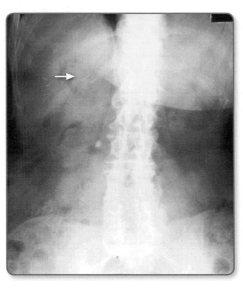

Figure 47.4 Pneumobilia. Gas is see~~n~~ in the right upper quadrant (arrow), within the biliary tree. This has been caused by a fistula developing between the gallbladder and duodenum. A radio-opaque gallsto~~ne~~ is also seen in the duodenum.

consisting primarily of bilirubin and calcium salts. Stones can also be of mixed composition.

The main differential here would be acute pancreatitis, however the history of a solitary large gallstone makes this less likely. Abdominal distention may be a feature of acute pancreatitis but patients are unlikely to be completely obstructed.

G Prehepatic

In the presence of a large haematoma which is resolving the most likely cause is the increased breakdown of haem. This produces unconjugated bilirubin. This is conjugated by hepatocytes and excreted with bile into the duodenum. In addition to serum bilirubin a range of tests can be used to determine the underlying cause of jaundice. Liver function tests classically include alkaline phosphatase, gamma-glutamyl transpeptidase and aminotransferase. While these are essentially markers of damage to hepatocytes and biliary epithelium, they are often useful in delineating the cause. This patient has an isolated raised bilirubin. This is most likely a prehepatic aetiology but disorders of bilirubin metabolism should be considered. In hepatocellular jaundice aminotransferase is likely to be greatly elevated, with alkaline phosphatise and gamma-glutamyl transpeptidase less markedly so. In cholestatic jaundice alkaline phosphatase and gamma-glutamyl transpeptidase are usually increased with aminotransferase less elevated. A coagulation screen (prothrombin time) can provide an indicator of synthetic liver function and will be prolonged in cases of considerable impairment. Especially in elderly patients it is important to consider medications that may cause jaundice.

D Mixed hepatic and posthepatic

This patient has the typical features of cholangitis. This is most likely caused by a gallstone within the common bile duct, known as choledocholithiasis. Patients developing cholangitis may deteriorate rapidly due to overwhelming sepsis. The classical symptoms of fever, jaundice and right upper quadrant tenderness are known as Charcot's triad. While choledocholithiasis is the commonest cause patients with biliary obstruction due to another cause may also develop these symptoms. The sepsis that has ensued following bile duct obstruction may result in a mixed liver function test picture (i.e. raised aminotransferase, gamma-glutamyl transpeptidase, and alkaline phosphatase) although the underlying cause is posthepatic.

G Prehepatic

A palpable spleen in the presence of jaundice suggests a haemolytic process; this is supported by the presence of pallor. The history suggests that anaemia has been a long-standing issue. The underlying aetiology may be autoimmune haemolytic anaemia or hereditary spherocytosis. The direct antiglobulin test can distinguish between the two; the former being positive and the latter negative. Autoimmune haemolytic anaemia is caused mainly by IgG or IgM antibodies directed against red blood cells. Hereditary spherocytosis is a condition which results in spherical rather than biconcave red blood cells. These spherical cells are more prone to haemolysis and given this patients are prone to gallstones. Splenectomy prevents anaemia and should be performed when symptomatic or when significant evidence of the disease is present.

8. A Abdominal ultrasound scan

This overweight, middle aged woman appears to be conforming to the classical picture of a patient with symptomatic gallstones. Biliary colic is caused by the gallbladder contracting against a gallstone in the neck of the gallbladder. This is usually intermitted with the patient generally pain free between episodes. The gallbladder may become inflamed with increasing constant pain in the right upper quadrant. Ultrasound scan would be the most appropriate first investigation and should provide an indication of the thickness of the gallbladder wall (suggesting inflammation), the presence of stones and the dimensions of the common bile duct. **Figure 47.5** provides a suggested management algorithm for patients with gallstone disease.

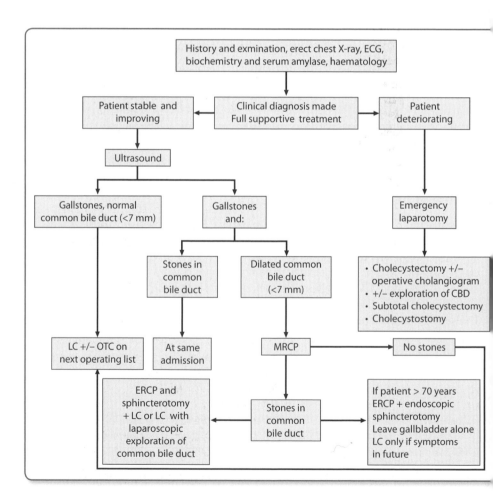

Figure 47.5 Algorithm showing suggested management of gallstone disease. LC, laparoscopic cholecystectomy; OTC, on table cholangiogram; CBD, common bile duct.

. E Magnetic resonance cholangiopancreatography

Sometimes the common bile duct may not be visualised by ultrasound, which is most often due to overlying bowel gas obscuring the view. As the patient has mildly deranged liver function tests a gallstone obstructing the bile duct should be contemplated. Magnetic resonance imaging in the form of magnetic resonance cholangiopancreatography can provide excellent views of the biliary tree and visualise filling defects which may represent a stone. The majority of gallstones are radiolucent and so would not be see on CT. Endoscopic retrograde cholangiopancreatography could be used to image the biliary system, but this is an invasive procedure exposing the patient to risks that would not necessarily be justified at this stage. In some centres the patient may go straight to laparoscopic cholecystectomy with intraoperative cholangiogram to assess for choledocholithiasis.

0. **F Operative cholangiogram**

This mildly derranged liver function tests in this case could indicate biliary obstruction. If the patient was symptomatic or if the derrangement was marked, it would be appropriate to delay surgery and arrange further investigation. Given the patient is currently well and pain free, it may be that has small stone has been passed through the common bile duct and no further intervention is required. However, it would be appropriate to perform intraoperative cholangiogram to investigate the possibility of a stone in the common bile duct. This procedure requires canulation of the biliary tree, usually via the cystic duct. It can be performed during laparoscopic or open procedures. If a stone is demonstrated, there are two main choices: (1) laparopscopic exploration of the common bile duct if the team is experienced in this technique or (2) complete the cholecystectomy laparoscopically and then electively perform endoscopic retrograde cholangiopancreatography and endoscopic papillotomy. **Figure 47.6** shows a cholangiogram performed during laparoscopic cholecystectomy with stone evident in the distal common bile duct.

1. **D Hepatocellular carcinoma**

This may arise spontaneously but more frequently occur on a background on liver cirrhosis. The tumour may either form a large single mass or occur as multiple foci throughout the liver. Patients may present with hepatomegaly, ascites and distant metastases. Deterioration may be rapid and patients usually present late. Some patients may be suitable for surgical resection but due to risks of decompensation patients with cirrhosis are not usually resected. In this instance the patient may be considered for liver transplantation. Chemoembolisation of large tumours may improve the preoperative condition of selected patients.

The main differential here is liver metastasis. However with the background of cirrhosis hepatocellular carcinoma is most likely.

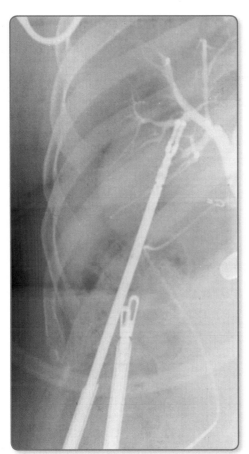

Figure 47.6 Operative cholangiogram at laparoscopic cholecystectomy. Findings include no flow of contrast into duodenum and stone (seen as filling defect) at the lower end of the common bile duct (Courtesy of Mr PW Fisher, Consultant Surgeon, Wick).

12. E Liver metastasis

This patient appears to have a malignant process underlying his current condition. The most likely cause for his right upper quadrant pain is hepatic metastases secondary to lung cancer. Increasing tumour bulk causes stretch on the liver capsule leading to pain. Metastatic hepatic malignancy is 20 times more common than primary liver malignancy. Common primary sites include the gastrointestinal tract, breast, lung, genitourinary system, melanoma, and sarcoma. However essentially all solid malignancies with metastatic potential may involve the liver.

13. C Primary biliary cirrhosis

This is an autoimmune disease of the liver characterised but progressive destruction of bile canaliculi eventually leading to fibrosis and cirrhosis. The disease classically affects middle aged women between the age of 30 and 65 years. Patients may present with fatigue, jaundice, itch and right upper quadrant pain. Late presentation may reveal the complications of cirrhosis and portal hypertensions such as ascites, varices and hepatic encephalopathy. Liver function tests show a cholestatic picture with abnormal immunological investigations. Immunology includes antimitochondrial antibodies (in 95% of patients), smooth muscle antibodies in 50%, IgM elevated in at least 80% of patients, and antineutrophil cytoplasmic antibody negative. Ursodeoxycholic acid may help reduce cholestasis and liver damage, cholestyramine can reduce itch. As the disease progresses liver transplantation may be the only option although the disease can recur in around 15% of patients. Primary biliary cirrhosis should be contrasted with primary sclerosing cholangitis which affects extrahepatic bile ducts, can lead to stricture formation and is associated with inflammatory bowel disease.

4. B Polycystic liver disease

Most patients with this condition are asymptomatic. It is often associated with polycystic kidney disease. Liver function is usually normal, but the hepatomegaly, potential bleeding into cysts, or obstruction of the venous or biliary drainage of the liver lead to complications. Most patients are managed conservatively unless symptoms are significant in which case laparoscopic deroofing of large cysts can be performed. Unusually, liver transplantation may be necessary where multiple cysts cannot be treated by resection.

Chapter 48

Surgery of small and large bowel

heme: Small intestine and appendix

tions for Questions 1–4:

A	Acute appendicitis	**E**	Ileocaecal tuberculosis
B	Acute small bowel ischaemia	**F**	Jejunal diverticulosis
C	Carcinoid tumour	**G**	Meckel's diverticulum
D	Crohn's disease	**H**	Small bowel lymphoma

r each of the following situations, select the single most likely diagnosis. Each option
ay be used once, more than once or not at all.

A 70-year-old man complains of severe acute abdominal pain all over the
abdomen followed by vomiting and blood-stained diarrhoea. Six weeks prior to
this episode he had a myocardial infarction. Examination reveals a patient who has
a blood pressure of 100 mmHg systolic, pulse rate of 120 beats per minute, atrial
fibrillation with cold extremities and tachypnoea. Abdominal examination reveals
generalised tenderness, rigidity and rebound tenderness.

A 45-year-old woman complains of alternating constipation and diarrhoea for 6
months. The diarrhoea takes the form of 4–6 loose motions a day often associated
with colicky abdominal pain and aching in the right iliac fossa. She has episodes
of feeling unwell. Recently, she noticed a couple of painful, bluish-red nodules on
her shin. Her general practitioner (GP) felt a vague mass in the right iliac fossa, and
diagnosed the lumps on her shin as erythema nodosum.

A 28-year-old woman complains of pain in the right iliac fossa of 18 hours duration.
The pain, initially started around the umbilicus, has now settled in the right lower
abdomen; it is exacerbated by coughing. It is associated with nausea, vomiting,
anorexia and several bouts of watery diarrhoea. On examination, she is afebrile with
tenderness, rigidity and rebound tenderness in her entire lower abdomen.

A 50-year-old woman complains of increasing diarrhoea of several weeks duration.
She is a sufferer of coeliac disease and has been on a gluten-free diet for almost 5
years. The present episode of diarrhoea is different from her usual bouts that she
experiences from her coeliac disease. Recently, she has started developing colicky
abdominal pain with episodes of fever and has noticed she has been losing weight.

Theme: Colon and rectum

Options for Questions 5–7:

A	Acute diverticulitis	G	Familial adenomatosis coli
B	Acute large bowel obstruction	H	Ischaemic colitis
C	Carcinoma of caecum	I	Pneumatosis intestinalis
D	Carcinoma of descending colon	J	Rectal prolapse
E	Carcinoma of rectum	K	Ulcerative colitis
F	Colovesical fistula		

For each of the following situations, select the single most likely diagnosis. Each option may be used once, more than once or not at all.

5. A 60-year-old man complains of alteration in his bowel habit having to wake up in the morning earlier than usual with an intense desire to open his bowels. He rushes to the toilet only to find that he passes considerable amount of wind, some watery stools and blood. He has lost some weight. His GP found that there are several masses in the left iliac fossa; rectal examination was normal.

6. A 60-year-old woman complains of undue shortness of breath when walking upstairs and carrying out her daily household work for the last couple of months. Her GP found that she had a mass in the right iliac fossa, haemoglobin was 7.5 g/dL and faecal occult blood tests (FOBs) were positive. An oesophagogastroduodenoscopy carried out in an open access endoscopy clinic was normal.

7. A 40-year-old woman complains of diarrhoea for 3 months. This takes the form of several loose motions a day (anything up to six), with slime and bright red blood. She feels lethargic with vague left-sided abdominal pain. She is anaemic without any abdominal signs; rectal examination shows blood and slime on the examining finger. Her C-reactive protein is 125 mg/L.

ıeme: Colon and rectum

tions for Questions 8–11:

A	Acute diverticulitis	G	Familial adenomatosis polyposis
B	Acute large bowel obstruction	H	Ischaemic colitis
C	Carcinoma of caecum	I	Pneumatosis intestinalis
D	Carcinoma of descending colon	J	Rectal prolapse
E	Carcinoma of rectum	K	Ulcerative colitis
F	Colovesical fistula		

r each of the following situations, select the single most likely diagnosis. Each option ıy be used once, more than once or not at all.

A 70-year-old slightly obese woman complains of pain in her left lower abdomen spreading to the rest of the abdomen for the past 10 days. She has had loose stools for 3 days. She has rigors and is pyrexial and has tenderness rigidity and rebound tenderness over the entire lower abdomen. Rectal examination reveals a tender mass felt in the pelvis through the rectal wall.

A 60-year-old man complains of frequency of micturition, suprapubic discomfort and passing very foul-smelling urine. He has been treated for repeated attacks of urinary tract infection by several courses of antibiotics. Recently, he has noticed passing air bubbles in urine. He has been constipated for many years. Clinical examination revealed no abnormality.

. A 68-year-old man complains of generalised colicky abdominal pain of 48 hours duration; in between the attacks of colic he is left with a dull ache. He has been constipated over the past few months, his last bowel action being 3 days ago. His abdomen is distended, mainly in the peripheral part, and tympanitic; the rectum is hollow.

. A 25-year-old man, recently moved to the area, presented to his new GP with loose stools with blood and mucus of 8 weeks duration. In the past, he was seen for regular camera examination of his large bowel once a year ever since he was a teenager. He is very concerned as his father died of cancer of the large bowel when he was 45 years old.

Theme: Anus and perianal region

Options for Questions 12–14:

A	Anal carcinoma	**F**	Perianal abscess
B	Condylomata acuminata	**G**	Pilonidal sinus
C	Fissure-in-ano	**H**	Pruritus ani
D	Fistula-in-ano	**I**	Solitary ulcer syndrome
E	Haemorrhoids		

For each of the following situations, select the single most likely diagnosis. Each option may be used once, more than once or not at all.

12 A 55-year-old man who has a renal transplant complains of 'piles'. He has noticed a lump around his anus which is constantly present, painful and bleeds on and off. This has been going on for the past 4–5 months. On examination, he has a fleshy ulcerated mass with raised and everted edges.

13 A 34-year-old man who is HIV positive complains of perianal itching and blood-stained discharge. On examination, he has wart-like lesions around the anus.

14 A 48-year-old man, a known patient of Crohn's disease, developed perianal pain with seropurulent discharge 6 weeks ago. When the discharge is significant, the pain is much less. It started when he felt an acute pain which was relieved, when there was a significant discharge.

Answers

B Acute small bowel ischaemia

This patient's clinical features of acute abdomen with bloody diarrhoea suggest acute small bowel ischaemia from a superior mesenteric artery embolus. Having had a myocardial infarction 6 weeks ago and suffering from atrial fibrillation as a result, this patient is prone to an arterial embolus. He has features of hypovolaemic and septic shock. In early stages of septic shock patients would have warm peripheries due to a hyperdynamic circulation; but this patient has cold extremities denoting severe shock. Mesenteric embolism is the cause of acute intestinal ischaemia in 25–30% of cases, (**Table 48.1**) the commonest site of origin being the heart (**Figure 48.1**).

The patient is resuscitated with intravenous fluids and antibiotics and heparinised. If time permits a selective superior mesenteric angiogram may be carried out. If an angiogram is being done, then radiological intervention (angioplasty/thrombolysis) may be considered. In most instances, laparotomy has to be done to inspect the bowel for viability. Depending upon the findings, the appropriate procedure is carried out – revascularisation such as embolectomy, reimplantation of the superior mesenteric artery into the aorta or bypass grafting from the aorta to the superior mesenteric artery. In case of gangrenous bowel, resection is the only choice.

Table 48.1	
Type of small bowel ischaemia	**Cause**
Arterial thrombosis	Atherosclerosis
	Thrombotic conditions
Arterial embolism	Atrial fibrillation
	Mural thrombus
	Vegetations
	Atherosclerotic plaque
Venous thrombosis	Hypercoagulable states
	Malignancy
	Inflammation
	Mechanical venous occlusion
Rare causes	Aortic dissection
	Cardiac bypass
	Interventional radiology

Table 48.1 Aetiology of small bowel ischaemia. (Adapted from Windsor ACJ and Heriot AG. The small Intestine. In: Burnand KG, Young AE, Lucas J. The New Aird's Companion in Surgical Studies, 3rd editon. Edinburgh: Churchill Livingstone, 2005.)

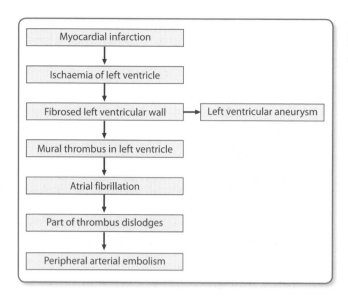

Figure 48.1
Pathophysiology of arterial embolism.

Depending upon the length of dead bowel, the patient may end up with short bowel syndrome and intestinal failure. This may require parenteral nutrition in the long-term (home parenteral nutrition).

2. D Crohn's disease

This woman with altered bowel habit, abdominal pain, generally feeling unwell, suggestion of a mass in the right iliac fossa and erythema nodosum has inflammatory bowel disease, with Crohn's disease being the most likely diagnosis. The perianal region should be thoroughly examined for other manifestations such as fistulae. The management would consist of confirmation of the diagnosis followed by definitive treatment.

A barium meal and follow through or small bowel enema is the first imaging technique. **Figure 48.2** shows gross narrowing of the terminal ileum as it enters the caecum – the classical 'string sign of Kantor'. Involvement of the ileum occurs in 60%. This should be followed by a colonoscopy to look for lesions in the large bowel which is affected in 30%; any suspicious lesions should be biopsied. The histology shows transmural inflammation with deep fissured aphthous ulcers. Classical non-caseating giant cell granuloma is seen in 60% (**Figure 48.3**). This disease can affect any part of the gastrointestinal system and is prone to various complications (**Table 48.2**).

These patients are ideally managed by a team consisting of a gastroenterologist, a colorectal surgeon and a dietitian. The mainstay of treatment is medical consisting of steroids, immunosuppressives such as azathioprine and infliximab (particularly in severe active perianal disease) and supportive therapy. Surgery is reserved for complications and should be as conservative as possible with various options available depending upon the findings – limited right hemicolectomy (**Figure 48.4**)

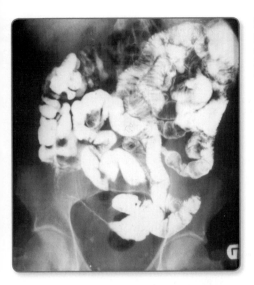

Figure 48.2 Barium meal and follow through showing a narrowed terminal ileum – the typical 'string sign of Kantor' in Crohn's disease.

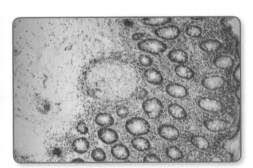

Figure 48.3 Histopathology in Crohn's disease: transmural inflammation with non-caseating granuloma.

local resections, strictureplasty, colectomy and ileorectal anastomosis and proctocolectomy.

A Acute appendicitis

This patient has some of the typical features of acute appendicitis – the visceral-somatic sequence of pain of periumbilical colic settling in the right iliac fossa combined with nausea, vomiting and anorexia. The diarrhoea would suggest a pelvic position of the appendix. The classical signs in acute appendicitis are not present in all patients. They are: the 'pointing sign', when the patient points to the umbilicus as the site of origin of the pain and the right iliac fossa as the site where the pain has settled; Rovsing's sign, when pressing in the left iliac fossa elicits pain the right iliac fossa due to the small bowel loops being pushed against the inflamed appendix; the 'psoas sign', when retrocaecal appendicitis can cause psoas spasm resulting in flexion of the hip for relief of pain; the 'obturator sign', when pain is elicited in the suprapubic area by flexing and internally rotating the hip causing the inflamed appendix to be in contact with the obturator internus.

Table 48.2

Local complications	Distant (metastatic) complications
• External fistulae:	*Infected*
– Enterocutaneous	Skin:
– Colocutaneous	• Pyoderma gangrenosum
– Enterovaginal	• Erythema nodosum
– Colovaginal	Eyes:
– Perianal	• Keratitis
• Internal fistulae:	• Episcleritis
– Enteroenteric	Joints:
– Enterocolic	• Septic arthritis
– Enterovesical	• Septicaemia
– Colovesical	• Psoas abscess
• Abscesses	*Non-infected*
• Stricture	• Polyarthropathy
• Carcinoma	• Venous thrombosis
• Haemorrhage	• Physical retardation
• Perforation	• Hepatobiliary disease
• Toxic megacolon	• Ureteric strictures

Table 48.2 Local and distant complications of Crohn's disease.

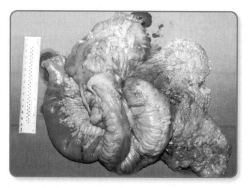

Figure 48.4 Right hemicolectomy specimen showing characteristic macroscopic features in Crohn's disease – thickened, oedematous ileum, mesenteric fat over-riding bowel wall, enteroenteric fistula.

The diagnosis of acute appendicitis is clinical. Because of the presence of the pelvic organs, women pose a greater challenge to the diagnosis. Whilst there are scoring methods and imaging techniques available to come to an accurate diagnosis, in practice, a diagnostic laparoscopy gives a definitive diagnosis. Emergency appendicectomy, laparoscopic or open, is the treatment of choice. Antibiotic treatment is started preoperatively with metronidazole and cefuroxime and continued postoperatively for 24 hours or longer if there has been generalised peritonitis.

. H Small bowel lymphoma

This patient who is a known sufferer of coeliac disease has developed colicky abdominal pain with increasing diarrhoea, a symptom distinctly different from her usual diarrhoea of coeliac disease. Patients with coeliac disease have an increased chance of developing small bowel lymphoma. Her colicky abdominal pain is suggestive of intermittent small bowel obstruction. The diagnosis can be confirmed by small bowel enema and CT scan. The treatment is small bowel resection and end-to-end anastomosis. Accurate staging of the disease is carried out followed by appropriate postoperative chemotherapy.

Often the diagnosis is made at laparotomy carried out as an emergency for intestinal obstruction or perforation. Lymphoma supervening on coeliac disease is of the T-cell type. There is another type which is a part of non-Hodgkin's B-cell lymphoma which is an annular ulcerative lesion and may present as obstruction, haemorrhage and perforation. These tumours are referred to as Mucosa Associated Lymphoid Tissue tumours (MALTomas).

. E Carcinoma of rectum

This 60-year-old man has severely altered bowel habit in the form of early morning spurious diarrhoea, tenesmus and feeling of incomplete evacuation of his bowels after several visits to the lavatory. This is typical of a low distal large bowel carcinoma. The masses felt in the left iliac fossa are inspissated faecal matter proximal to an annular growth causing impending obstruction. He needs a sigmoidoscopy and biopsy followed by a barium enema which may show a 'napkin-ring' appearance (**Figure 48.5**). The patient has an annular carcinoma in the rectosigmoid. Always a synchronous carcinoma (**Figure 48.6**), which occurs in up to 10%, should be excluded by a colonoscopy. However, in this patient it would not be possible to negotiate the colonoscope beyond the growth.

The carcinoma should be accurately staged by a contrast-enhanced CT scan, MRI of the pelvis and endoluminal ultrasound. After confirmation of the diagnosis and staging, definitive treatment is instituted after discussion in a multidisciplinary team. In this patient the surgical treatment should be anterior resection (**Figure 48.7**) with total mesorectal excision. Dependent upon the local spread of the growth, preoperative radiotherapy may be given. Postoperative adjuvant chemotherapy may be required depending on the Dukes' staging and histological grading. In very low rectal growths which are within 2–3 cm of the anal verge, an abdominoperineal excision of the rectum (**Figure 48.8**) will have to be done. In general for carcinoma of the rectum, the vast majority of patients will have a restorative resection.

. C Carcinoma of the caecum

This woman suffers from anaemic hypoxia and is unable to do her daily, routine activities without becoming breathless. She is obviously bleeding from her lower gastrointestinal tract as her faecal occult blood test is positive and oesophagogastroduodenoscopy is negative. With no alteration in her bowel

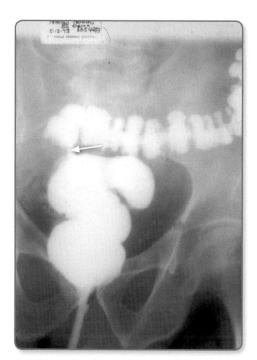

Figure 48.5 Barium enema of the upper rectum showing a 'napkin-ring' deformity (arrow) typical of annular carcinoma.

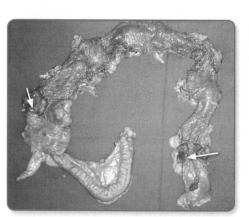

Figure 48.6 Specimen from a sub-total colectomy showing synchronous carcinoma (arrows).

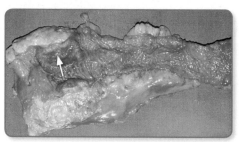

Figure 48.7 Specimen showing anterior resection for carcinoma of the upper rectum (arrow).

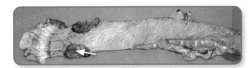

Figure 48.8 Specimen of abdomino-perineal resection showing carcinoma of lower rectum (arrow).

habit and a mass in the right iliac fossa, a carcinoma of the caecum should be suspected. A barium enema (**Figure 48.9a**) shows an irregular filling defect in the caecum, typical of a polypoid carcinoma. Caecal carcinoma can also present as an emergency with acute distal small bowel obstruction due to obstruction to the ileocaecal junction by the growth; another emergency presentation is when the condition masquerades as 'acute appendicitis' because of obstruction to the lumen of the appendix by the cancer. In such cases, the diagnosis of caecal carcinoma should be strongly suspected because the patient would be anaemic, which is not a feature of acute appendicitis.

Although confirmation of the diagnosis by a colonoscopic biopsy may be carried out, with such a classical picture this would be academic and a waste of resources. A contrast CT scan should be the next imaging technique. After staging, a right hemicolectomy (**Figure 48.9b**) is carried out with ileotransverse anastomosis. Even in the presence of liver secondaries, a right hemicolectomy should be the treatment as excision of the carcinoma is the best palliation. If the postoperative staging shows a Dukes' C cancer, then adjuvant chemotherapy is given.

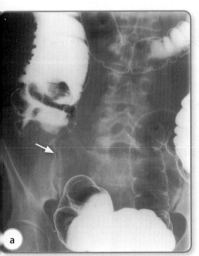

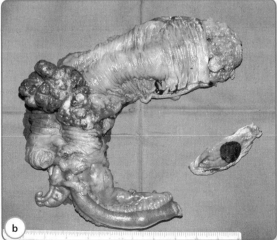

Figure 48.9 (a) Barium enema showing an irregular filling defect (arrow) in the caecum, typical of a polypoid carcinoma. (b) Specimen from the same patient after right hemicolectomy; there is polypoid carcinoma of the caecum; coincidental cholecystectomy is also seen.

7. K Ulcerative colitis

This young woman presents with clinical features of ulcerative colitis – several loose motions a day with blood and slime, lethargy, left-sided abdominal pain, raised inflammatory markers and anaemia. She requires a full colonoscopy and biopsy to confirm the diagnosis. The colonoscopic findings are red, inflamed mucosa that bleeds easily on touch, purulent discharge, small ulcers and regenerative nodules called pseudopolyps. Biopsy shows increased inflammatory cells confined to the mucosa with numerous crypt abscesses and depletion of goblet cells. The barium enema will show complete loss of haustration, granular mucosa, narrow contracted colon likened to a 'lead-pipe' (**Figure 48.10a**); in the lateral view (**Figure 48.10b**) there is increase in the retrorectal or presacral space. The disease is categorised as mild, moderate and severe depending upon the clinical features.

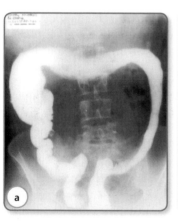
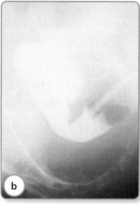

Figure 48.10 (a) Barium enema showing complete loss of haustration, granular mucosa, and narrow contracted colon, likened to a 'lead-pipe'. (b) Barium enema showing an increase in the retro-rectal or pre-sacral space in severe ulcerative colitis.

The mainstay of treatment is medical with steroids and 5-aminosalicylic acid (5-ASA) derivatives, given both systemically and locally as enemas. These patients are prone to developing complications (**Table 48.3**). Surgery is considered under certain circumstances (**Table 48.4**). The incidence of cancer increases with the duration of the disease. Therefore, patients who have had the disease for more than 10 years are kept under annual colonoscopic surveillance and biopsy to look for dysplasia or carcinoma. Patients who have a stricture (**Figure 48.11a**) should be meticulously colonoscoped and biopsied for an underlying carcinoma. Various types of operations are available and used according to the clinical situation: Proctocolectomy and ileostomy (**Figure 48.11b**), restorative proctocolectomy and ileoanal pouch, colectomy and ileorectal anastomosis.

8. A Acute diverticulitis

This 70-year-old woman has the clinical features of acute diverticulitis – pain in the left lower abdomen, passage of loose stools, fever, nausea and abdominal distension with tenderness, rigidity and rebound tenderness in the left iliac fossa. Moreover, on rectal examination a tender mass is felt in the pouch of Douglas through the rectal

Table 48.3

Local complications	Systemic (remote or distant) complications
• Acute dilatation or toxic megacolon (10%)	• Arthritis
• Perforation (2%)	• Ankylosing spondylitis
• Massive haemorrhage (3%)	• Skin lesions :
• Benign stricture (10%)	– Erythema nodosum
• Inflammatory polyposis	– Pyoderma gangrenosum
• Carcinoma (5%)	• Eye lesions
• Anorectal complications (15%):	• Liver and biliary tract disease:
– Fissure	– Sclerosing cholangitis
– Anorectal abscess and fistula	• Stomatitis
– Rectovaginal fistula	• Oesophagitis

Table 48.3 Local and systemic complications of ulcerative colitis.

Table 48.4

Indications for emergency/urgent operations	Failure of medical treatment during an acute exacerbation
	Perforation
	Acute toxic megacolon
	Severe haemorrhage
Indications for elective operations	Intractability and chronic invalidism
	Risk (or actual development) of malignant change
	Retardation of growth and development
	Local anorectal complication
	Remote or systemic complications

Table 48.4 Indications for emergency/urgent and elective operations for ulcerative colitis.

wall – the inflamed mass of sigmoid diverticulitis. Routine haematological tests should show polymorphonuclear leucocytosis and increase in inflammatory markers.

After blood cultures are taken, she is treated with intravenous metronidazole and cefuroxime, intravenous fluids and analgesics. The diagnosis is confirmed by ultrasound or CT. Once the patient has recovered, thorough imaging is carried out by barium enema and colonoscopy. The latter may not be possible if there is a significant stricture seen on barium enema (**Figure 48.12**) which may be an

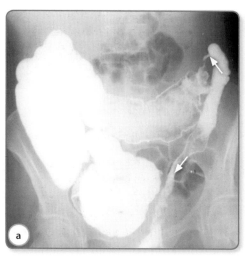
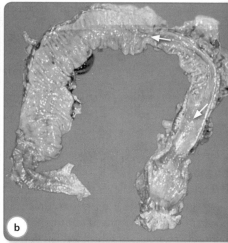

Figure 48.11 (a) Barium enema showing two strictures in ulcerative colitis (arrows); both turned out to be carcinoma. (b) Specimen of panproctocolectomy from the same patient, showing two carcinomas (arrows).

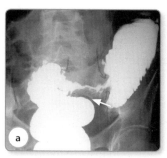
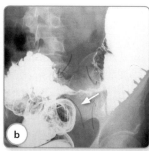

Figure 48.12 (a) and (b) Barium enema showing stricture of sigmoid colon from diverticular disease (arrows).

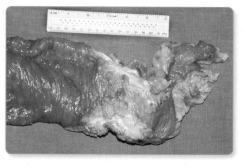

Figure 48.13 Specimen from sigmoid resection for diverticular stricture, from the same patient as in Figure 48.12.

aftermath of diverticulitis. Nevertheless it is important to do colonoscopy and biopsy to exclude the possibility of an unexpected carcinoma within the diverticular segment. An elective sigmoid resection (**Figure 48.13**) is carried out to prevent recurrence of complications (**Table 48.5**). If the acute diverticulitis does not settle, it may result in a pericolic abscess.

Table 48.5

Types of diverticular disease	Notes	Complications
Diverticulosis	Asymptomatic Symptomatic	Fistulae: • Colovesical • Coloenteric • Colocutaneous • Colovaginal • Colocolic
Painful diverticular disease	Due to excessive segmentation	Obstruction (mimics carcinoma)
		Abscess
Acute diverticulitis	Also referred to as left-sided appendicitis	Perforation (purulent or faecal peritonitis) Haemorrhage (almost always stops with conservative management)

Table 48.5 Types of diverticular disease and a summary of complications.

A pericolic abscess is confirmed by US or CT and then drained percutaneously by the radiologist. Once the patient has recovered from this, the sequence of subsequent management is the same as above. In the Western population 60% of those over the age of 60 years have diverticular disease, the sigmoid colon being affected in 90%.

F Colovesical fistula

This patient has the clinical features of repeated attacks of urinary tract infection, particularly pneumatinuria, a classical method of presentation of colovesical fistula. Some patients may be astute enough to complain of faecaluria. Colovesical fistula most commonly occurs from diverticular disease, other causes being Crohn's colitis and colorectal carcinoma. In view of this patient's long-standing constipation, diverticulitis should come to mind as the cause of his problem.

This patient requires a barium enema to confirm the diagnosis of diverticular disease and gas in the urinary bladder (**Figure 48.14**) or rarely barium in the urinary bladder (**Figure 48.15**). A flexible sigmoidoscopy or colonoscopy and biopsy must be carried out to exclude an unsuspected carcinoma in the midst of the diverticular segment. Full colonoscopy may not be possible in view of the strictured sigmoid colon, a common occurrence.

After a full course of antibiotics laparotomy is performed. In diverticular disease the affected sigmoid colon is pinched off or separated from the bladder, the hole in the bladder (which sometimes may not be seen due to the induration and inflammation) is sutured and the sigmoid colon resected with an end-to-end anastomosis; in colonic Crohn's a small portion of the bladder wall is excised with the bowel and the bladder closed; in colonic carcinoma a good part of the bladder wall is excised in continuity with the sigmoid colon (as a partial cystectomy) followed by end-to-end anastomosis. In all cases an indwelling catheter is left for about 10 days.

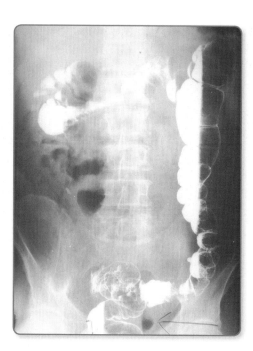

Figure 48.14 Barium enema showing air in the urinary bladder (arrow).

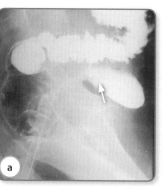

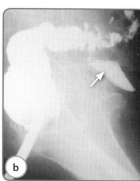

Figure 48.15 (a) and (b) Barium enema showing barium in the urinary bladder and colovesical fistulous track (arrows)

---

10. B Acute large bowel obstruction

This patient has the features of acute closed-loop large bowel obstruction – colicky abdominal pain with persisting dull ache in between colics, increasing constipation, peripheral abdominal distension and a hollow rectum. As he has not vomited, his problem is one of closed-loop obstruction where there is a competent ileocaecal valve with no distension of the small bowel. With a history of increasing constipation over the previous few months, the cause should be presumed to be a left colonic carcinoma until proven otherwise.

This patient now needs to be resuscitated. Once stabilised, the next step is imaging to establish the site and cause of obstruction. After supine and erect plain abdominal X-rays (**Figure 48.16**), imaging can be done in various ways depending upon the facilities available: urgent Gastrografin enema, flexible sigmoidoscopy or

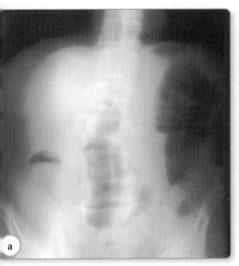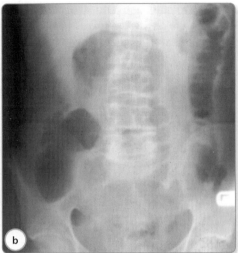

a   b

Figure 48.16 Plain abdominal X-rays showing acute closed-loop large bowel obstruction. (a) X-ray taken in an erect position, which reveals multiple fluid levels. (b) X-ray taken in a supine position, which shows that the caecum, transverse colon and descending colon are massively distended.

colonoscopy, CT colonography; lower gastrointestinal endoscopy has the advantage of a biopsy.

Once optimised and the cause and site of obstruction determined, definitive treatment is instituted. The choices are as follows:

- Initial stenting of the obstruction during contrast enema followed by biopsy, staging and a one-stage resection and anastomosis
- One-stage resection and anastomosis with on-table intraoperative colonic irrigation
- Sub-total colectomy or extended right hemicolectomy (depending upon the site of the growth) with ileocolic anastomosis (**Figure 48.17**) – a one-stage procedure

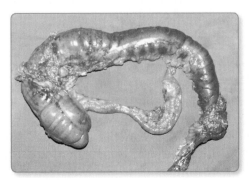

Figure 48.17 Specimen from a sub-total colectomy for acute closed-loop large bowel obstruction, resulting from descending colon carcinoma.

- Two-stage procedure: Hartmann-type resection with end colostomy; second-stage procedure for restoration of bowel continuity after 2–3 months
- If the obstruction is due to a right colonic carcinoma, a right hemicolectomy with ileotransverse anastomosis

11. G Familial adenomatous polyposis

This young man with loose stools combined with blood and mucus and colicky abdominal pain with a family history of large bowel cancer should arouse the suspicion of familial adenomatous polyposis. The fact that his father died at a young age of cancer and he was under annual colonoscopic surveillance in his previous place of residence, since he was a teenager makes the diagnosis very probable. He needs urgent imaging with full colonoscopy and a barium enema with genetic studies carried out. An oesophagogastroduodenoscopy is also carried out to exclude polyps in the duodenum and a barium meal and follow through to detect any small bowel polyps.

If the diagnosis is established the patient should be offered surgical treatment in the form of:

- Colectomy and ileorectal anastomosis if the rectum is spared. Such patients should have regular 6-monthly flexible sigmoidoscopy for any polyps which should be fulgurated and biopsied. If cancer supervenes, the ileorectal anatomises and rectal stump is excised with a permanent ileostomy.
- Restorative proctocolectomy with ileoanal anastomosis.

The condition is inherited as an autosomal dominant inherited disease from mutation of the adenomatous polyposis colic gene which has been identified on the short arm of the chromosome 5. At risk family members should be offered genetic counselling, testing and colonoscopic surveillance from their early teens until the age of 20. If by then no polyps appear then they are offered a colonoscopy check every 5 years until the age of 50.

12. A Anal carcinoma

When patients complain of 'piles' it is important to ask the patient to explain in detail the actual symptom as the lay person refers to any symptom around the anus as 'piles'. This patient says that he can feel a painful lump that is constantly present and bleeds. The fact that the lump is always present and does not reduce should arouse the suspicion that it is not piles. Moreover, as a renal transplant patient he has a 100 times increased risk of developing anal carcinoma. Other predisposing causes are human papilloma virus infection, anal intraepithelial neoplasia, HIV infection and homosexual men with anal sexual practices. The physical findings of an ulcerated mass with raised everted edges are clinically diagnostic of squamous cell carcinoma. The disease should be confirmed, staged and treated.

Confirmation is carried out by biopsy under general anaesthetic. At the same time an examination under anaesthetic, a useful method of clinical staging, is carried out. A CT scan and MRI should complete the staging. Chemoradiotherapy is the mainstay of treatment.

3. B Condylomata acuminata (anal warts)

This young man has anal warts also known as condylomata acuminata. This condition is more common in those with human papilloma virus and HIV. Pruritus, discharge, bleeding and a painful wart-like growth are the typical clinical features. A cauliflower-like excrescence will be seen (**Figure 48.18**). Associated warts in the genital tracts may be present. Biopsy is done to confirm the diagnosis and exclude malignancy. Treatment is a combination of surgical excision and application of 25% podophyllin.

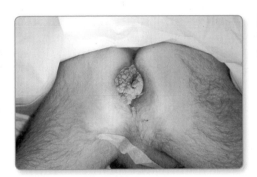

Figure 48.18 Condylomata acuminata, which has a fleshy, cauliflower-like excrescence.

4. D Fistula-in-ano

This patient, who is a sufferer from Crohn's disease, has perianal symptoms suggestive of fistula-in-ano which has occurred as a complication. The history suggests that 6 weeks ago he had a perianal abscess that naturally burst resulting in his fistula.

He now needs the fistula thoroughly evaluated. Clinical assessment of the function of the anal sphincter by resting tone and voluntary squeeze is made; this is complemented by more accurate assessment by anal manometry and endoanal ultrasound. Finally an MRI and examination under anaesthesia using a probe is essential to look for secondary extensions. It must be established whether the internal opening is above the anal sphincter (high anal fistula) or below the anal sphincter (low anal fistula) as the type of surgical treatment will depend upon that finding.

A high anal fistula will require a staged procedure of fistulotomy and use of a Seton (a length of non-absorbable suture material) so as to avoid incontinence. In complicated cases using the technique of an anorectal advancement flap may be indicated. A low anal fistula may be treated by fistulectomy. The use of fibrin tissue glue to plug and seal the track is under evaluation.

In this particular patient the underlying Crohn's disease must be kept under control medically. If intractable, the role of immunotherapy by using infliximab (a tumour necrosis factor alpha antagonist) should be considered.

Chapter 49

Endocrine and breast

Theme: The thyroid gland

Options for Questions 1–3:

A	Anaplastic carcinoma	E	Lateral aberrant thyroid
B	Colloid goitre	F	Multinodular goitre
C	Differentiated thyroid cancer	G	Physiological goitre
D	Grave's disease	H	Toxic multinodular goitre

For each of the following situations, select the single most likely diagnosis. Each option may be used once, more than once or not at all.

1. A 52-year-old woman presents with a multinodular goitre, which was diagnosed 10 years ago. Recently, she complains of severe palpitation. On examination, the only abnormality is a pulse rate of 112 beats per minute.

2. A 32-year-old woman presents with a solitary thyroid nodule of 2 months duration. On clinical examination a 2 cm nodule is found in the left lobe. She is euthyroid. Ultrasound (US) demonstrates a mixed solid and cystic lesion. US-guided fine-needle aspiration cytology from the solid part of the lesion reads 'malignancy cannot be excluded'.

3. A 60-year-old woman with a large multinodular goitre of 20 years duration complains of hoarseness of voice, dysphagia and dyspnoea lasting 6 weeks. She also has stridor and a sensation of heaviness and choking in her throat.

Theme: Hypercalcaemia/hyperparathyroidism

Options for Questions 4–6:

A	Familial hypocalciuric hypercalcaemia	E	Parathyroid hyperplasia
		F	Secondary hyperparathyroidism
B	Hyperthyroidism	G	Sarcoidosis
C	Hypercalcaemia of malignancy	H	Pheochromocytoma
D	Parathyroid adenoma	I	Tertiary hyperparathyroidism

For each of the following situations, select the single most likely diagnosis. Each option may be used once, more than once or not at all.

4. A 72-year-old woman presents with marked thirst, aches and pains all over her body and a feeling of nausea. Routine blood biochemistry shows a serum calcium of 2.9 mmol/L. She underwent a mastectomy 6 years ago for carcinoma.

5. A 30-year-old man complains of lethargy, abdominal pain and generally feeling unwell for the past couple of months. He has had two typical attacks of ureteric colic, once on each side. On routine biochemistry his serum calcium is found to be 3.1 mmol/L.

6. A 50-year-old woman who suffered from chronic renal failure for many years underwent a renal transplant 1 year ago. She felt very well after her transplant for a few months. Thereafter, she started feeling lethargic and generally unwell although her renal function remained stable. Her serum calcium is 2.9 mmol/L, and she has a raised serum phosphate.

Theme: The adrenals/endocrine disorders

Options for Questions 7–9:

A   Addison's disease
B   Conn's syndrome
C   Cushing's syndrome
D   Multiple endocrine neoplasia
E   Pheochromocytoma

For each of the following situations, select the single most likely diagnosis. Each option may be used once, more than once or not at all.

7. A 45-year-old woman presents with headaches, generalised muscle weakness, tiredness, polydypsia and polyuria of 7 months duration. She also has resistant hypertension. Her serum potassium is 2.2 mmol/L with metabolic alkalosis.

8. A 38-year-old man presents with paroxysmal headaches, palpitations and sweating. He has attacks of dyspnoea and bitterly complains of feeling generally unwell and weak. His general practitioner has noted that he has intermittent episodes of labile hypertension.

9. A 40-year-old woman presents with recurrent attacks of ureteric colic that have been treated conservatively. Since the age of 30 years, she has been diagnosed with duodenal ulcers, which are also treated conservatively and she has been on continuous medical treatment. Recently, she has been embarrassed by the onset of milk secretion from her breasts. She is found to have hypercalcaemia.

Theme: The breast

Options for Questions 10–12:

A   Abscess
B   Aberration of normal development and involution
C   Carcinoma
D   Fat necrosis
E   Fibroadenoma
F   Mondor's disease
G   Phyllodes tumour

For each of the following situations, select the single most likely diagnosis. Each option may be used once, more than once or not at all.

0. A 22-year-old woman presents after finding a painless lump in her left breast 4 weeks ago. The lump moves about very freely and she is concerned about cancer. On examination she has a mobile firm 2 cm discrete lump in her left breast.

1. A 38-year-old woman complains of generalised pain in her right breast, often associated with her periods. She sometimes feels a lump, the size of which tends to vary. On examination, she has a tender lump in the upper outer quadrant of her right breast.

2. A 55-year-old woman complains of a lump in her left breast that appeared about 4 months ago and has been rapidly growing. It is painful. On examination, she has a mobile, slightly tender, 12 cm irregular lump, the surface of which is bosselated with the overlying skin stretched and about to ulcerate.

Answers

1. H Toxic multinodular goitre

This woman with a long-standing goitre has developed features of secondary thyrotoxicosis. These patients present with cardiovascular symptoms, as in this patient who has tachycardia. They do not exhibit any of the features of Graves' disease such as eye signs. This is the outcome of autonomous overproduction of thyroxine by the multinodular goitre. The nodules may be inactive, the thyroid overactivity coming from the internodular tissue. In some instances one or more of the nodules may be overactive. The toxicity is due to autonomous thyroid tissue. It is uncertain why previous non-functioning nodules should start to over-function. One theory is that there may be mutations of growth factor receptors. This condition is sometimes called Plummer's syndrome.

The patient is investigated by a radioisotope iodine scan. She is treated medically and once stabilised, surgery is considered.

2. C Differentiated thyroid cancer

This young woman, presenting with an euthyroid solitary nodule, has a differentiated thyroid cancer (papillary or follicular or one of their variants) unless otherwise proven. Ultrasound of the nodule shows a solid and cystic lesion whilst the result of the fine-needle aspiration cytology was equivocal. In this situation this patient requires a hemithyroidectomy to obtain proper histology. Before this is done, the patient should have a chest X-ray and MRI of the neck to detect lymphadenopathy.

The facility of frozen section, if available, is most welcome. This is because should the frozen section show a follicular carcinoma, then the surgeon proceeds to total thyroidectomy. If it shows papillary carcinoma, the appropriate surgery can be carried out depending upon the scoring of the cancer and choice of the individual surgeon (total or hemi-thyroidectomy with node dissection). In papillary carcinoma, branching papillae and cells with empty nuclei ('Orphan Annie' cells) are seen with calcospherites (calcium laden microscopic masses also called psammoma bodies). Follicular carcinoma can only be diagnosed in the presence of vascular and capsular invasion – hence the need for histology.

3. A Anaplastic carcinoma

This woman has the typical features of an anaplastic (undifferentiated) carcinoma – a long-standing goitre with recent onset of tracheal compression and recurrent laryngeal nerve infiltration. This type of thyroid cancer constitutes 10% of thyroid cancers and occurs most often in areas of endemic goitre. It spreads by local infiltration, lymphatics and blood stream. The diagnosis is confirmed by fine-needle aspiration cytology or core biopsy; the tumour shows spindle-shaped and giant cells with polypoid nuclei and numerous mitoses. After staging the disease with a CT scan and chest X-ray, external beam radiotherapy is the treatment of choice. Respiratory embarrassment may require tracheal decompression by isthmusectomy. The prognosis is extremely poor, with the majority of patients succumbing to the disease within 6 months of the diagnosis being made.

C Hypercalcaemia of malignancy

This woman, who underwent a mastectomy for carcinoma 6 years ago, now has generalised features of hypercalcaemia. This is a paraneoplastic complication arising from skeletal metastases. It affects 10% of all cancer patients. In a minority hypercalcaemia may occur without any bony metastases. The cause of malignant hypercalcaemia is the secretion of a parathormone-like peptide by the tumour. It also occurs from osteoclastic activity; other causes may be the production of prostaglandins, vitamin D metabolites, tumour growth factor-α (TGF-α) and tumour growth factor-β (TGF-β). The treatment is to palliate the patient by rehydration and the use of bisphosphonates.

D Parathyroid adenoma

This man has the features of hypercalcaemia. The classical description of 'stones, moans, abdominal groans and psychic moans' are an exception rather than a rule. Most often this condition is discovered by hypercalcaemia on routine biochemical screening for some unrelated complaint. Patients may develop symptoms from a peptic ulcer or suffer from recurrent attacks of pancreatitis, acute or chronic. Clinically usually there are no signs.

These patients need to be thoroughly investigated. Corrected serum calcium level is calculated. If elevated, serum parathormone level is assayed. A raised serum calcium in the presence of elevated parathyroid hormone confirms primary hyperparathyroidism. The cause in 90% of such patients is a parathyroid adenoma. While there are many methods of localising the adenoma, at present US and technetium-labelled sestamibi scan are the two modalities of choice. The latter is particularly important to exclude an adenoma in an ectopic gland such as in the mediastinum. Once localised, the adenoma is excised.

I Tertiary hyperparathyroidism

This patient who has had a renal transplant after suffering from chronic renal failure for many years has tertiary hyperparathyroidism. This condition arises after many years of chronic renal failure resulting in hypocalcaemia and increased serum phosphate. This causes increased secretion of PTH resulting in functional hyperplasia of the parathyroids. Normally the condition is reversed after renal transplantation.

However, occasionally hyperfunction continues in an autonomous manner even after renal transplantation. This results in continued parathyroid hyperplasia. In such instances one or more of the glands may become autonomous producing an adenoma. This requires parathyroidectomy for the adenoma or hyperplasia as the case may be.

7. B Conn's syndrome

This patient has Conn's syndrome or primary aldosteronism as evidenced by refractory hypertension and features of severe potassium depletion – generalised muscle weakness and fatigue. Polyuria and polydypsia result from inability of the kidney to concentrate the urine. The commonest cause is an unilateral adenoma less than 3 cm in diameter arising from the adrenal cortex. Bilateral nodular hyperplasia may be the cause in a minority of cases. Pathologically the tumors are yellow in colour; the cells are arranged in rods, clear and rich in lipid resembling zona fasciculata.

The biochemical diagnosis is confirmed by: persistently low serum potassium, high urinary potassium excretion, and a ratio of plasma aldosterone plasma renin activity greater than 50. An aldosterone suppression test and aldosterone to cortisol ratio in blood from selective adrenal vein catheterisation are other tests carried out. A CT scan will localise lesions more than 1 cm whereas MRI is necessary for smaller or bilateral lesions. Treatment is excision of the adenoma which can be done laparoscopically.

8. E Pheochromocytoma

This patient has the key features of a pheochromocytoma – labile hypertension with palpitation, sweating and headache resulting from episodic catecholamine release from the tumour. This may be precipitated by physical activity. Undetected for a long time, there may be harmful effects of catecholamine on the heart collectively referred to catecholamine cardiomyopathy. The tumour is often referred to as the '10% tumour' because 10% are bilateral, 10% occur in children, 10% are extra-adrenal, 10% are malignant and 10% are inherited.

Initially the biochemical diagnosis is made by two separate 24-hour urinary levels of metanephrines, catecholamines and vanillylmandelic acid. This is followed by localisation of the tumour. For this MRI is the investigation of choice particularly to localise a tumour in an extra-adrenal site. It is also a safer investigation than a CT scan because use of contrast during CT may provoke a hypertensive crisis. Although the treatment is surgical, the overall management has to be a team effort between the cardiologist, anaesthetist, surgeon and radiologist.

9. D Multiple endocrine neoplasia (MEN 1 syndrome)

This woman has hypercalcaemia, peptic ulcer and galactorrhoea. This should alert one to the diagnosis of multiple endocrine neoplasia syndrome 1 consisting of primary hyperparathyroidism (pHPT), gastrinoma (pancreatic endocrine tumour) and a prolactinoma (pituitary tumour). Hypercalcaemic symptoms are usually the initial presentation. This is due to parathyroid hyperplasia for which she needs to be investigated. A gastrinoma producing Zollinger–Ellison syndrome is the cause of her recurrent and refractory peptic ulcer. Serum gastrin estimation and the secretin test followed by localisation of the tumour within the gastrinoma triangle are done. CT scan, MRI, and endoscopic and intraoperative ultrasound are the localisation techniques. The pituitary tumour is a prolactin-secreting microadenoma (prolactinoma). As it is a small tumour, it does not produce pressure symptoms but causes endocrine dysfunction; in some patients there may be no endocrine disturbance. Diagnosis is confirmed by elevated blood prolactin levels and localisation done by MRI.

Treatment is surgical for the parathyroid dysfunction and gastrinoma. The prolactinoma is treated medically by dopamine agonist and regularly monitored. Multiple endocrine neoplasia (MEN) syndrome is of two types: MEN2A consisting of familial medullary thyroid carcinoma (MCT), pHPT and phaeochromocytoma; MEN2B comprises of MCT, phaeochromocytoma, oral mucosal neuromas, intestinal ganglioneuromatosis with a marfanoid habitus.

. E Fibroadenoma

This young woman has a typical fibroadenoma – a small, firm, painless, freely mobile lump which tends to slip under the finger very easily; hence it is called a 'breast mouse'. Occasionally, a fibroadenoma may grow to a large size – when more than 5 cm in diameter it is referred to as a giant fibroadenoma, a condition more commonly seen in patients from the African continent. It arises from a single lobule which undergoes hyperplasia and is well encapsulated. Pathologically there are two types – pericanalicular (hard) and intracanalicular (soft), both being indistinguishable clinically. Their distinction is histological, the former having more stromal tissue and the latter more epithelial elements. Juvenile fibroadenomas occur in adolescents and may grow to a large size.

Diagnosis usually in a one-stop breast clinic is confirmed by triple assessment – clinical examination, imaging by ultrasound and pathological confirmation by fine-needle aspiration cytology or core biopsy. After confirmation and reassurance of the benign nature of the lesion, if the patient desires, it is excised. Very rarely lobular carcinoma or ductal carcinoma in situ may occur in a fibroadenoma exhibiting marked epithelial hyperplasia. In such cases, the prognosis is good.

. B Aberration of normal development and involution

This woman suffers from aberration of normal development and involution (ANDI), a term coined by Cardiff Breast Clinic to encompass several terms used in the past to denote various aspects of benign breast disease such as fibroadenosis, chronic mastitis, benign mammary dysplasia, cystic mastopathy and fibrocystic disease. This condition affects one-third of women between the ages of 20 and 50 years. It occurs as a result of the effect of cyclical pattern of the female hormones on breast tissue. This is influenced by menstrual cycle, pregnancy, the contraceptive pill and hormone replacement therapy. The clinical changes are a reflection of these hormonal changes on the tissues of the breast – lobules, ducts, stroma and epithelium lined by apocrine cells. Cysts form wherein the fluid is thin and dark giving a blue hue – hence the term 'blue-dome' cyst. The main pathological features are: nonproliferative fibrocystic change, apocrine metaplasia, proliferative fibrocystic change and florid epithelial hyperplasia, the latter being precancerous.

The management should follow the usual triple assessment of clinical examination imaging by ultrasound and/or mammography and pathological diagnosis by fine-needle aspiration cytology or core biopsy. Reassurance, medical treatment with drugs, aspiration of cysts and close follow-up is the essence of treatment.

12. G Phyllodes tumour

This woman has a phyllodes tumour also called serocystic disease of Brodie (described by Sir Benjamin Brodie in 1840) and cystosarcoma phyllodes (although is not cystic and very rarely sarcomatous). The name of the tumour is derived from the Greek word 'phyllo' meaning 'leaf' and macroscopically the tumour has a leaf-like appearance. The clinical features in this woman may easily be mistaken for an advanced carcinoma. It is a benign tumour which may have a very low malignant risk, the latter showing hypercellular stroma. Some tumours are termed borderline.

Imaging by mammography will show a well circumscribed or lobulated lesion; US shows hyperechoic areas within a hypoechoic mass. Treatment in the majority is enucleation or wide local excision depending upon the size. Mastectomy may be necessary when the tumour is massive or in case of malignancy.

Chapter 50

Vascular surgery

Theme: Abdominal aortic aneurysms

Options for Questions 1–3:

A   Aortocaval fistula
B   Aortoenteric fistula
C   Infected aortic graft
D   Myocardial infarction
E   Occlusion of marginal artery of Drummond

F   Ruptured abdominal aortic aneurysm
G   Ureteric colic

For each of the following cases, select the single most likely diagnosis. Each option may be used once, more than once or none at all.

A 73-year-old man presents with left sided flank pain, associated with haematuria and breathlessness. His blood biochemistry reveals markedly raised creatinine and urea levels. On examination, he has severe pain over his flank regions, worse on the left and is feeling hot but has no pyrexia. He is normotensive.

A 69-year-old man underwent a ruptured abdominal aortic aneurysm repair 2 years ago and is admitted with pain in his epigastrium with pyrexia. His white cell count is raised and his haemoglobin is 87 g/L. He has lost almost 15 kg in weight over the last 3 months with loss of appetite.

A 57-year-old woman undergoes repair of an elective abdominal aortic aneurysm. Postoperatively, she has a prolonged ileus followed by rectal bleeding. The white cell count is raised and she has tachycardia and abdominal pain, worse on the left side of the abdomen.

Theme: Arteriovenous fistulae

Options for Questions 4–6:

A	Anastomotic stenosis	E	Steal phenomenon
B	High output cardiac failure	F	Thrombosis of brachial cephalic
C	Ischaemic monomelic neuropathy		fistula
D	Phlebitis within a functioning fistula	G	Upstream stenosis of cephalic vei

For each of the following cases, select the single most likely diagnosis. Each option ma
be used once, more than once or none at all.

4. A 33-year-old woman attends the dialysis unit with a 2-day history of increasing
breathlessness and lower limb oedema. She undergoes her routine dialysis
through a functioning right arm fistula which is uncomplicated. Her breathlessne
persists and a duplex scan of the fistula confirms that there is good flow in the
cephalic vein in excess of 2.8 litres per minute.

5. A 43-year-old woman attends dialysis and her fistula is noted to be very tense wi
high venous pressures. Creatinine clearance is reduced and the patient has been
feeling increasingly lethargic.

6. A 67-year-old man presents with a newly created left brachial cephalic fistula
complaining of pain in the arm and a cold left hand. The patient has normal
neurological function. Two months later, during dialysis, his symptoms are much
worse. He wears a glove on his left hand which helps his symptoms.

Theme: Peripheral vascular disease

Options for Questions 7–9:

A	Bilateral external iliac stenosis	E	Popliteal aneurysm
B	Critical limb ischaemia	F	Popliteal entrapment
C	Intermittent claudication	G	Spinal claudication
D	Leriche syndrome		

For each of the following cases, select the single most likely diagnosis. Each option ma
be used once, more than once or none at all.

7. A 56-year-old man presents with bilateral buttock claudication at 100 metres and
impotence. He is a heavy smoker. His symptoms have got worse over the past 6
months. On examination, he is found to have weak bilateral femoral pulses but a
full compliment of pulses down both legs.

8. A 68-year-old man attends his GP with a 5-week history of pain in his right calf,
associated with numbness in his foot during exercise. Typically the pain comes o
after walking 50 metres, but sooner when he is walking uphill. On examination, h

has good bilateral femoral pulses but no pulses distal to his femorals bilaterally. He smokes 40 cigarettes a day and has no other past medical history.

A 49-year-old diabetic man is referred to the vascular surgeons with a 7-month history of worsening claudication in both legs. On examination, he has good bilateral femoral pulses and popliteal pulses but no distal pulses. His right foot has a 'punched out' ulcer over the 1st metatarsophalangeal joint on the plantar aspect. He also has a necrotic 5th toe. He denies any pain.

heme: Vascular investigations

ptions for Questions 10–12:

A Arterial duplex scan	**E** Magnetic resonance venogram
B CT angiogram	**F** Resting and post-exercise ankle
C Lymphangiogram	brachial pressure index
D Magnetic resonance angiography	**G** Venous duplex scan

r each of the following cases, select the single most appropriate investigation. Each tion may be used once, more than once or none at all.

. A 28-year-old woman presents with extensive, recurrent left leg varicose veins. She has a strong family history of varicose veins. Six years ago, she underwent injection sclerotherapy to her varicose veins. Now she presents with intermittent swelling of her left leg and marked haemosiderin deposition around her gaiter area.

. An obese 61-year-old woman with renal failure (estimated glomerular filtration rate < 15 mL/min) presenting with claudication affecting her right buttock and calf. She is known to have extensive calcification of her arteries and has a weak right femoral pulse.

. A 55-year-old man presents with calf claudication at 200 metres and normal peripheral pulses.

Answers

1. A Aortocaval fistula

The classical presentation of an aortocaval fistula is haematuria from back pressure in the renal vein giving rise to renal failure. The kidneys become congested and give rise to flank pain. If the fistula is of a significant size, the patient can develop symptoms of high output cardiac failure giving rise to breathlessness. There is often a 'machinery murmur' present on auscultation.

2. C Infected aortic graft

Aortic graft infection following aneurysm repair varies from <1% (elective aneurysm repair) up to 4% (ruptured aortic aneurysm repair). Any patient with a history of aortic surgery presenting with nonspecific and progressive symptoms of anaemia, weight loss and pyrexia with epigastric pain should be assumed to have an aortic graft infection unless proven otherwise. A contrast CT scan or a white cell count-labelled scan establishes the diagnosis.

3. E Occlusion of marginal artery of Drummond

The marginal artery (of Drummond) is the main connection between the inferior mesenteric and superior mesenteric arteries. The majority of patients shall exhibit this connection. In aneurysm surgery, the inferior mesenteric artery is often sacrificed, especially if it is blocked or has brisk back-bleeding. If the artery is patent but does not bleed, then it should be reimplanted to avoid ischaemia of the left colon. In this patient, the ileus, bleeding per rectum and the raised white cell count indicates bowel ischaemia.

4. B High output cardiac failure

The symptoms here relate to a fistula which has an extremely high flow rate. Over half of this patient's cardiac output is going through the fistula, giving rise to high output cardiac failure. The breathlessness and lower limb oedema point to cardiac failure as a result of the high fistula flow. Patients who have severe left ventricular dysfunction can develop an exacerbation of their cardiac failure with much lower fistula flow rates.

5. G Upstream stenosis of cephalic vein

Upstream cephalic vein stenosis will result in a very firm fistula which does not collapse on elevation of the arm. This is due to the arterial inflow being normal but the outflow compromised due to a narrowing of the cephalic vein (usually at or beyond the deltopectoral groove). During dialysis, the stenosis would prevent the patient from achieving adequate dialysis resulting is a reduced creatinine clearance and symptoms of uraemia.

E Steal phenomenon

This patient demonstrates classical steal phenomenon where most of the blood from the brachial artery is going through the fistula and very little flow into the forearm and hand. The ischaemic pain is typically worse during dialysis as this can further reduce the perfusion to the hand. Several methods can be employed to address this complication. In extreme cases when there is gangrenous change in the digits, the fistula often needs to be tied off.

D Leriche syndrome

The triad of Leriche syndrome (buttock claudication, absent or reduced femoral pulses and impotence in men) is likely here. The lesion is in the common iliac artery and this then affects flow into both the internal and external iliac arteries. Palpable distal pulses indicates his disease is localised to the aortoiliac segment.

C Intermittent claudication

This relates to the symptoms of intermittent claudication which classically are worse when walking uphill. The numbness in the foot is related to the fairly short history and is likely to improve with the development of collaterals. He is a smoker and clinically has superficial femoral artery occlusions or stenosis. The right leg is worse than the left, which at present is asymptomatic, only because the patient does not walk far enough continuously to subject himself to claudication in his left leg.

B Critical limb ischaemia

This patient has critical limb ischaemia. Although he denies any pain, this is likely due to severe neuropathy. Ulceration and gangrene with evidence of vascular disease (in this case within the crural vessels) is a serious situation that is likely to require urgent attention. Most neuropathic ulcers in diabetics have an ischaemic component to them.

0. G Venous duplex scan

Any varicose vein investigations should start with a venous duplex. It can comment on the degree of venous reflux and the anatomy of the veins. It is operator dependant but is an excellent first line investigation.

1. B CT angiogram

A CT scan would be the most appropriate investigation. An arterial duplex, especially at the level of the aortoiliac segment in an obese patient is difficult. Also, calcification is likely to cause an acoustic shadow with duplex scanning, even in the crural vessels. Renal failure is a contraindication for MRI that use gadolinium due to the risk of nephrogenic systemic fibrosis. ABPI pressures shall be spuriously high due to calcification.

12. F Resting and post-exercise ankle brachial pressure index

A patient who has a convincing history of claudication but normal palpable pulses may require pre- and post-exercise resting and post-exercise ankle brachial pressure index (ABPI). It is not uncommon for a high-grade iliac stenosis to give rise to 'normal' palpable pulses and resting ankle pressures. During exercise, there is often a drop in the ABPI signifying that the patient has a stenosis, not easily assessed during rest.

Chapter 51

Genitourinary surgery

Theme: Urological investigation

Options for Questions 1–3:

A	Bone scan	D	Plain intravenous urography
B	Kidney, ureters and bladder X-ray	E	Renal tract ultrasound scan
C	Non-contrast CT kidney, ureters and bladder	F	Triple phase contrast enhanced CT abdomen and pelvis

For each of the following situations, select the single most appropriate investigation. Each option may be used once, more than once or not at all.

1. A 29-year-old man presents with sudden onset of left loin pain which radiates to his left testis. He has tenderness in the left loin but an otherwise unremarkable examination. Urinalysis reveals microscopic haematuria only. Full blood count and renal function are normal. Renal colic is suspected.

2. A 35-year-old man presents to the emergency department having been stabbed with a kitchen knife in the left loin. He is haemodynamically stable but has passed frank haematuria. His abdomen is soft and non-tender. He has no significant past medical history.

3. A 25-year-old woman is referred to the urology department with recurrent urinary tract infections. A flexible cystoscopy is undertaken to ensure the patient does not have a bladder stone or fistula and to assess for urethral stenosis. The cystoscopy is normal. She requires further investigation to exclude a renal cause of her infections.

Theme: Urolithiasis

Options for Questions 4–6:

A	Conservative management	D	Percutaneous nephrolithotomy
B	Extracorporeal shockwave lithotripsy	E	Rigid ureteroscopy and stone fragmentation
C	Nephrectomy	F	Ureteric stent insertion

For each of the following situations, select the single most appropriate treatment. Eac[h] option may be used once, more than once or not at all.

4. A 32-year-old woman has right loin to groin pain with fevers. She has associated nausea and vomiting. Inflammatory markers are raised and she has a polymorphonuclear leucocytosis. Renal function is normal. She has no significan[t] past medical history. Imaging confirms a 7 mm distal right ureteric calculus with proximal hydronephrosis. She is commenced on analgesia, intravenous hydratio[n] and antibiotics but she continues to spike fevers.

5. A 49-year-old man, a football coach, has recurrent episodes of left loin pain which is controlled with diclofenac. A CT confirms the diagnosis of urolithiasis with a 7 mm right upper pole calculus with a density of 600 Hounsfield units. It is visible on plain abdominal X-ray.

6. A 47-year-old man with recurrent urinary tract infections is found to have a left staghorn calculus on CT kidneys, ureters and bladder. A dimercapto-succinic acid renogram confirms the split function to be 45% on the left and 55% on the right.

Theme: Scrotal swellings

Options for Questions 7–8:

A	Direct inguinal hernia	D	Indirect inguinal hernia
B	Epididymal cyst	E	Testicular tumour
C	Hydrocele	F	Varicocele

For each of the following situations, select the single most likely diagnosis. Each optio[n] may be used once, more than once or not at all.

7. A 27-year-old man presents with a 6-month history of scrotal swelling. There is no associated pain. He has no systemic upset. He does suffer from chronic constipatio[n]. The swelling is reducible and has a cough impulse. It is distinct from the testis.

8. A 64-year-old man with a recent diagnosis with a left renal tumour attends for his preoperative assessment and mentions to the junior doctor that he has a recent le[ft] scrotal swelling. It is a soft swelling, more obvious on standing but is not painful and feels separate to the testis. It does not trans-illuminate.

Theme: Bladder cancer

Options for Questions 9–10:

A	Course (six doses) of intravesical Bacillus Calmette–Guérin	D	Radical pelvic radiotherapy
B	Cystectomy	E	Transurethral resection of bladder tumour
C	Percutaneous needle biopsy	F	Conservative management

For each of the following situations, select the single most appropriate treatment. Each option may be used once, more than once or not at all.

A 57-year-old woman is referred by her general practitioner after 2 days of frank painless haematuria. She is otherwise well with significant co-morbidities. At haematuria clinic she has an ultrasound which is normal and a flexible cystoscopy which reveals a papillary tumour on the right lateral bladder wall.

10. A 69-year-old man with a history of ulcerative colitis and G3pT1a bladder cancer has his initial course of intravesical Bacillus Calmette–Guérin therapy. At follow-up cystoscopy there is a recurrent tumour which is resected. There is a mobile mass palpable on examination under anaesthetic. Pathology of the re-resection reveals disease progression to at least G3pT2a disease. Staging CT chest, abdomen and pelvis reveals no evidence of metastatic disease.

Theme: Prostate cancer

Options for Questions 11–12:

A	Active surveillance		ultrasound
B	Androgen deprivation	E	Radical prostatectomy
C	Cryotherapy	F	Radical radiotherapy
D	High intensity focussed		

For each of the following situations, select the single most appropriate treatment. Each option may be used once, more than once or not at all.

11. A 65-year-old man with Gleason 3 + 3 = 6 prostate cancer and a presenting prostate-specific antigen of 8 µg/L. He has had previous radiotherapy for testicular cancer but is otherwise very fit. He is keen on a radical treatment for this prostate cancer.

12. A 90-year-old man presents with urinary retention, a stony hard prostate which is fixed, and a prostate-specific antigen of 567µg/L. He has a bone scan which confirms sclerotic bone metastases.

Theme: Bladder outlet obstruction

Options for Questions 13–14:

    A   Finasteride (5-α-reductase inhibitor)
    B   Observation
    C   Open prostatectomy
    D   Tamsulosin (α-blocker)
    E   Transurethral resection of prostate

For each of the following situations, select the single most appropriate treatment. Each option may be used once, more than once or not at all.

13. An 81-year-old man presents to the emergency department with poor urinary flow, passing very little in the urine over the last few days, and nocturnal incontinence. He is very fit with minimal past medical history. He has a palpable bladder, a large (90 g) but smooth prostate. The bladder scanner reveals >999 mL residual volume. He is catheterised and has a residual volume of 1.5 L. His urea and electrolytes show a creatinine of 627 mg/dL (the baseline value 2 weeks previously was 65 mg/dL).

14. A 70-year-old man has severe lower urinary tract symptoms. He has been on tamsulosin and finasteride for 18 months with no improvement. On rectal examination, the prostate is very large and transrectal ultrasound confirms the volume to be 130 cm^3. Flexible cystoscopy is normal with the exception of a large occlusive prostate. His urinary flow rate is impaired. He wishes further treatment.

Answers

. C Non-contrast CT kidney, ureters and bladder

Non-contrast CT kidney, ureters and bladder (CTKUB) is the gold standard investigation for diagnosis of urinary tract calculi with a sensitivity >97%, while plain intravenous urography and kidney, ureters and bladder X-ray have sensitivities of 85 and 50% respectively. CTKUB has the advantage that intravenous contrast is not required thus avoiding associated complications and CT may diagnose other causes of flank pain.

. F Triple phase contrast-enhanced CT abdomen and pelvis

Triple phase CT is the imaging of choice for suspected renal injury. This allows accurate assessment of the degree of parenchymal, collecting system and vascular disruption. Indications for imaging include any penetrating renal injury or blunt injury with at least one of the following conditions (i) frank haematuria, (ii) microscopic haematuria and any haemodynamic instability, (iii) pre-existing anatomical abnormality, (iv) paediatric patients or (v) a significant mechanism of injury. Most cases of renal injury are managed conservatively. Interventional radiology and selective embolisation for ongoing bleeding can be used and occasionally surgical intervention is required.

. E Renal tract ultrasound scan

An ultrasound is the investigation of choice to ensure there are no upper urinary calculi or associated hydronephrosis. An ultrasound is ideal in this young female patient as is it non-invasive and there is no exposure to X-rays.

. F Ureteric stent insertion

An infected, obstructed kidney is a urological emergency and prompt decompression is important for resolution of sepsis. This can be done by either nephrostomy or ureteric stent insertion. Following resolution of sepsis the patient can have definite stone management. Stones <1 cm may pass spontaneously but with these complications, it is likely to be impacted and require active intervention. Extracorporeal shockwave lithotripsy, and ureteroscopy and stone fragmentation are possibilities in the proximal ureter; ureteroscopy and stone fragmentation is more appropriate in the distal ureter.

. B Extracorporeal shockwave lithotripsy

This patient has a symptomatic stone, which therefore requires treatment. Renal stones can be treated with extracorporeal shockwave lithotripsy (ESWL), flexible ureteroscopy and stone fragmentation or percutaneous nephrolithotomy (PCNL). ESWL would be the treatment of choice for most renal stones <1 cm, with a stone-free rate of approximately 85%. It is less effective for larger stones (>1 cm), harder stones (>1000 HU), stones in the lower pole of the kidney and distal ureter and in those with obesity. In such cases flexible ureteroscopy and stone fragmentation may be an alternative. Note rigid ureteroscopy is not possible in the kidney as ureteroscopic deflection is required for stone localisation. PCNL is generally reserved for patients who have stones resistant to ESWL or ureteroscopy, large stones >2 cm or staghorn calculi.

6. D Percutaneous nephrolithotomy (PCNL)

A staghorn calculus should be treated if the patient if fit enough. Left untreated mortality renal related mortality as a result of the stone is 30%. Standard treatment would be PCNL. This is the most effective form of treatment for complete stone clearance, which will preserve renal function as well as preventing infection. In case when the kidney is non-functioning, there is no need to preserve the kidney for function and the patient is best served by nephrectomy.

7. D Indirect inguinal hernia

A hydrocele often does not allow palpation of the testis if large and transilluminate without a cough impulse, unlike the hernia presented here. This is an indirect hernia as it follows the inguinal canal into the scrotum. Surgical repair is indicated to prevent complications. Chronic constipation is a risk factor and this should be managed appropriately to prevent recurrence.

8. F Varicocele

A varicocele is a dilatation of the veins (pampiniform plexus) around the testis. It is more common on the left as these veins combine to form the testicular vein which drains perpendicularly into the left renal vein. On the right the testicular vein drains into the vena cava. Varicoceles are typically idiopathic. They can be described as 'a bag of worms' on examination and often reduce in size or disappear on lying flat. They are largely asymptomatic. In this case, the varicocele is a likely complication of the known renal cancer which may involve the left renal vein and obstruct testicular venous drainage.

9. E Transurethral resection of bladder tumour

Initial treatment of bladder cancer is transurethral resection which allows local staging. In those patients which superficial disease is suspected a single dose of mitomycin C is given postoperatively to prevent disease recurrence. At diagnosis 50% patients have superficial disease (pTa); 20% have superficially invasive (pT1) and 30% have muscle invasive disease (pT2-4). In those patients with pTa or pT1 disease trans-urethral resection of bladder tumour may be definitive treatment although risk of disease recurrence and progression can be stratified pathologically and further intravesical immunotherapy (Bacillus Calmette–Guérin) or chemotherapy (mitomycin C) given.

0. B Cystectomy

This man has muscle invasive disease with no evidence of metastasis. Local endoscopic treatment or intravesical chemotherapy and immunotherapy will not be sufficient for disease control. Options include radical radiotherapy or cystectomy. Although there are no randomised controlled trials and the evidence is debated by some, cystectomy may have a survival benefit over radiotherapy for those fit enough to undergo such major surgery. In this case inflammatory bowel disease would also make radiotherapy less attractive.

1. E Radical prostatectomy

This man is most likely to have localised prostate cancer (low prostate-specific antigen and moderately differentiated prostate cancer). As such, his treatment options are active surveillance, brachytherapy, radical radiotherapy and radical prostatectomy. In view of previous pelvic radiotherapy he would not be suitable for further radiotherapeutic treatment. As such the only suitable treatment available to choose from here is radical surgery. Radical prostatectomy can be performed by open, laparoscopic or robotic means. The more minimally invasive treatments offer reduced blood transfusion requirements and more rapid hospital discharge.

2. B Androgen deprivation

This patient has metastatic prostate cancer; tissue is not required for confirmation. Men with this condition should be offered androgen deprivation therapy in the form of luteinising hormone releasing hormone agonist injections (usually every 3 months), with initial androgen receptor blocker treatment for 3 weeks to prevent testosterone flare. This therapy will prevent pathological fracture rates and reduce the prostate-specific antigen (PSA) in the vast majority of patients. Eventually the prostate cancer will escape control (PSA will rise) and an androgen receptor blocker will be required in addition to a luteinising hormone releasing hormone agonist. Once the PSA rises again, so-called castration-resistant prostate cancer (CRPC) has developed. At this stage in younger, higher performance patients chemotherapy can provide approximately 3 months survival advantage. Median survival in CRPC is 12–18 months.

3. E Transurethral resection of prostate

This patient has chronic urinary retention due to his increasing difficulty passing urine, with nocturnal incontinence (pathognomic of this condition) and the residual volume of >800 mL. This man has high pressure chronic retention in view of his new onset renal failure. As such he should not be treated with conservative or medical treatment, otherwise this problem will reoccur. He should have a transurethral resection of prostate, long term catheter or possibly intermittent self catheterisation, if he is motivated to do so.

14. C Open prostatectomy

This man has severe lower urinary tract symptoms secondary to bladder outflow obstruction. Medical therapy has been unsuccessful. Surgical treatment is indicated. As the prostate is large (> 100 g) open prostatectomy is the procedure of choice.

Chapter 52

Transplantation

Theme: Types of transplant graft

Options for Questions 1–4:

A	Autograft	D	Piggy-back graft
B	Allograft	E	Split graft
C	Isograft	F	Xenograft

For each of the following situations below, select the single most likely graft type. Each option may be used once, more than once or not at all.

1. A 65-year-old man has end-stage liver disease due to alcohol induced cirrhosis. Following appropriate work up a liver transplant is performed using the right lobe of his son's liver. Postoperatively both patients progressed well.

2. A 50-year-old woman of rare blood type requires a major surgical procedure. Two weeks prior to the procedure the patient donates blood which is stored in the event that it is required in the perioperative period.

3. A 75-year-old man has been under follow-up for severe aortic stenosis. He is known to have a calcified bicuspid aortic valve. Recently, he has experienced syncopal episodes on exertion and developed mild angina. The decision is made that he should undergo aortic valve replacement with a porcine valve.

4. A 58-year-old man with severe heart failure has been on the waiting list for cardiac transplantation. Prior to transplantation it was decided that the donor heart may not provide sufficient cardiac function alone and so the decision is made to leave the patient's heart in situ, with additional support provided by the donor heart.

Theme: Principles of transplantation

Options for Questions 5–7:

A Brainstem dead	**D** Living unrelated
B Cross-species	**E** Non-heart beating
C Living related	

For each of the following situations, select the single most likely option. Each option may be used once, more than once or not at all.

5. A 49-year-old man with chronic renal failure of unknown aetiology has been on long term dialysis and awaits kidney transplantation. At clinic review the patient is keen to discuss options for transplantation and is concerned about receiving a transplant from an accepted donor source which is associated with the least favourable outcome.

6. A 58-year-old man with alcohol-related cirrhosis of the liver presents with acute-on-chronic liver failure. Given the severity of his condition he requires urgent liver transplantation. After waiting for several days, organ transplantation is performed from a donor source which is most commonly used for this type of transplantation.

7. A 79-year-old man was involved in a road traffic accident 2 months previously, where he had suffered a serious head injury. He has remained unconscious since, requiring respiratory support. After much consideration the patient is assessed by two independent physicians to consider the suitability for organ donation.

Theme: Basic principles of transplant immunology

Options for Questions 8–10:

A Acute rejection	**D** Hyperacute rejection
B Acute-on-chronic rejection	**E** Super acute rejection
C Chronic rejection	

For each of the following situations, select the single most likely rejection type. Each option may be used once, more than once or not at all.

8. A 55-year-old man received a renal transplant 2 months previously for renal failure of unknown aetiology. After initially functioning well his renal function has now deteriorated considerably.

9. A 64-year-old man received a renal transplantation for diabetic nephropathy 3 years previously. Over the past 18 months his creatinine clearance has been slowly deteriorating. He has noticed his urine output has reduced recently.

10. A 67-year-old woman with decompensated chronic liver failure undergoes liver transplantation. Soon after the vasculature is anastomosed the organ becomes congested and dusky. The transplant surgeon is concerned about the viability of the organ.

heme: Renal replacement therapy

ptions for Questions 11–14:

A	Fluid resuscitation	D	Peritoneal dialysis
B	Haemodialysis	E	Peritoneal filtration
C	Haemofiltration		

or each of the following situations, select the single most likely therapy. Each option ay be used once, more than once or not at all.

1. A 78-year-old woman patient has developed renal failure secondary to long standing hypertension. She has been placed on the transplant waiting list but requires renal replacement therapy until a donor kidney becomes available.

2. A 39-year-old professional man has developed renal failure. He is diabetic but this has been well-controlled, despite the deterioration in renal function. He requires renal replacement therapy but hopes to maintain his career during the wait for a donor organ.

3. A 60-year-old diabetic woman is recovering on the intensive care unit following major abdominal surgery. Several days following the procedure has developed significant fluid overload in the context of oliguria and hyperkalaemia.

4. An 89-year-old woman is reviewed on the orthopaedic ward 4 days following hemiarthroplasty for fracture neck of femur. She is found to be severely dehydrated. Blood tests are sent urgently which show markedly elevated urea and creatinine with a potassium level of 6.0 mEq/L.

Answers

1. B Allograft

This refers to graft tissue from a donor of the same species. Liver transplantation is performed for a range of acute, chronic and malignant conditions **Table 52.1**. While the majority of organs originate from deceased donors, living donor liver transplantation is becoming more frequent. Here the right (or sometimes left) lobe of the donor's liver is removed (55–70% of total liver volume) with the remaining liver regenerating over several weeks to months.

Split graft refers to the division of a single donated liver to serve two patients.

Table 52.1	
Reason for liver transplant	**Cause**
Acute hepatic failure	Viral hepatitis
	Paracetamol overdose
	Other drug/toxin induced acute liver failure
Chronic hepatic failure	Hepatitis B or C cirrhosis
	Primary biliary cirrhosis
	Primary sclerosing cholangitis
	Biliary atresia
	Alcoholic cirrhosis
	Autoimmune chronic active hepatitis
	Budd–Chiari syndrome
	Hemochromatosis
Malignancy	Non-resectable hepatoblastoma which is chemo-sensitive
	Hepatocellular carcinoma according to the Milan criteria
	Epithelioid haemangioendothelioma
	(Note: metastatic liver disease is NOT an indication for transplantation)
Inborn errors of metabolism	Crigler–Najjar Type 1
	Primary oxalosis
	Urea cycle defects
	Familial amyloid polyneuropathy

Table 52.1 Indications for liver transplantation.

. A Autograft

Patients with rare blood groups may be able to donate blood preoperatively to enable transfusion if required intraoperatively. This may reduce complications associated with blood transfusion in these patient groups but its use is dependent on the centre.

During major abdominal surgery, such as aortic aneurysm repair, where high blood loss can occur a system to reinfuse blood lost into the abdominal cavity can be employed. A number of systems exist, capable of filtering and washing red cells prior to reinfusion.

Other examples of an autograft include bone graft to aid repair of complex fractures and tissue transfer for plastic surgery procedures.

. F Xenograft

This refers to transplantation across species. Porcine valves offer a range of advantages over mechanical valves including greater durability and no requirement for anticoagulation. Valves are treated to remove all immunogenic material. Bovine and human valves can also be used.

In the over 70 age group aetiology of aortic stenosis is predominantly degenerative, with other causes including bicuspid valve, postinflammatory and hypoplastic. Patients with severe aortic stenosis can develop shortness of breath, syncopal episodes, angina and progress to frank heart failure. The heart function may be preserved due to compensatory hypertrophy as the stenosis progresses. However at a certain point decompensation may occur resulting in heart failure. Given this, heart failure may not ensue until the latter stages; timely intervention prior to this is often warranted. Echocardiography is used to provide an indicator of severity of stenosis and left ventricular systolic function. Symptomatic patients benefit from valve replacement, although in asymptomatic patients the value may be less clear.

. D Piggy-back graft

This is also known as heterotopic transplantation. The recipient's heart remains in situ and the donor heart is transplanted by joining the aorta to the recipient's aorta, superior vena cava to the recipient's right atrium and the aorta to the recipient's aorta. The left atria are merged. Piggy-back transplantation may be performed if the function of the donated heart is thought to be inadequate by itself or if the patient suffers from pulmonary hypertension. The majority of cardiac transplantation is performed using the orthotopic technique where the recipient's heart is removed and replaced with the donated heart in its normal anatomical location.

. E Non-heart beating

In the context of a predictable cardiac arrest in a controlled setting such as intensive care unit non-heart beating donors may be considered for renal transplantation. However organs from this donor source who do not meet the criteria for brainstem death confer the worst prognosis. Minimising the length of time between cardiac arrest and organ retrieval is crucial to optimise long-term graft viability. Alive relative and alive unrelated donors offer the best graft outcomes given suitable tissue and blood typing match.

Cross-species transplantation is not currently a viable option and certainly not considered a treatment option.

6. A Brainstem dead

Patients who fulfil the criteria for brainstem death and are ventilated in the intensive care unit may be considered for organ donation. At present this is commonest source of donated livers. It is preferable to non-heart beating donors as brainstem dead donors have a shorter warm ischaemic time, which corresponds to a more favourable outcome. With recent developments in techniques to treat organs in transit as well as improved immunosuppressive regimens outcomes are improving.

Living related donations have increased in recent years and they are often associated with the best outcomes.

7. A Brainstem dead

Criteria for brainstem death vary around the world. In some countries the condition is not recognised due to cultural or religious reasons. In the UK two suitably qualified physicians must perform a series of neurological tests in the correct context for the diagnosis to be made (**Table 52.2**).

Table 52.2
Preconditions
1. No doubt that the patient's conditions due to irreversible brain damage of known aetiology 2. No evidence that this state is due to depressant drugs 3. Primary hypothermia must be excluded 4. Potential reversible circulatory, metabolic and endocrine disturbances must be excluded 5. Reversible causes of apnoea, such as muscle relaxants and cervical cord injury must be excluded
Definitive criteria
1. Fixed pupils 2. No corneal reflexes 3. Absent oculovestibular reflex 4. No response to supraorbital pressure 5. No cough reflex to bronchial stimulation or gagging response to pharyngeal stimulation 6. No respiratory effort in response to disconnection of the ventilator to ensure elevation of the arterial partial pressure of carbon dioxide to at least 6.0 kPa (6.5 kPa in patients with chronic carbon dioxide retention)

Table 52.2 Criteria for brainstem death.

8. A Acute rejection

Acute rejection usually presents within 3 months but can occur up to 6 months following organ transplantation. It is detected by graft dysfunction. Acute rejection is a T-cell mediated process, with lymphocyte infiltration in the interstitium and later the vessel walls. It is likely to occur in all allografts to some extent based on mismatched human leukocyte antigens. Given the fact that human leukocyte antigens are polymorphic it is extremely unlikely that a perfect match will occur.

The diagnosis can be confirmed by biopsy, although is difficult to distinguish from acute tubular necrosis or drug nephrotoxicity. The incidence of acute rejection can be reduced by maintenance immunosuppressive regimens and if/when acute rejection does occur it may be reversible with episodic use of high dose steroids.

9. C Chronic rejection

This can occur anytime from months to years following transplantation and is defined as an alloimmune response leading to gradual deterioration in organ function. It involves both humoral and cell mediated responses.

At biopsy renal tubular atrophy, glomerular basement membrane thickening and vascular changes may be noticed. There is no treatment and chronic rejection is not reversible. Fortunately, it is becoming less common with the use of variable immunosuppressive drug regimens tailored to the patient.

In addition to the phenomenon of immune mediated rejection other major factors which determine long-term graft function include donor age, preservation/reperfusion related graft injury, tissue quality and posttransplant stressors in the recipient such as infection, drug toxicity and comorbidity. A constellation of these factors can contribute to chronic allograft dysfunction, where the underlying alloimmune response seen in chronic rejection is less evident. Chronic allograft nephropathy is characterised by renal insufficiency, progressive vasculopathy and non-specific pathology occurring at least 3–6 months following renal transplantation. In the clinical setting the term 'chronic rejection' is often applied to late graft dysfunction of any cause, without evidence of underlying immune response.

10. D Hyperacute rejection

Hyperacute rejection can occur immediately or within minutes to hours of transplantation. It occurs where there are preformed antibodies in the serum of the recipient against donor antigens, eliciting a humoral immune response. Antibodies attach to class 1 antigens on the vascular endothelium leading to complement activation, intravascular coagulation and subsequent impaired tissue perfusion. Thrombotic occlusion then leads to graft necrosis and loss of the graft.

Antibodies involved in hyperacute rejection include ABO blood group antigens, histocompatibility antigens and vascular endothelial antigens. The treatment for hyperacute rejection is immediate removal of the organ. Patients undergo ABO blood typing and human leukocyte typing prior to transplantation with the aim of reducing the possibility of hyperacute rejection but this feared complication may still occur. Patients who have had multiple pregnancies, multiple blood transfusions or previous transplants are more likely to have developed antibodies to transplant antigens.

11. B Haemodialysis

A percutaneous large bore cannula is sited to enable access to a central vein. Blood is pumped into the dialysis machine where a semi-permeable membrane separates the blood from the dialysis fluid. The blood and dialysis fluid run in different directions, known as counter current circulation. Diffusion of substances occurs across the membrane. Haemodialysis requires the patient to attend the haemodialysis centre around three times per week. For patients with work or childcare commitments this can be a considerable burden, and peritoneal dialysis may be more appropriate.

12. D Peritoneal dialysis

Here dialysis fluid is infused into the peritoneal cavity via an access port in the abdominal wall. The osmotic pressure within the dialysis fluid leads to ultrafiltration due to osmotic pressure and diffusion to replace the renal excretory functions. Peritoneal dialysis can be performed independently by the patient at home, rather than having to attend a dialysis centre and may prove a more practical solution. In patients with poorly controlled diabetes peritoneal dialysis is contraindicated due to the risk of infection.

Peritoneal filtration is not a recognised practice.

13. C Haemofiltration

This is a short-term solution for the management of renal failure. Haemofiltration relies on a positive hydrostatic pressure enabling water and solutes to pass across a semipermeable membrane. Fluid is replaced in isotonic form to account for water and electrolytes removed. The rate of solute removal is related to the pressure gradient applied, which can be adjusted to account for the clinical situation. Haemofiltation is mainly used in the critical care environment where temporary support of renal function can be provided.

Haemodialysis and peritoneal dialysis are long-term options which would not be appropriate here as the patient's renal function will hopefully recover.

14. A Fluid resuscitation

The commonest cause of postoperative renal dysfunction progressing to renal failure is prerenal. Hypovolaemia caused by blood loss or dehydration is implicated in the vast majority of cases. This patient is clearly fluid deplete requiring urgent rehydration with intravenous fluids. The raised potassium level is concerning, likely indicating ineffective renal elimination of potassium. Cardiac arrhythmias may be triggered by hyperkalaemia, generally at higher levels than seen in this case, but regardless an ECG should be performed.

ECG signs of hyperkalaemia include peaked (or tented) T waves and reduction in the size of P waves. Severe hyperkalaemia can cause a widening of the QRS complex, eventually evolving to a sinusoidal shape prior to death. A potassium level of 6 mmol/L should reduce with fluid supplementation in the context of hypovolaemia, but if this is persistent treatment includes nebulised salbutamol or dextrose/insulin infusion. Local protocols should be followed.

In this case renal function should improve with fluid replacement therapy. If no improvement in renal function is seen after fluid replacement temporary haemofiltration may be considered as discussed above. Haemodialysis is more permanent option which would not be suitable here as the patient's renal function is likely to recover.

Chapter 53

Head and neck

Theme: Face

Options for Questions 1–3:

A Actinic keratosis
B Basal cell carcinoma
C Cutaneous T-cell lymphoma
D Infected sebaceous cyst
E Malignant melanoma

F Merkel cell carcinoma
G Periorbital cellulitis
H Rhinophyma
I Seborrhoeic keratosis
J Squamous cell carcinoma

For each of the following situations, select the single most likely diagnosis. Each option may be used once, more than once or not at all.

A 28-year-old woman holiday courier notices a uniform brown lesion on her right forehead 2 months ago. Over the past 4 weeks she reports the lesion to have increased in size, and the colour to have changed. On examination, there is a 1 cm brown pigmented lesion on the right forehead. The degree of pigmentation varies across the lesion and the border is indistinct. There is a palpable right cervical lymph node.

A 74-year-old woman, who is retired farmer's wife, presents with a lesion on the left side of the nose. It has been present for 18 months and has gradually increased in size. There is no associated pain, however minor trauma results in bleeding. On examination, there is a 1 cm pearly lesion overlying the left nasal skin. There is no palpable cervical lymphadenopathy.

An 8-year-old girl with a 1-day history of swelling around the right eye, with a background history of recent upper respiratory tract infection, right facial pain and right nasal discharge.

Theme: Oral cavity and tongue

Options for Questions 4–6:

A	Assessment of HIV status	G	Incisional tissue biopsy
B	CT scanning	H	Lateral neck X-ray
C	Epstein–Barr virus serology	I	MRI scanning
D	Excision tissue biopsy	J	Oral swab for microscopic analysis
E	Fine needle aspiration biopsy	K	Saliva sample for microscopic
F	Human papilloma virus serology		analysis

For each of the following situations, select the single most appropriate investigation. Each option may be used once, more than once or not at all.

4. A 64-year-old man presents with a 6-week history of loose teeth and ulceration of the gum. He has an 80 pack-year history of cigarette smoking. Examination reveals a 2 cm ulcerated lesion over the left mandible and no palpable lymph nodes in the neck.

5. A 75-year-old woman presents with a 3-month history of oral discomfort. Her past history includes non-insulin dependent diabetes mellitus and chronic obstructive pulmonary disease, for which she uses a steroid inhaler. On removal of her dentures, examination reveals white plaques involving the hard palate and buccal mucosa. Gentle brushing dislodges the plaques to reveal reddened mucosa.

6. A 59-year-old man presents with a neck mass. He has a 50 pack-year history of smoking. Examination of the neck reveals a 2 cm firm mass in the anterior triangle without fixation to the skin. Examination of the mouth reveals poor dentition without any identifiable primary lesion.

Theme: Nose and sinuses

Options for Questions 7–10:

A	Acute sinusitis	F	Nasal fracture
B	Chronic sinusitis	G	Nasal polyposis
C	Congenital syphilis	H	Nasal septal deviation
D	Midline T cell lymphoma	I	Squamous cell carcinoma
E	Nasal foreign body	J	Wegner's granulomatosis

For each of the following situations, select the single most likely diagnosis. Each option may be used once, more than once or not at all.

7. A 45-year-old man presents with a 1-year history of anosmia (loss of sense of smell) and bilateral nasal obstruction. He has a history of asthma. Examination of the nose reveals bilateral obstruction with greyish masses visible on both sides of the nasal cavity.

A 23-year-old woman who works as a teacher presents with a 2-week history of right sided rhinorrhoea (nasal discharge) and facial pain, which followed a recent viral upper respiratory tract infection. On examination, she is pyrexial (38.5°C) with tenderness over the left cheek, periorbital and frontal regions, with green discharge visible in the right nostril.

A 45-year-old woman presents with symptoms of nasal obstruction and discharge. She has renal and pulmonary dysfunction. Examination reveals a nasal septal perforation and significantly abnormally thickened erythematous nasal mucosa.

). A 4-year-old boy presents with a 1-month history of unilateral nasal discharge. He is well, but has profuse discharge from the left nostril which is foul-smelling.

heme: Salivary glands

ptions for Questions 11–13:

A	Auriculotemporal nerve	E	Parotid duct
B	Facial nerve	F	Parotid gland
C	Lingual nerve	G	Sublingual gland
D	Minor salivary gland of the hard palate	H	Submandibular duct
		I	Submandibular gland

or each of the following situations, select the single most primary structure involved. ach option may be used once, more than once or not at all.

1. A 55-year-old woman presents with recurrent pain and swelling inferior her right mandible. The symptoms are related to eating and have been present for 3 months. On examination she has no palpable abnormality in the neck, however a hard 5 mm mass is palpable in the right floor of mouth.

2. A 72-year-old man presents with a 3-year history of a slowly enlarging mass inferior to the left ear. The mass is painless, and there is no history of weight loss. On examination there is an 8 cm mass overlying the left angle of mandible. The overlying skin is normal and facial nerve function is not affected.

3. A 72-year-old man presents with a 3-month history of a rapidly enlarging mass over the right cheek. The mass is painful and is associated with weakness of the right face. Examination confirms a mass over the angle of the right mandible which is 5 cm, firm with indurated overlying skin and associated weakness of the muscles of facial expression on the right side of the face.

Theme: Ear disease

Options for Questions 14–15:

    A   Acute mastoiditis
    B   Bullous myringitis
    C   Cholesteatoma
    D   Chronic otitis media with effusion

    E   Otitis externa
    F   Squamous cell carcinoma of postnasal space

For each of the following situations, select the single most likely diagnosis. Each option may be used once, more than once or not at all.

14. A 6-year-old boy presents with a 1-week history of fever and right ear pain, which has not responded to antibiotics. On examination he is well, but has a temperature of 38.5°C. Examination of his left ear is normal, but the skin behind the right ear is erythematous and fluctuant. Examination of the ear canal shows a bulging, red ear drum.

15. A 76-year-old man, a smoker, presents with a 1-month history of left sided deafness. Examination of the ears shows normal ear canals, with a fluid level visible on the left ear drum.

Answers

E Malignant melanoma

This presentation suggests malignant melanoma. Although less common than basal cell or squamous cell carcinoma, melanoma accounts for more deaths. Caucasians who are exposed to excess sunlight are most at risk. The increase in size represents the radial growth phase, where malignant melanocytes are limited to the superficial layers of the skin. The vertical growth phase results in tumour cells invading down through the skin towards the blood and lymphatic vessels of the dermis, increasing the likelihood of metastasis. It is this vertical growth described by Clark and Breslow scales which are used to classify these malignancies. The presence of palpable lymphadenopathy is suggestive of metastasis which should be investigated with imaging (CT) and confirmed using fine-needle aspiration sampling. The results of these investigations will be used to guide treatment.

B Basal cell carcinoma

Basal cell carcinoma is the most common malignancy of the skin. It grows slowly, is locally invasive, and rarely metastasises. It is most often diagnosed in patients over the age of 40 years and is related to sun exposure, therefore such lesions are often seen on the head and neck. Examination features include a pearly or waxy appearance, although lesions can be whitish, pink or brown (see Figure 54.4). Biopsy may be required to differentiate such a lesion from squamous cell carcinoma which tends to be faster growing, and have a greater tendency to metastasise. Excision of basal cell carcinoma with an adequate clear margin results in cure, however such margins can be difficult to achieve without significant functional and cosmetic impact around the face. Advanced reconstructive techniques including rotation flaps can be employed to reduce the postoperative morbidity suffered by such patients.

G Periorbital cellulitis

This child has typical history of periorbital cellulitis. This is a condition which is related to infection of the paranasal sinuses. Typically infection in the ethmoid sinuses spreads laterally to involve the periosteum of the medial orbital wall. Often this condition is limited to the soft tissue anterior to the orbital septum (preseptal) but when it results in pus collecting within the orbit, it can cause a rise in orbital pressure which can in turn compromise function of the optic nerve. Assessment includes examination of movement of the eye, visual acuity and colour vision which is the first aspect of vision to be affected. In situations where the eyelids are too oedematous to allow full examination, CT scanning of the sinuses, orbits and brain are indicated. Potential complications include blindness, intracranial sepsis and cavernous sinus thrombosis.

4. G Incisional tissue biopsy

The most likely diagnosis here is squamous cell carcinoma. The disease is strongly associated with smoking, and tends to present in patients in their 60s and 70s. Confirmation of the diagnosis is best achieved with an incisional biopsy. Treatment will depend on the size of the primary lesion (determined by examination and imaging), the presence of nodal metastases and any evidence of distant metastases (usually pulmonary). Although excisional biopsy would allow a diagnosis to be made, it would be likely to require a major operation including sacrifice of part of the mandible. It would be inappropriate to undertake such major surgery without first confirming the diagnosis and staging the disease to allow treatment planning.

5. J Oral swab for microscopic analysis

Oral candidiasis often presents with pain. Examination reveals the characteristic white plaques which can be removed by brushing with a moist swab. Predisposing factors include diabetes, dentures, as well as corticosteroid and antibiotic use. Treatment would include oral solutions containing nystatin, or for resistant cases, systemic therapy such as fluconazole. In addition to these treatments this patient should be advised in regards to oral hygiene, and also encouraged to rinse her mouth following use of her steroid inhaler to remove residue from the oral mucosa. Although oesophageal candidiasis is related to HIV infection and considered an AIDS defining illness, oral candidiasis is common and not an indication for assessment of HIV status.

6. E Fine-needle aspiration biopsy

Patients with a significant history of smoking are at risk of head and neck cancer. Although a primary lesion in the mouth would be expected in such a patient, the absence of one does not exclude squamous cell carcinoma. The most appropriate investigation would be fine-needle aspiration of the neck node, This would ideally be done under ultrasound guidance to maximise the chance of a diagnostic sample. Although Epstein–Barr virus and human papilloma virus have both been shown to be related to cancers of the head and neck, serology would not be diagnostic and so are less useful than cytology in this case. Having made a diagnosis of small cell carcinoma, cross-sectional imaging would be appropriate, and in most cases CT scanning is employed. It is quick, cheap and more readily available than MRI, although in cases where dental amalgam results in significant artefact on CT scanning, MRI can be particularly useful.

7. G Nasal polyposis

This patient presents with the classical symptoms of nasal polyps. Inflammation of the sinonasal mucosa results in oedematous tissue which eventually bunches out to obstruct the airway, thereby interfering with smell. There is thought to be an allergic component, and nasal polyps are common in asthmatics. Symptoms tend to be bilateral, and indeed unilateral nasal polyps should be considered as malignant until proven otherwise. Examination of inflammatory nasal polyps reveals insensate greyish polypoid mucosa, although in extreme cases where mucosa approaches the nasal vestibule the superficial mucosa may become hypertrophic. Treatment of these patients starts with steroids, often topically applied in an attempt to shrink the polyps. Although surgery may be used for non-responders, it does not cure the condition, but rather debulks tissue which reduces symptoms and allows for more effective delivery of steroids to affected mucosa.

A Acute sinusitis

Acute sinusitis occurs when the sinus ostia (drainage pathways of the sinuses in to the nose) become blocked. This tends to result from infection. The sinus then becomes a closed system and mucus which builds up can become infected. Patients present with pain, fever and ipsilateral nasal discharge. Although the maxillary sinus is most commonly affected, the relationship of the sinus drainage pathways means that a pan-sinusitis often develops. Such patients were classically investigated with plain X-ray imaging, however such films add little to management and with the advent of low radiation dose CT scanning, cross-sectional imaging has replaced standard X-rays as the investigation of choice. Treatment includes decongestion of the nasal mucosa and antibiotic therapy, with surgical drainage reserved for the occasional patient that does not respond. Complications of acute sinusitis are rare but can be life-threatening and include the spread of infection to the cranial cavity and orbit.

J Wegener's granulomatosis

Wegener's granulomatosis is a vasculitis which can affect many systems, but commonly involved are renal and pulmonary with associated airway problems. The mucosa of the nose can be affected by granulomas which over time can result in perforation of the nasal septum, and collapse of the dorsum of the nose. Although this can also occur in congenital syphilis, she is in the wrong age group. Malignancy would also be possible, and although unlikely a biopsy could be performed to exclude small cell carcinoma or T-cell lymphoma. Wegener's is most commonly treated with systemic steroids and surgical input is rarely required for nasal symptoms. The upper airway can also be affected at the level of the subglottis, which can result in airway obstruction from inflamed mucosa. Although it is rare, this is an occasional indication for tracheostomy.

0. E Nasal foreign body

This presentation is typical for a nasal foreign body. Often a child will inserts the object and does not inform the parents. Such objects can remain without symptoms and signs for long periods before resulting in infection with associated discharge. Organic materials and sponge result in a particularly offensive smell. Treatment requires removal, either with or without general anaesthetic depending on cooperation of the child. Specific foreign bodies including batteries and magnets applied to both sides of the nasal septum require urgent removal, whereas incidental foreign bodies such as this can be removed on the next available theatre list.

11. H Submandibular duct

This patient presents with symptoms which are typical of submandibular duct obstruction. The examination findings confirm the presence of a stone within the duct which is causing obstruction. A plain X-ray of floor of the mouth confirms the diagnosis (**Figure 53.1**). Although the submandibular gland swells within its capsule causing pain, the pathology is located within the duct. The sublingual gland drains directly in to the floor of mouth via multiple smaller ducts and so would not be affected by submandibular duct obstruction. The submandibular gland produces a constant flow of saliva however during mastication, saliva production increases, hence the association of symptoms with eating.

Salivary stones most commonly affect the submandibular rather than the parotid duct. This may relate to the fact that drainage against gravity tends to result in salivary stasis. Floor of mouth X-ray (shown below) will demonstrate submandibular stones in 80% of cases. Transoral resection under local or general anaesthetic with marsupialisation of the duct to prevent subsequent stenosis should allow removal of this stone. The duct runs in close proximity to the lingual nerve; in fact the two loop around one another and care must be taken not to damage the nerve both in transoral and transcervical approaches to the submandibular duct.

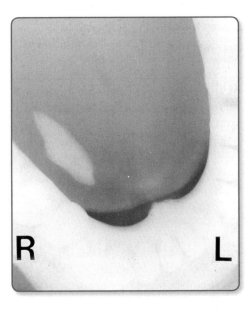

Figure 53.1 Floor of mouth X-ray demonstrating a radio-opaque stone in the right submandibular duct.

2. F Parotid gland

Although many students expect parotid lesions to present in the cheek, the most common site to find a small parotid lesion is inferior to the ear lobe in the tail of the parotid. This elderly man presents with symptoms which suggest a benign neoplasm of salivary tissue. The most common diagnosis here would be pleomorphic adenoma, although Warthin's tumour (also called papillary cystadenoma lymphomatosum) would be in the differential diagnosis also. Both of these tumours more commonly affect the parotid than the submandibular salivary gland. Malignancy of the parotid is less likely, particularly in the absence of features such as pain, facial nerve dysfunction and overlying skin changes.

Investigation of salivary masses starts with fine-needle aspiration biopsy, and many clinicians would also order cross-sectional imaging (ideally MRI). Although fine-needle aspiration biopsy is not 100% accurate, a biopsy suggesting malignancy would alter preoperative work up, consent, and the extent of surgical resection.

3. F Parotid gland

This man presents in a similar fashion to the preceding case but with some specific differences. The mass is growing rapidly, is painful and associated with both skin change and facial nerve dysfunction. These are all hallmarks of malignancy. Although the facial nerve is involved, this is much more likely to be parotid pathology than a primary of the facial nerve. The most commonly involved structure would be the parotid gland itself, which can be affected by conditions including mucoepidermoid carcinoma, adenocarcinoma, adenoid cystic carcinoma and carcinoma ex-pleomorphic adenoma (**Figure 53.2**). Although primary parotid pathology should be suspected, this could also represent a metastatic intraparotid

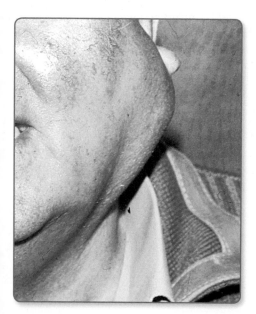

Figure 53.2 Classical parotid swelling.

lymph node, which highlights the need for a full head and neck examination with particular reference to the skin of the scalp, the lymphatic drainage of which includes these nodes. The next stage in management here would involve fine-needle aspiration cytology followed by imaging of the lesion (probably with MRI) and the neck to identify any involved cervical lymph nodes.

14. A Acute mastoiditis

This child has acute mastoiditis with a subperiosteal abscess. Acute otitis media is very common, with up to 80% of children experiencing at least one episode. Acute mastoiditis used to be common and potentially fatal, however with modern antibiotics and surgical management, it is less common and rarely fatal. In the event that an episode of acute otitis media does not resolve without complication, the tympanic membrane may rupture, allowing the pus under pressure to escape. The mastoid air cells drain in to the middle ear, and infection of the middle ear space results in mucosal oedema which can obstruct this outflow. The closed system which results from this obstruction may harbour infection that will ultimately discharge, either into the soft tissues over the bone as in this case, or superiorly in to the cranial cavity, putting the child at risk of meningitis or intracranial abscess.

Investigation of this child should involve contrast enhanced CT to visualise the mastoid air cell system and to identify any intracranial abscess. Management is guided by imaging, but assuming there is no collection in the brain, incision and drainage of the collection should be performed. The mastoid air cells may also be addressed, to improve drainage in to the middle ear at the same operation in an attempt to prevent further episodes.

15. F Squamous cell carcinoma of postnasal space

Unilateral deafness in an elderly patient who smokes is a red flag for cancer. The ear drains in to the postnasal space via the Eustachian tube. If occluded, the serous fluid produced by the middle ear mucosa is trapped and will lead to a conductive hearing loss. This patient requires nasendoscopy to exclude a lesion in the postnasal space. Assuming there is an abnormality, urgent biopsy should be arranged with imaging to stage local, regional and distant disease.

Chronic otitis media with effusion, or glue ear, has some similar features. This affects children who present with a hearing loss related to fluid within the middle ear cleft. Treatment ranges from reassurance to insertion of ventilation tubes (grommets) and adenoidectomy to improve Eustachian tube function depending on the degree and duration of disability.

Chapter 54

Surgical conditions
of the skin

heme: Surgical technique for skin closure

tions for Questions 1–4:

A	Allograft	**E**	Porcine xenograft
B	Delayed primary closure	**F**	Primary closure
C	Free flap	**G**	Secondary intention
D	Full thickness skin graft	**H**	Split skin graft

r each of the following cases, select the single most appropriate technique for
rgical closure. Each option may be used once, more than once or not at all.

A 35-year-old woman presents with a 3 × 4 cm pilonidal abscess. The patient is
taken to theatre for an incision and drainage procedure to be performed.

A 56-year-old woman presents with a 1 × 0.7 cm pigmented lesion on her left
cheek. On examination, there is very little laxity in the surrounding skin.

A 75-year-old woman presents with a 5 × 5 cm clean non-healing wound from a left
pre-tibial laceration when she fell at home 3 weeks ago. The GP practice nurse has
been managing it with a vacuum dressing. She has no other past medical history
of note. On examination, she has easily palpable biphasic pedal pulses and a
capillary refill time of 2 seconds.

A 45-year-old woman is referred to the plastic surgical clinic with a 16 × 12 cm full
thickness burn on her left hip. This occurred when she was scalded by hot water
2 weeks ago.

Theme: Lumps and bumps

Options for Questions 5–7:

A	Dermatofibroma	E	Lipoma
B	Congenital dermoid cyst	F	Sebaceous cyst
C	Fibroepithelial polyp	G	Seborrhoeic keratosis
D	Keratoacanthoma	H	Solar keratosis

For each of the following cases, select the single most likely diagnosis. Each option m be used once, more than once or not at all.

5. A 32-year-old woman presents with a 5 × 7 cm soft, lobulated, hemispherical, slightly fluctuant, painless lump on her back just medial to her right scapula. The overlying skin appears normal.

6. A 36-year-old woman presents with a painless, pink to brown pigmented, firm 1 × 1 cm nodule on her leg 8 cm above the medial malleolus. It is attached to the underlying skin.

7. A 47-year-old man presents with a long-standing non-tender intradermal lump o his scalp. He describes that it has previously become red, tender and enlarged an discharged yellow, cheesy material. On examination, a central punctum is seen.

Theme: Skin and systemic disease

Options for Questions 8–10:

A	Acanthosis nigricans	E	Pretibial myxoedema
B	Erythema ab igne	F	Pyoderma gangrenosum
C	Erythema multiforme	G	Pyogenic granuloma
D	Neurofibroma	H	Spider naevi

For each of the following cases, select the single most likely related skin manifestatio Each option may be used once, more than once or not at all.

8. A 67-year-old man with known diabetes and peripheral vascular disease attends vascular clinic for routine follow-up. On examination, a skin finding is noted.

9. A 33-year-old woman with known ulcerative colitis attends colorectal clinic for routine follow-up. On examination, a skin lesion in noted.

10. A 45-year-old man with known chronic liver failure presents to the emergency department with abdominal pain. On examination, a skin finding is noted.

Theme: Premalignant and malignant skin lesions

Options for Questions 11–12:

A   Basal cell carcinoma
B   Bowen's disease
C   Keratoacanthoma
D   Malignant melanoma
E   Seborrhoeic keratosis
F   Solar keratosis
G   Squamous cell carcinoma

For each of the following cases, select the single most diagnosis. Each option may be used once, more than once or not at all.

11. A 52-year-old man, a farmer, presents with a firm, skin-coloured 1.5 × 2 cm lesion on his left cheek. It has a darker crusty centre. He reports that it first appeared 10 weeks ago and increased in size quickly over the first 3 weeks. However, it appears to be slowly regressing over the latter 6 weeks.

12. A 64-year-old woman presents with a 1-year history of a raised, asymptomatic 1 cm nodule on the left side of her forehead. The lesion has an irregular, rolled, pearly edge and a depressed, ulcerated centre with an adherent crust. The patient has no past medical history of note but is an avid gardener.

Answers

1. G Secondary intention

This is a contaminated wound with frank pus. It should be curetted, irrigated, pack and allowed to heal by secondary intention. The wound is left open and heals from the base upward by a combination of granulation, epithelialisation and contractio These wounds need regular wound care and pack changes. They take longer to he with poor cosmesis. However, if the wound is closed primarily before the pus has adequately drained, the abscess will recur and the wound will likely breakdown.

2. D Full thickness skin graft

Full thickness skin grafts are ideal for small facial wounds not amenable to primary closure or local flaps. A full thickness skin graft (Wolfe grafts) contains the epiderm dermis and adnexal structures. These grafts heal with good cosmesis and thinner scars. They are better colour matched and undergo less contracture than split thickness skin grafts. Donor sites are less painful and can be closed primarily. A go blood supply, clean bed and adequate nutrition are essential for graft take.

3. H Split skin graft

Pretibial lacerations are commonly seen in patients with thin skin – elderly, patients on steroids. These injuries are usually large and are not usually amenable to primary closure. Split thickness skin grafts are commonly used for these injuries, either primar or in patients with poorly healing wounds. Split thickness skin grafts (Thiersch grafts) consist of the epidermal layer and a variable thickness of dermis. Split thickness skin grafts can be used to cover large areas and, as it is usually quite thin, it tends to confo to underlying contours well. However, these grafts tend to contract as they heal and result in poorer cosmesis with poor matching of colour and texture.

4. H. Split skin graft

Large full thickness or deep dermal burns may require excision and split skin grafti as they are unlikely to heal by secondary intention. For full thickness burns on a sm area, regular dressing with non-adherent dressing may be sufficient. Superficial dermal burns tend to heal well without scarring within 2 weeks (if kept clean and n infected). Silver sulphazidine is sometimes used on deep burns to reduce infection.

5. E. Lipoma

Lipomas are the commonest soft tissue tumours, affecting 1% of the population. Th are hamartomas of mature fat cells and are typically asymptomatic lumps, which occur in areas where fat normally occurs (hence, rarely seen on the palms, soles or scalp). They can very in size from a few centimetres to giant lipomas (**Figure 54.1**).

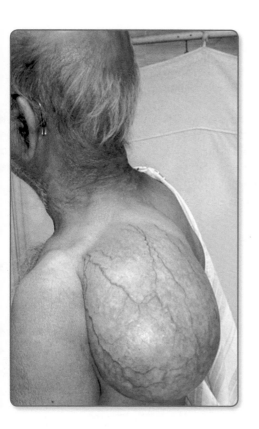

Figure 54.1 Giant lipoma.

A Dermatofibroma

Dermatofibromas (fibrous histiocytomas) is a benign neoplasm of dermal fibroblasts. They may occur anywhere but are most commonly seen on the lower limbs of young to middle-aged females. The aetiology is unclear – it is probably secondary to an abortive immunoreactive process (previously thought to be secondary to minor trauma, e.g. insect bites but this theory has now fallen out of favour).

F Sebaceous cyst

Sebaceous cysts (epidermal cysts/pilar cysts) are very common skin lesions that arise within skin itself (intradermal). They occur on hair-bearing surfaces (not palms/soles) and contain sebum/keratinous debris. They can vary in size and consistency but are usually non-tender raised lumps. A punctum is seen in 50% of these cysts.

A Acanthosis nigricans

Acanthosis nigricans refers to a poorly defined area of velvety hyperpigmentation that occurs in skin folds – axilla, neck groin. It is associated with endocrinopathies (diabetes mellitus, polycystic ovarian syndrome, acromegaly, thyroid disease), obesity and internal malignancy (most commonly, gastric carcinoma).

9. F Pyoderma gangrenosum

Pyoderma gangrenosum (**Figure 54.2**) is a deep nodulo-pustular ulcer with a pustular surface and tender reddish blue overhanging necrotic edges. The ulcers can be large and chronic, and typically occur on the lower limbs. The condition is thought to be immune-mediated and is associated with inflammatory bowel disease (ulcerative colitis > Crohn's disease), Wegener's granulomatosis, myeloma, autoimmune hepatitis and rheumatoid arthritis.

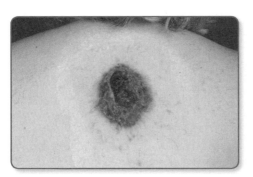

Figure 54.2 Pyoderma gangrenosum in a patient with ulcerative colitis.

10. H Spider naevi

Spider naevi are red lesions seen on the surface of the skin, which blanch on pressure. There is a central arteriole with radiating vessels around it – resembling the legs of a spider. There are seen in healthy individuals but the presence of five or more usually indicate underlying pathology. The most common pathological cause for spider naevi is liver disease. Other causes include pregnancy and oral contraceptive pill.

11. C Keratoacanthoma

Keratoacanthomas (**Figure 54.3**) are epidermal tumours derived from hair follicles. They are characterised by a central keratin plug, rapid growth over 2–4 weeks and spontaneous resolution over 2–12 months leaving a depressed scar. They are associated with exposure to sunlight and typically occur on the face, neck and hands. Clinically and histologically, keratoacanthomas are difficult to differentiate from squamous cell carcinomas (SCCs). Hence, they are often reported as a variant of a well-differentiated SCC. However, unlike keratoacanthomas, SCCs tend to be slower-growing, progress into ulcers and do not resolve spontaneously.

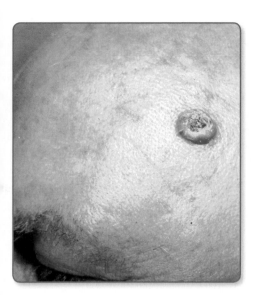

Figure 54.3 Keratoacanthoma.

2. A Basal cell carcinoma

Basal cell carcinomas are the commonest type of skin cancer and are typically seen in fair-skinned individual in sun-exposed areas. They are usually slow-growing tumours which rarely metastasise but are locally invasive and can cause significant destruction to surrounding tissue if allowed to develop (**Figure 54.4**).

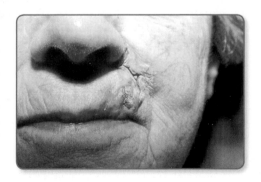

Figure 54.4 Basal cell carcinoma.

Chapter 55

Hand disorders

heme: Differential diagnosis of hand disorders

tions for Questions 1–4:

A	Bouchard's nodes	F	de Quervain's tenosynovitis
B	Boutonnière deformity	G	Rheumatoid nodule
C	Carpal tunnel syndrome	H	Swan neck deformity
D	Ganglion	I	Trigger finger
E	Dupuytren's contracture	J	Wrist osteoarthritis

r each of the following cases, select the single most appropriate diagnosis. Each
tion may be used once, more than once or not at all.

A 50-year-old woman, with a background of diabetes, presents with a history
of difficulty in extending her left ring finger at the level of the proximal
interphalangeal joint. Full extension of the finger is possible when she uses her
other hand to stretch out the finger, with a pop felt. Her symptoms are worse in the
morning. On examination, she has a tender nodule with some associated swelling
over the flexor aspect of the affected finger.

A 43-year-old woman presents with pain and tenderness over the dorsoradial
aspect of her right wrist and thumb. On examination, she has tenderness and
crepitus in the region of the tendons of the first extensor compartment with a
positive Finkelstein's test.

A 46-year-old man with a background of epilepsy presents with progressive fixed
flexion contractures of the ring and little fingers in both hands. On examination
painless nodules and thick cords can be felt on the palmar aspects of both hands
and the table top test is positive bilaterally.

A 53-year-old woman presents with a known diagnosis of rheumatoid arthritis.
On examination the patient is found to have ulnar deviation of the fingers in both
hands, tender swellings at the level of the proximal interphalangeal joints, with
a flexion deformity of the proximal interphalangeal joint and a hyperextension
deformity of the distal interphalangeal joint of the right middle finger.

Theme: Hand trauma

Options for Questions 5–8:

A	Flexor tenosynovitis	F	Zone 1 flexor tendon injury
B	Mallet finger	G	Zone 2 flexor tendon injury
C	Mallet thumb	H	Zone 3 flexor tendon injury
D	Ulnar collateral ligament injury	I	Zone 4 flexor tendon injury
E	Volar plate injury		

For each of the following cases, select the single most appropriate diagnosis. Each option may be used once, more than once or not at all.

5. A 22-year-old man presents with pain, swelling and deformity to the right little finger following an impact with a cricket ball leading to a forced flexion injury. On examination, there is swelling and tenderness at the level of the distal interphalangeal joints in the right little finger, with a correctable flexion deformit at that level. Radiographs are normal.

6. A 31-year-old woman presents with an injury to her left thumb following a fall whilst skiing. She is found to have tenderness, swelling and ecchymosis over the region of the left thumb thenar eminence and metacarpophalangeal joint, with a decreased range of movement throughout the digit. There is instability of the metacarpophalangeal joint on stress testing, particularly on radial deviation of th thumb. Standard radiographs reveal no fracture.

7. A 54-year-old woman presents for her six week review following a dorsally displaced right distal radius managed conservatively in a Colles' cast. On removal of the cast the fracture site is non-tender and she has a moderate range of movement at the wrist. However, the patient is complaining of an inability to extend her ipsilateral thumb at the level of the inter-phalangeal joint. Radiograph demonstrate no new injury.

8. A 42-year-old man presents following an accident work with a kitchen knife. On examination he has an incised wound over the palmar aspect of the left index finger at the level of the proximal interphalangeal joint. On examination, the patient is unable to flex the proximal interphalangeal joint of the left index finger when the other fingers are held in extension. The patient also has decreased sensation and sweating over the radial aspect of the digit, but there is no gross vascular deficit found.

heme: Upper limb nerve lesions

ptions for Questions 9–12:

A   Cheiralgia paresthetica
B   Carpal tunnel syndrome
C   Cubital tunnel syndrome
D   Palmar branch of the median
    nerve
E   Posterior interosseous nerve
    compression

F   Pronator teres syndrome
G   Saturday night palsy
H   Supinator tunnel syndrome
I   Ulnar tunnel syndrome

or each of the following cases, select the single most appropriate diagnosis. Each
ption may be used once, more than once or not at all.

A 30-year-old woman presents with a 2-year history of worsening paraesthesia
in the medial one and half digits, with associated weakness, in the left hand.
On examination, she has a cubitus valgus deformity secondary to an ipsilateral
supracondylar fracture as a child. She has a positive Froment's test but with no
evidence of clawing in the hand.

). A 58-year-old woman presents with an 8-month history of progressive pain and
paraesthesia affecting the lateral three and half digits of her right hand, with her
symptoms often worse at night. On examination, she has signs of muscle wasting
to the thenar eminence and a positive Tinel's test.

. A 42-year-old alcoholic man presents to the emergency department in police
custody wearing handcuffs. He is complaining of a loss of sensation on the
dorsoradial aspect of the right hand and wrist. There is no evidence of any motor
deficit.

2. A 41-year-old woman presents with an 18-month history of pain and tenderness
over the proximal volar aspect of the left forearm, with associated tingling and
weakness of the left hand. On examination, there is paraesthesia affecting the
lateral fingers and palm of the hand with an associated weakness of the pincer
movement.

Answers

1. I Trigger finger

Trigger finger or thumb is characterised by fibrotic thickening of affected tendon sheaths leading to stenosis that ultimately results in the affected flexor tendon being caught within the retinacular pulley system, most commonly at the first annular (A1) pulley. Associated risk factors include middle age, female sex, rheumatoid arthritis, diabetes mellitus and gout. The ring and middle fingers and thumb are most frequently involved.

Diagnosis is made on clinical evaluation with patient complaining of pain, swelling and difficulty moving the affected digit, with symptoms often worse in the morning. On examination, a tender nodule may be felt on the palmar aspect of the affected digit, and it will remain locked in flexion when passive extension of all digits is attempted. Extension is possible with further effort or with passive force applied, with a pop and triggering of the finger.

Treatment is with conservative (analgesia, physiotherapy, steroid injection) or surgical (release, tenosynovectomy) measures.

2. F de Quervain's tenosynovitis

De Quervain's tenosynovitis was initially described in 1895 by Swiss surgeon Fritz de Quervain. It is characterised by sheath inflammation and stenosis, of the tendons of the first extensor compartment (extensor pollicis brevis, abductor pollicis longus). Peak incidence is between 30–50 years of age with a female predominance. The cause is not known, though associations with repetitive overuse and inflammatory arthritis are proposed.

Patients often present with pain, tenderness and swelling of the affected thumb and wrist (dorsoradial). Finkelstein's test is diagnostic as it reproduces the pain in the region of the first extensor compartment. The patient flexes the thumb across the palm, makes a fist and then performs passive ulnar deviation of the wrist. Differential diagnosis includes osteoarthritis of the wrist and/or thumb carpometacarpal joint, which would be found on plane radiographs.

Treatment is either non-operative (rest and avoidance, nonsteroidal anti-inflammatory drugs, splints, steroid injection) or operative (division and release of affected tendon sheaths). Potential complications of surgical treatment are recurrence and neurapraxia of the superficial branch of the radial nerve.

3. E Dupuytren's contracture

Dupuytren's disease was initially documented in 1831 by Parisian surgeon Baron Guillaume Dupuytren, who described the treatment for the disorder. It is characterised by nodules in the palm of the hand, development of cords, progressive fibrotic thickening of the palmar and digital fascia with hyperplasia and contracture (change of collagen from type I to type III), ultimately resulting in fixed flexion deformities of the affected fingers. The incidence rises sharply after 40 years of age and males (10:1) are more commonly affected. Risk factors include:

- Genetics (autosomal dominant)
- Trauma
- Epilepsy, e.g. phenytoin therapy
- Diabetes mellitus
- AIDS/HIV
- Alcohol excess and liver disease/cirrhosis
- Associated disorders:
  - Ledderhose disease (plantar fibromatosis)
  - Peyronie's disease (penile fibromatosis)
  - Garrod's knuckles

The disease often presents in both hands with a symmetrical pattern. The ring and little fingers are most frequently affected (**Figure 55.1**) and pain is rare. The Hueston tabletop test is considered positive when a dorsal aspect of an open hand cannot be placed flat on the table, and is used as an indication for surgery. Treatment includes conservative, collagenase therapy (non-invasive enzyme fasciotomy), fasciotomy, fasciectomy or dermofasciectomy. Complications include recurrence (~30%), infection, neurovascular injury, haematoma, stiffness and complex regional pain syndrome.

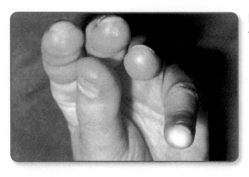

Figure 55.1 Dupuytren's contracture of the little finger.

4. B Boutonnière deformity

Rheumatoid arthritis frequently leads to symptoms involves the joints and soft tissue of both hands. Inflammation and repeated trauma leads to flexor and extensor tendon damage, with potential deformities including:

- **Boutonnière deformity** is characterised by distal interphalangeal joint hyperextension and proximal interphalangeal joint flexion. Initial disruption of the central slip of the extensor tendon leads to separation and volar subluxation of the lateral bands, followed by dorsal subluxation of the proximal phalanx head. The deformity persists due to contracture of the volar plate, collateral ligaments and oblique retinacular ligament. Stages of the deformity include extension lag followed by flexion contracture.

- **Swan neck deformity** is characterised by proximal interphalangeal joint hyperextension with metacarpophalangeal joint and distal interphalangeal joint flexion and can originate from flexor digitorum superficialis rupture or extensor digitorum communis shortening.
- **Ulnar and volar deviation of the fingers** is secondary to synovial inflammation of the wrist joint and metacarpophalangeal joints.
- **Z-thumb deformity** is often seen due to rupture of the flexor pollicis longus tendon, which in turn is associated with abnormalities within the carpus.

5. B Mallet finger

A mallet finger usually occurs following a direct blow to an actively extended finger causing a hyper flexion injury, e.g. attempting to catch a cricket ball. This results in rupture of the distal extensor digitorum tendon slip from its insertion on the distal phalanx, with associated avulsion fractures from the dorsal base possible. Examination demonstrates tenderness and swelling in the region of the distal phalanx, with an inability to actively extend flexed at the distal interphalangeal joint (passive extension possible). Anteroposterior, lateral and oblique radiographs of the affected digit reveal any bony abnormality. Management is with Mallet splint immobilisation (distal interphalangeal joint held in hyperextension) for 6–8 weeks. If there is subluxation of the distal interphalangeal joint or a large amount of the articular surface involved (>50%), fixation with an extension blocking K-wire may be required.

6. D Ulnar collateral ligament injury

The ulnar collateral ligament originates from the head of the thumb metacarpal and inserts on the proximal phalanx of the thumb. Rupture of the ulnar collateral ligament is also known as gamekeeper's thumb (chronic) or skier's thumb (acute). Following a complete rupture, ~80% cases will have a Stener lesion (interposition of the aponeurosis of adductor pollicis muscle between the insertion and the ruptured free edge of the ligament).

Injury commonly occurs following a fall onto an outstretched hand leading to forced abduction of an extended thumb. On examination, there will be tenderness (ulnar aspect), swelling and possible ecchymosis at the thumb metacarpophalangeal joint and thenar eminence, with a restricted range of movement and evidence of instability. Radiographs of the thumb are to exclude an avulsion fracture from the base of the proximal phalanx, with radial stress views (following infiltration of local anaesthetic) demonstrating instability of the metacarpophalangeal joint.

Treatment is with:

- Immobilisation with a thumb spica (partial rupture)
- Operative repair (complete rupture, Stener lesion, avulsion fracture)

C Mallet thumb

A mallet thumb is characterised by rupture of the insertion of the extensor pollicis longus tendon at the distal phalanx of the thumb (originates from the middle third of the dorsal ulna surface). Associated avulsion fractures can occur. Causes of a mallet thumb are:

- Acute trauma
- Distal radius fracture
  - Late complication (3–12 weeks post injury) due to radial tubercle disruption or fracture fragment
- Rheumatoid arthritis, SLE
  - Degeneration as the tendon passes over Lister's tubercle

Examination will reveal tenderness and swelling in the region of the distal phalanx following an acute injury. All patients will have an inability to actively extend flexed at the interphalangeal joint of the thumb, but with passive extension often possible. Thumb radiographs are necessary to exclude an associated fracture. Management is with:

- Immobilisation
- Direct operative repair
- Free tendon transfer (e.g. extensor indicis)

G Zone 2 flexor tendon injury

Flexor tendon injuries are divided into zones (Verden zones) that guides treatment and prognosis (**Tables 55.1** and **55.2, Figure 55.2**). Zone 2, also known as 'no man's land'.

Treatment is with repair, with concomitant repair of the neurovascular structures that are frequently involved.

Table 55.1			
Zone	**From**	**To**	**Contents**
1	Mid-point middle phalanx	Finger tip	Flexor digitorum profundus
2	Distal palmar crease (A1 pulley)	Mid-point middle phalanx	Flexor digitorum profundus, flexor digitorum superficialis (sheath)
3	Distal edge carpal tunnel	Distal palmar crease (A1 pulley)	Flexor digitorum profundus, flexor digitorum superficialis
4	Proximal edge carpal tunnel	Distal edge carpal tunnel	Carpal tunnel
5	Forearm and wrist	Proximal edge carpal tunnel	Volar compartment

Table 55.1 Flexor tendon injury zones in the fingers.

Table 55.2

Zone	From	To
1	Interphalangeal joint	Finger tip
2	A1 pulley (Proximal phalanx)	Interphalangeal joint
3	Thenar muscles	Distal palmar crease
4	Proximal edge carpal tunnel	Distal edge carpal tunnel
5	Musculotendinous junction	Proximal edge carpal tunnel

Table 55.2 Flexor tendon injury zones in the thumb.

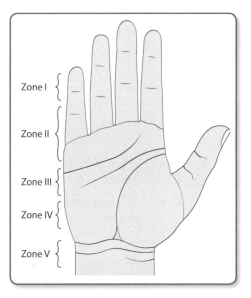

Figure 55.2 Flexor tendon injury zone

9. C Cubital tunnel syndrome

Cubital tunnel syndrome is the second most frequent neuropathy of the upper limb and is due to a lesion of the ulnar nerve at the level of the elbow. Potential causes/ sites include:

- Arcade of Struthers
- Medial epicondyle
  - Medial epicondylitis
- Osborne's ligament
- Anconeus epitrochlearis
- Flexor carpi ulnaris aponeurosis
- Tumours or ganglions
- Trauma and deformity
  - Cubitus varus or valgus post supracondylar fracture
  - Burns

Clinical signs and symptoms are due to proximal ulnar nerve compression with pain and paraesthesia of the medial one and a half digits. Intrinsic muscle weakness and/or atrophy can be found with a positive Froment's sign (adductor pollicis weakness leads to compensatory thumb IPJ flexion). Hand clawing may occur, however, the more proximal the lesion, the less pronounced is the clawing due to the loss of innervation to flexor digitorum profundus medial two digits (ulnar paradox). Therefore, with ulnar tunnel syndrome there is compression of the ulnar at the wrist (Guyon's canal) and thus more pronounced clawing of the hand as innervation to flexor digitorum profundus is preserved. Provocation tests include Tinel's test (tapping over nerve as runs posterior to medial epicondyle) and prolonged elbow flexion test. Nerve conduction studies can confirm the diagnosis. Management options include:

- Non-operative
  - Activity modification, splints, anti-inflammatories, steroid injection
- Operative
  - Decompression (open or endoscopic)
  - Medial epicondylectomy
  - Anterior transposition

. B Carpal tunnel syndrome

The anatomy of the carpal tunnel is discussed on p. 19. Carpal tunnel syndrome is the most common compressive neuropathy of the upper limb and is due to microvascular compression and neural ischaemia to the median nerve as it passes posterior to the flexor retinaculum of the carpal tunnel. Risk factors include:

- Increasing age (peak incidence middle age)
- Gender (females)
- Obesity, smoking, alcoholism
- Co-morbidities, e.g. diabetes mellitus, hypothyroidism, acromegaly
- Fluid retention, e.g. pregnancy, combined oral contraceptive, congestive cardiac failure
- Inflammatory arthritis, e.g. rheumatoid arthritis
- Trauma, e.g. distal radius fracture, lunate fracture/dislocation
- Occupation (possible links with repetitive movements)

Clinical signs and symptoms are due to median nerve compression within the carpal tunnel, with common findings pain (worse at night, shake hand to relieve) and paraesthesia of thumb, index, middle and the radial half of the ring fingers. Sensation over the radial palm of the hand is preserved as this is innervated by the palmar cutaneous branch of the median nerve. Thenar muscle atrophy and weakness are late signs. Provocation tests include Phalen's test (flex ipsilateral wrist for 1–2 minutes) and Tinel's test (tapping over nerve at volar wrist crease). Nerve conduction studies are often used when the diagnosis is unclear. Management options include:

- Non-operative
  - Activity modification, splints, anti-inflammatories, steroid injection
- Operative
  - Carpal tunnel release and decompression (open or endoscopic)

11. A Cheiralgia paresthetica

Cheiralgia paresthetica, also known as Wartenberg syndrome, is a neuropathy of the superficial sensory branch of the radial nerve. Causes can either be compression (or forearm pronation between extensor carpi radialis longus and brachioradialis) or trauma (external compression from watch or handcuffs). Patients present with pain, burning sensation and paraesthesia over the radio-dorsal aspect of the wrist and hand, but with no motor abnormality present. Provocation tests include Tinel sign (tapping over nerve) or resisted forearm pronation for approximately one minute. Treatment options are:

- Non-operative
  - Activity modification, splints, anti-inflammatories
- Operative
  - Decompression

12. F Pronator teres syndrome

Pronator teres syndrome is caused by compression of the median nerve as it passes between the heads of pronator teres on entering the forearm. This disorder is part of the group of disorders known as pronator syndrome. Other potential sites of compression include the:

- Ligament of Struthers
- Bicipital aponeurosis
- Flexor digitorum superficialis aponeurotic arch

The key clinical signs for differentiating pronator syndrome from carpal tunnel syndrome are:

- The loss of sensation over the radial palm of the hand due to the involvement of the palmar cutaneous branch of the median nerve
- Pain at the level of the elbow and/or at the proximal volar forearm
- Phalen's and Tinel's signs at the wrist should be negative
- Weakness of the muscles of the forearm flexor compartment would indicate anterior interosseous nerve involvement
- Provocation test positive on resisted forearm pronation

Management options include:

- Non-operative
  - Activity modification, splints, anti-inflammatories
- Operative
  - Decompression of affected site

Chapter 56

Surgical disorders of the brain

Theme: Intracranial lesions

Options for Questions 1–3:

A	Extradural haematoma	D	Intracranial tumour
B	Subarachnoid haemorrhage	E	Hydrocephalus
C	Chronic subdural haematoma	F	Cerebral abscess

For each of the following situations, select the single most likely diagnosis. Each option may be used once, more than once or not at all.

1. A 60-year-old man complains of increasing generalised headache associated with nausea and vomiting for 3 days. He feels feverish and has double vision. In the past he has suffered from and been treated for recurrent sinusitis. He has had type 1 diabetes for 30 years and recently has been on steroids for asthma. On examination, he is pyrexial with a temperature of 39°C and on funduscopy has early papilloedema.

2. A 25-year-old man is brought into the accident and emergency department from the football pitch with gradual drowsiness. During the course of play he collided with another player at the goalmouth while heading the ball. He was momentarily unconscious but continued playing for some time after the incident. His Glasgow coma score is 14, the pupils are equal and reacting to light and he has no papilloedema.

3. A 70-year-old man is admitted following a seizure that lasted for 10–15 minutes. On admission his Glasgow coma score is 15. He complains of recent headaches with vomiting. Six years ago, he underwent a radical right nephrectomy for hypernephroma.

Theme: Intracranial lesions

Options for Questions 4–6:

A Extradural haematoma	**D** Intracranial tumour
B Subarachnoid haemorrhage	**E** Hydrocephalus
C Chronic subdural haematoma	**F** Cerebral abscess

4. A 45-year-old man is admitted with sudden onset of very severe occipital headache which he describes as though somebody has given him a hammer blow to the back of the head. He has vomiting and marked photophobia and is very drowsy. On examination, he has some neck stiffness and occulomotor (3rd nerve) palsy. His blood pressure is 180/100 mmHg and pulse rate 60 beats per minute.

5. An 80-year-old woman has been intermittently drowsy for a few days. She is on antiplatelet agents. During one of these drowsy occasions she fell out of bed and banged her head. At times she is forgetful, wanders about on the ward and is often found to be very sleepy. On examination, she is slow in her answers to questions. She has a Glasgow coma score of 15.

6. A 45-year-old woman complains of gradual hearing loss and tinnitus of 4 – 6 months duration. She has noticed dizziness and feels an illusory sense of her body revolving. She also has right-sided temporal headache which is often associated with vomiting. On examination, she has some facial weakness and numbness in the distribution of the 7th cranial nerve.

Answers

. F Cerebral abscess

This patient who has long-term type 1 diabetes (and hence is immunocompromised) has features of raised intracranial pressure – headache, nausea and vomiting, and visual disturbances – with signs of infection. Past history of sinusitis gives a clue as to the source of cerebral infection. The condition starts with cerebritis followed by the formation of a core of necrotic tissue which becomes encapsulated within a couple of weeks. As the lesion forms a capsule, pyrexia and raised inflammatory markers may be absent.

On CT scan a ring-enhancing mass lesion is typical of an abscess. Image-guided surgical aspiration under intravenous antibiotic cover is the mainstay of treatment. Aspiration may have to be repeated and the antibiotics continued for 6 weeks. Rarely excision of the abscess wall may be necessary. Steroids may be used in severe oedema but with caution as their use may conflict with the efficacy of antibiotics. Because of the high chance of epilepsy in the long-term, prophylactic anticonvulsant treatment is instituted.

Subdural empyema is less common but more serious and carries a higher mortality. It occurs as a result of acute mastoiditis and rhinosinusitis.

. A Extradural haematoma

This young man has the typical features of a rapidly forming extradural haematoma (EDH). Presence of a lucid interval is pathognomonic of the diagnosis although this symptom may not always be present. Being the thinnest part of the cranium, the squamous part of the temporal bone is most commonly fractured with tear of the underlying middle meningeal artery resulting in the haematoma. The classical presentation of EDH of head injury followed by lucid interval with later rapid deterioration in the Glasgow coma score is seen only in a minority of patients. If missed, the condition will progress to contralateral hemiparesis, unconsciousness and ipsilateral pupillary dilatation due to uncal herniation.

On CT scan a biconvex hyperdense lesion is seen between the calvaria and the brain. The treatment is prompt evacuation of the EDH by a craniotomy preferably carried out by a neurosurgeon.

. D Intracranial tumour

This 70-year-old man has been admitted as an emergency with an epileptic fit from which he has recovered. There is an immediate past history of early morning headache with vomiting, symptoms of raised intracranial pressure. Previous history of radical nephrectomy for renal cell carcinoma is very significant as cerebral metastasis should be considered as the cause of his fit. A thorough neurological examination should be done, followed by a contrast CT scan.

Adenocarcinoma of the kidney metastasizes by the blood stream to the lungs, bones and brain. It is well-known that blood borne metastasis may manifest many years after successful removal of a primary renal cell carcinoma. Cerebral metastasis is the commonest brain tumour and is known to occur in 25% of cancer sufferers. Multiple lesions are treated by steroids and irradiation. When there is a significant period of recurrence-free interval between removal of the primary and appearance of the secondary, surgical removal of a solitary cerebral metastasis has much to recommend it provided there is no other evidence of the disease.

4. B Subarachnoid haemorrhage

The history of a sudden onset of a severe headache typically described as a hammer blow at the back of the head is characteristic of subarachnoid haemorrhage (SAH) from rupture of a cerebral aneurysm. The patient has the other typical features – meningism, photophobia and 3rd nerve palsy; the latter is due to rupture of an aneurysm in the posterior communicating artery, which is in close proximity to the occulomotor nerve, which is compressed by the haematoma. The immediate past history from his wife of occipital and cervical headache is even more suggestive of the diagnosis.

A CT scan confirms the diagnosis in the vast majority if carried out early. If the CT scan is negative a lumbar puncture is carried out. In elective patients with a convincing history and negative lumbar puncture and CT scan, a CT angiogram or cerebral digital subtraction angiogram is done. The treatment is endovascular coiling carried out by an interventional radiologist or craniotomy and clipping by a neurosurgeon.

The commonest cause of non-traumatic SAH is cerebral aneurysm. Clinically SAH is graded according to the World Federation of Neurological Surgeons system. The complications of rupture of cerebral aneurysms are: rebleeding, delayed ischaemic neurological deficit, hydrocephalus and hyponatraemia from cerebral salt wasting.

5. C Chronic subdural haematoma

This elderly patient who is prone to episodes of drowsiness had a fall from her bed. Although she is aware of her surroundings, she has headaches and is not always in control of her faculties. The history of minor head injury in a patient on antiplatelet drugs and problems with cognition should alert one to a diagnosis of chronic subdural haematoma unless otherwise proven. There may be seizures and focal neurological deficits. Patients on anticoagulants are also prone to chronic subdural haematoma.

A CT scan is the imaging of choice. The appearances are variable: an acute bleed is seen as a hyperdense lesion, a subacute bleed shows an isodense lesion whereas a chronic bleed is hypodense. In some cases there may be a combination of acute-on-chronic bleed. The treatment is evacuation by making burr holes which can be carried out under local anaesthetic in the elderly patient with co-morbidity.

. D Intracranial tumour

This woman has clinical features of raised intracranial pressure with focal neurological deficits suggestive of a tumour in the vicinity of the 8th cranial (vestibulocochlear) nerve. She has tinnitus, deafness and vertigo, symptoms that confirm the suspicion. Facial numbness and weakness point to compression of the 5th (trigeminal) and 7th (facial) cranial nerves. The diagnosis is an acoustic neuroma that arises at the cerebellopontine angle. As it enlarges laterally it may cause erosion of the internal auditory meatus while medially it may extend into the subarachnoid space causing hydrocephalus. In late cases there may be compression of the brainstem and tonsillar herniation which is lethal.

The tumour is a schwannoma, a benign tumour, arising from the schwann cells of the vestibular component of the 8th cranial nerve. It is slow growing and accounts for 8% of primary intracranial tumours. The imaging of choice is gadolinium-enhanced MRI. Excision by open surgery is the treatment of choice. Preservation of facial and auditory nerve function will depend upon the size of the tumour and the preoperative disability. Usually when unilateral, the condition is sporadic. If bilateral, it is a component of neurofibromatosis Type II which may include meningioma, glioma or neurofibroma.

Chapter 57

Differences between the paediatric and adult surgical patient

---

Theme: Anatomy

Options for Questions 1–4:

A	Greater body surface area to body mass ratio than the adult	D	Muscle mass is less than the adult
B	Head is proportionally smaller than in an adult	E	Narrowest part of the paediatric airway is at the level of the cricoid cartilage
C	Larynx is higher and more anterior in the neck than the adult	F	Tongue is small relative to the oropharynx

For each of the following situations, select the single most likely answer. Each option may be used once, more than once or not at all.

1. A 3-year-old boy develops respiratory difficulties during the administration of inhalational anaesthesia prior to a minor surgical procedure. The boy is otherwise healthy, with no history of previous respiratory difficulties.

2. A 6-year-old girl is found to be hypothermic during intraoperative monitoring. The surgeon is undertaking adenoidectomy, but there have been numerous delays in theatre and the procedure is taking much longer than planned.

3. An 8-year-old girl is involved in a road traffic accident resulting in intra-abdominal injury. She was a rear seat passenger wearing a seat belt. Her mother was sitting next to her and was also wearing a seat belt but is uninjured.

4. A 7-year-old boy requires a lengthy surgical procedure under general anaesthetic. The patient has no significant past medical history. A cuffed endotracheal tube was used and the anaesthetist is concerned about the risk of pressure necrosis developing due to prolonged intubation.

Theme: Common surgical disorders of the paediatric patient

Options for Questions 5–8:

A   Appendicitis
B   Inguinal hernia
C   Intussusception
D   Oesophageal atresia

E   Pyloric stenosis
F   Torsion of the testis
G   Undescended testes

For each of the following situations, select the single most likely diagnosis. Each option may be used once, more than once or not at all.

5.   A 12-year-old boy presents with acute right iliac fossa pain. On further questioning it is found that the pain initially began in the scrotum but now radiates into the scrotum. The abdomen is examined, revealing a soft and apparently non tender abdomen.

6.   A 6-week-old boy presents dehydrated and withdrawn. Parents describe forceful vomiting which has increased in severity over the past 7 days. Intermittent vomiting had been present since 2 weeks old. Vomiting occurs immediately after or during feeds.

7.   A 7-month-old girl presents with 10 days of increasingly severe episodes of colic, during which she draws up her legs and screams. Over the past 24 hours, she has been vomiting bile stained fluid.

8.   A 10-month-old boy presents with an intermittent lump in her left groin which was noticed by her parents when she is crying. The lump always disappears when relaxed, but appears to be increasing in size when crying. The infant is otherwise well with no suggestion of gastrointestinal upset.

Theme: Neonatal surgical abnormalities

Options for Questions 9–11:

A   Biliary atresia
B   Diaphragmatic hernia
C   Exomphalos
D   Gastric outlet obstruction
E   Gastroschisis

F   Haemolytic disease of the newborn
G   Meckel's diverticulum
H   Oesophageal atresia
I   Tracheal atresia

For each of the following situations, select the single most likely diagnosis. Each option may be used once, more than once or not at all.

9.   A newborn female infant is noted to be drooling and coughing. The midwife is concerned. Spontaneous vaginal delivery was uncomplicated. No abnormalities

had been detected at the 20 weeks ultrasound scan and the pregnancy was unremarkable.

A newborn male infant is noted to have respiratory difficulty and an obvious sunken appearance to the anterior abdominal wall is seen. Prenatal ultrasound scan had demonstrated polyhydramnios but no cause for this had been identified.

A 2-week-old girl is noticed to be jaundiced at the postnatal midwife review. The mother reports pale stools and dark urine over the past few days. The infant has been a little irritable but otherwise well. On examination the infant is afebrile; the abdomen is soft and appears to be non-tender. The liver and spleen appear enlarged

eme : Paediatric oncology

tions for Questions 12–14:

A Germ cell tumour
B Hepatoblastoma
C Hepatocellular carcinoma

D Rhabdomyosarcoma
E Wilms' tumour

: each of the following situations, select the single most likely diagnosis. Each option y be used once, more than once or not at all.

A 4-year-old previously healthy boy presents with fever, abdominal swelling and blood stained urine.

A 16-year-old girl presents with lump arising from her right thigh. The mass has gradually increased in size over the previous 4 weeks and is non-tender. She is otherwise well and there is no significant past medical history.

A 2-year-old boy presents with an obvious swelling at the base of his spine. His parents report that this has gradually increased in size over the past month, but does not appear to cause any discomfort. Past medical history is unremarkable. On examination there is a firm, immobile mass in the sacral region which appears non-tender.

Answers

1. C Larynx is higher and more anterior in the neck than the adult

One of the consequences of the larynx being positioned at the level of C3/C4, compared to C4/C5 in the adult, is that the tongue is in closer proximity to the palate. This risks airway obstruction, particularly in the setting of inhalational anaesthesia. Other anatomical predispositions to airway difficulties include a large tongue relative to the oropharynx, vocal cords are at a more antero-caudal angle and the epiglottis is inclined more posteriorly.

2. A Greater body surface area to body mass ratio than the adult

Due to increased body surface area, children are more susceptible to heat loss, especially when they are exposed during surgical procedures or resuscitation. In addition, due to higher basal metabolic rate children have a higher respiratory rate and can become hypoxic more quickly. Children also have a proportionally larger head compared to adults which contributes to greater potential for heat loss.

3. D Muscle mass is less than the adult

In addition to less muscle mass, children generally have less fat, with closer proximity of chest and abdominal organs to the site of impact. In particular the liver and spleen are proportionally larger than in adults Injury to these organs can go unrecognised leading to significant blood loss. Combined with the enhanced ability to compensate for intravascular depletion this can result in late recognition haemodynamic compromise.

4. E Narrowest part of the paediatric airway is at the level of the cricoid cartilage

This can risk pressure necrosis at the level of the cricoid if a cuffed endotracheal tube is used. It should be noted that in the adult the narrowest part of the airway is at the level of the vocal cords.

5. F Torsion of the testis

As well as highlighting the potential variable presentation of surgical disorders this case brings to light possible difficulties in history taking in the paediatric patient. On first impression the patient may have been triaged as a 'right iliac fossa pain' for repeat abdominal examination considering appendicitis. However with a full history of the presenting complaint it is clear the diagnosis lies elsewhere. It is important that examination of the scrotum is included in the abdominal examination. In the case of possible testicular torsion considering the diagnosis early is key, with urgent intervention to save the testes as appropriate. In testicular torsion pain is usually present for less than 6 hours. While no consistent causative factors have been identified a number of risk factors should be considered. Risk factors may include a malformation of the processus vaginalis where the mesorchium terminates early resulting in mobile testes within the tunica vaginalis, bell clapper deformity and pubertal changes. Other potential risk factors include physical activities or cold weather where the cremasteric contraction may induce torsion and anatomical abnormalities such as cryptorchidism (undescended testes are at higher risk of torsion). On examination of the scrotum the affected testes may have a horizontal lie, and the cremasteric reflex may be absent. The testes are usually not particularly swollen. In terms of investigation, Doppler ultrasound scan is very good at determining the presence or absence of torsion.

Patients require prompt diagnosis and treatment. This is a surgical emergency. If treated within 6 hours there is a high chance of saving the testes, but this falls to 50% between 6 and 12 hours. In younger boys (<10 years) testicular torsion is responsible for 30% of presentations with an acute scrotum. The hydatid of Morgagni (present in around 90%) can become contorted and present with similar pain. This may be difficult to differentiate clinically and surgical exploration is likely to be indicated.

E Pyloric stenosis

Infants with pyloric stenosis usually present within the first 8 weeks of life. The pylorus is thickened causing gastric outlet obstruction with non-bilious, projectile vomiting. Patients usually present dehydrated with a hypochloraemic metabolic alkalosis. The underlying aetiology is unknown although there may be a genetic background as children with parents of the condition are more likely to be sufferers. It is more common in boys than girls and is rare past 6 months of age. On examination a 'pyloric olive' may be palpable in the epigastrium. Diagnosis is made by ultrasound scan which demonstrates the thickened pylorus. **Figure 57.1** demonstrates pyloric stenosis seen at barium meal, which is no longer the investigation of choice.

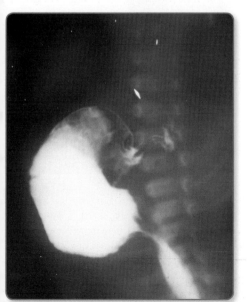

Figure 57.1 Barium meal in a 4-week-old boy showing congenital hypertrophic pyloric stenosis. Nowadays ultrasound is the investigation of choice.

7. C Intussusception

This is the invagination of one part of the intestine into another. Infants present with intermittent severe cramping abdominal pains or colic. During an episode the child may scream, draw up their legs, or fall asleep between episodes. Later in the course the infant may develop bilious vomiting and 'redcurrant jelly stools' or rectal bleeding. In approximately one-third of patients the intussuscepted segment is palpable as a sausage shaped mass. Late complications include perforation and peritonitis. In infants the majority occur in relation to a viral infection where the lead point is an enlarged Peyer's patch. In older patients the underlying aetiology is likely to be pathological, including a tumour, polyp or Meckel's diverticulum. Ultrasound scan may show a typical 'target sign'. Small bowel obstruction is seen on abdominal X-ray. If the patient is unstable laparotomy is indicated given the potential for bowel ischemia or perforation. In the stable patient a barium enema which shows a 'crab-claw' deformity confirms the diagnosis (**Figure 57.2**); the procedure could also be used to relieve the intussusception. A successful outcome is indicated by reflux of barium into the terminal ileum.

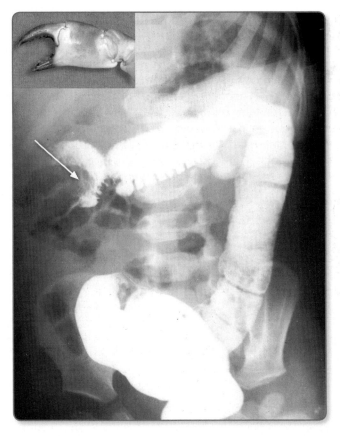

Figure 57.2 Barium enema showing typical crab claw appearance (see the crab claw, inset) in ileocaecocolic intussusception in a baby.

B Inguinal hernia

In children, inguinal herniae are invariably indirect and more often occur on the right side due to the later descent of the right testes. There is a male preponderance. In females the lump is present in the upper part of the labia majora. Risk of incarceration is high in infants (less than 1-year-old) and so surgery should be undertaken within around 2 weeks, as an 'urgent elective' case. After one year of age the risk of incarceration is reduced and surgery may be less urgent.

Inguinal hernia repair is a common operation in young children, especially ex-premature infants and low birth weight babies. In the latter patients the abdominal wall is weak and the normal obliteration of the sac has not occurred.

In terms of management, in the case of the irreducible hernia gentle pressure may be applied in an attempt to reduce the hernia. Attempting reduction with firm pressure under anaesthesia is contraindicated. However evidence of intestinal obstruction or suggestion of ischemia necessitates early surgery.

H Oesophageal atresia

This is a congenital defect whereby the oesophagus terminates before reaching the stomach, leading to two blind ending pouches. The condition may be associated with a fistula to the trachea (tracheoesophageal fistula). The condition is noticed and treated soon after birth. Rarely an emergency procedure is required as nutritional supplements and fluids can be provided parenterally allowing for further investigations to exclude other abnormalities. Associated defects may include cardiac, spinal and/or renal abnormalities. The presence of multiple abnormalities in this context is known as VACTERL syndrome (vertebral column, anorectal, cardiac, tracheal, oesophageal, renal and limbs). Oesophageal atresia can be diagnosed from around 26 weeks gestation by ultrasound scan. Treatment is surgical, usually requiring primary anastomosis or occasionally colonic transposition if the two sections of oesophagus cannot be approximated. Infants with tracheal atresia present with stridor. Although present from birth tracheal atresia may not cause significant symptoms until later in life.

). B Diaphragmatic hernia

This sunken appearance to the anterior abdominal wall is also known as a 'scaphoid abdomen'. It takes its appearance due to the position of upper abdominal viscera which have moved into the thorax secondary to a large diaphragmatic hernia. Around 50% of diaphragmatic hernias are detected on prenatal ultrasound scan and polyhydramnios may be detected. The condition is associated with a variable degree of pulmonary hypoplasia and in severe cases left ventricular hypoplasia may also be seen. **Figures 57.3** and **57.4** demonstrate X-ray findings of diaphragmatic hernia with and without contrast.

The commonest type of congenital diaphragmatic hernia is Bochdalek's hernia which is a posterolateral defect. Other types include Morgagni's, a rare anterior diaphragmatic defect, and diaphragm eventration where an otherwise intact diaphragm is displaced within the chest.

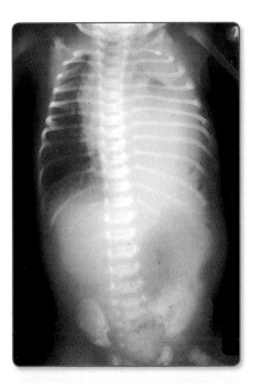

Figure 57.3 Plain X-ray in a neonate showing no left lung shadow and no left dome of diaphragm – congenital diaphragmatic hernia.

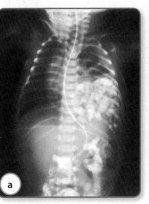
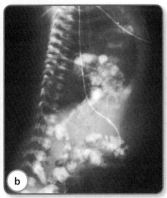

Figure 57.4 Barium meal showing left congenital diaphragmatic hernia (a) Anteroposterior view and (b) lateral view.

Initial management includes the placement of an orogastric tube and intubation to protect the airway followed by surgical intervention as appropriate.

11. A Biliary atresia

The aetiology of biliary atresia is unknown. It is characterised by an inflammatory condition leading to destruction of the extrahepatic bile ducts. Infants present with signs of obstructive jaundice and hepatosplenomegaly. The majority of presentations are isolated (known as the postnatal form), but up to a third may be associated with other abnormalities such as situs inversus or polysplenia/asplenia (known as the fetal/embryonic form). Treatment is surgical and may involve biliary enteric anastomosis, portoenterostomy or liver transplantation. An important differential diagnosis of jaundice in this context is a choledochal cyst. This results in a functional distal biliary obstruction caused by a congenital weakness in the wall of the biliary tree. Infants may present in the first year of life. A mass in the right upper quadrant may be palpable but otherwise it is indistinguishable from biliary atresia. Other causes of jaundice in this patient group include physiological jaundice which can occur due to hepatic immaturity or breastfeeding. Rhesus haemolytic disease of the new born would present with jaundice soon after birth without signs of biliary obstruction. Other medical causes are numerous and include ABO incompatibility, glucose-6-phosphate dehydrogenase deficiency, hypothyroidism, congenital spherocytosis and congenital/acquired infections.

2. E Wilms' tumour

This renal tumour represents the most common primary malignant renal tumour of childhood (approximately 8% of solid tumours). Up to 10% of tumours are bilateral. Potential for lung metastases and involvement of the renal vein and vena cava should be investigated with CT and ultrasound scanning respectively. First presentation usually relates to a large abdominal mass which is easily palpable. Patients may also experience abdominal pain, fever, nausea/vomiting, haematuria in approximately 20% and occasionally hypertension. Most are chemosensitive, with patients undergoing preoperative chemotherapy followed by delayed resection. Often the kidney can be preserved where there is a pseudocapsule around the tumour. If the tumour is not completely microscopically excised radiotherapy may be applied. For early stages survival is greater than 90%. Neuroblastoma is a differential diagnosis for malignant cause of abdominal swelling. It usually effects a younger age group (<2). Neuroblastoma tends to encase vascular structures, rather than invade.

3. D Rhabdomyosarcoma

This is a rare tumour which generally arises from skeletal muscle. Incidence is highest in children aged 1–5 and 15–19 years old. A combination of surgery and either pre- or postoperative chemotherapy and/or radiotherapy is used depending on tumour subtype and extent. Cure is dependent on the type, location and extent of tumour, although survival is usually long-term.

4. A Germ cell tumour

Germ cell tumours originate from primordial or pluripotential germ cells. The commonest type of germ cell tumour is a sacrococcygeal teratoma. Presentation is usually with an obvious mass in the sacral region, although some can be entirely presacral with no obvious external mass. Presacral tumours may present with lower gastrointestinal or urinary symptoms.

The preferred treatment is surgical resection, which should include the sacrum and coccyx. While the majority of germ cell tumours are benign the malignant potential requires long-term oncological follow-up.

Index